# South Asian Perspectives in Mental Health and Psychology

**Series Editors**

S. M. Yasir Arafat, Bangladesh Specialized Hospital Limited, Dhaka, Bangladesh

Sujita Kumar Kar, Department of Psychiatry, King George's Medical University, Lucknow, Uttar Pradesh, India

This series of books is an endeavor to gather and present a comprehensive understanding of the various aspects of mental health that are relevant to people living in South Asia. The books aim to provide in-depth guidance and practical solutions to the mental health challenges that are unique to these areas. The content covers a wide range of topics, including but not limited to, climate change and its impact, prison mental health, perinatal mental health, social psychiatry, mental health and disorder among the elderly population, psychiatry education and training, suicide, SDGs and mental health, trauma, addiction, and social isolation. The books also emphasize the importance of early intervention and provide resources for seeking help. The ultimate goal of this series is to empower individuals and communities to take proactive steps toward enhancing their mental wellbeing. The proposed books will fill the existing unmet need in the region with huge populations in low and middle-income country (LMIC) settings.

South Asia, home to about 2 billion people, is a region of diverse cultures, languages, and religions. It caters to about 25% of the global population. This densely populated region faces a myriad of challenges, both natural and man-made. The frequent occurrence of natural disasters, such as earthquakes, floods, and landslides, threaten the lives and livelihoods of millions of people. War, terrorism, and political instability have caused significant disruptions to the region's socio-political fabric. Poverty, migration, and tropical infectious diseases remain major challenges that hinder progress towards sustainable development. Climate change exacerbates these challenges, causing widespread environmental degradation, food insecurity, and water scarcity. Despite these obstacles, South Asian people have shown remarkable resilience and strength in the face of adversity.

Mental health issues in the South Asian region significantly contribute to the global burden of mental illnesses. However, the region faces plenty of challenges such as high stigma, low mental health literacy, poor budgetary allocation, high out-of-pocket expense for mental health services, lack of adequate infrastructure, and limited human resources are significant barriers in mental healthcare. The majority of research on mental health issues is produced by the western countries which may not fit all in the South Asian culture, albeit evidence is needed to test. There is a paucity of research and evidence-based strategies that are region-specific. This series of books is an attempt to compile the important dimensions of mental health that will benefit the regional people.

Sujita Kumar Kar • S. M. Yasir Arafat
Vikas Menon • M. Kishor • Mohan Isaac
Editors

# Teaching and Training in Psychiatry in South Asia

Springer

*Editors*
Sujita Kumar Kar
Department of Psychiatry
King George's Medical University
Lucknow, Uttar Pradesh, India

S. M. Yasir Arafat
Department of Psychiatry
Bangladesh Specialized Hospital Limited
Dhaka, Bangladesh

Vikas Menon
Department of Psychiatry
Jawaharlal Institute of Postgraduate Medical Education and Research (JIPMER)
Puducherry, Pondicherry, India

M. Kishor
Department of Psychiatry
JSS Medical College & Hospital,
JSS Academy of Higher Education & Research
Mysuru, Karnataka, India

Mohan Isaac
Department of Psychiatry
University of Western Australia (UWA),
School of Psychiatry and Clinical Neurosciences
Perth, WA, Australia

ISSN 3059-3646 ISSN 3059-3522 (electronic)
South Asian Perspectives in Mental Health and Psychology
ISBN 978-981-95-1844-9 ISBN 978-981-95-1845-6 (eBook)
https://doi.org/10.1007/978-981-95-1845-6



This Springer imprint is published by the registered company Springer Nature Singapore Pte Ltd.
The registered company address is: 152 Beach Road, #21-01/04 Gateway East, Singapore 189721, Singapore

# Foreword

In early March 1968, the World Health Organization (WHO) convened a meeting of leading mental health specialists representing most of the important teaching institutions in countries included in the South-East Asia Region of the WHO. A chief goal of the meeting was to obtain information about the way in which psychiatry was taught in the Region and to agree on recommendations concerning the further development of psychiatric education.

The experts presented the situation in their countries and agreed on a series of recommendations. One of them was that it will be useful to have regular reviews of development of education and its improvement or difficulties. The experts departed and did, for a few years, correspond and circulate materials related to education of psychiatry in their countries. After a while, despite efforts by some of the experts and the WHO, the connections weakened and the hope to develop a regular exchange of information so as to learn from each other fell into the background.

There were other efforts to review the situation and to enable all to benefit from mutual help and learning. Thus, for example, leaders in psychiatric education from nine Asia Pacific countries prepared country reports and met in 2018 to discuss and identify implementable solutions to improve training in psychiatry. The meeting of experts and their consultations identified numerous gaps that needed to be addressed and produced ideas to enhance the quality of education in psychiatry in Asia. The report and recommendations of the meeting were widely read and used (Isaac et al. 2018).

More recently, there were further commendable efforts by teachers of psychiatry. Thus, for example, in India, the Indian Teachers of Psychiatry (IToP) forum (www.indianteachersofpsychiatry.com) has initiated the application of a series of innovative and sustainable measures to enhance the quality of training in psychiatry. It is to be hoped that similar ventures will take place soon in countries of South Asia.

The book edited by Kar, Arafat, Menon, Kishor, and Isaac provides useful information and will facilitate collaboration and contacts among those concerned with education in psychiatry at this time when the rising prevalence of mental disorders and availability of medication and other ways of dealing with mental illness make it imperative to ensure that medical graduates receive adequate education in psychiatry.

We should be grateful to the editors of this volume who with their colleagues produced a book which does not only provide useful information but can also serve as a basis to cordial and useful collaboration among mental health professionals in the South Asian region and between them and the world.

President, Association for the Improvement of Mental Health Programs,
Former Director of the mental health program of the World Health Organization (WHO) and former president of the European and the World Associations of Psychiatry
Geneva, Switzerland

Norman Sartorius

# Preface

Teaching and training serve as essential pillars of the educational process. Traditionally, psychiatric education emphasized knowledge transmission, but there is a notable shift toward cultivating practical skills that enable students and professionals to effectively apply their knowledge in real-life contexts. Recently, numerous countries have embraced competency-based medical education frameworks, leading to a thorough reformation of psychiatric teaching and training structures and content. This change aims not only to standardize psychiatry education across various environments but also to address the distinctive regional trends and requirements of each region.

Over the past few decades, the curriculum for psychiatry teaching and training has experienced substantial changes. Key developments include the introduction of Competency-Based Medical Education, which emphasizes the practical application of skills and knowledge, and adaptations prompted by the COVID-19 pandemic, which necessitated innovative educational approaches. As a result, many institutions have implemented structural changes and innovative practices in psychiatric education to promote effective learning experiences for students.

South Asia, a home to approximately 2 billion people, presents a distinct educational challenge due to its cultural diversity and social homogeneity. Despite the vast population, there is a surprising lack of scholarly resources that thoroughly compare and contrast psychiatric teaching and training across the South Asian region. To bridge this gap, this new book has been designed, which aims to be the first comprehensive resource of its kind. It will serve as a vital tool for psychiatric educators, academic faculty, and policymakers in South Asia, as well as in other low- and middle-income settings.

The book commences with a comprehensive chapter that traces the evolution of psychiatry education from its inception in various parts of the world. This historical context provides a framework for understanding current practices and methodologies. Following this, the book features detailed country-specific chapters that explore psychiatric teaching and training in each of these South Asian nations. These chapters examine the current curricula for undergraduate medical education, their historical development, available postgraduate training programs for specialist psychiatrists, and the range of training opportunities currently offered. Furthermore, each chapter identifies potential challenges facing psychiatric education in the country and discusses future directions for the field.

In addition to country-specific insights, the book delves into emerging methodologies in psychiatry teaching that are gaining traction in South Asia. Topics include the adoption of online teaching platforms, the implementation of competency-based medical education, and the introduction of innovative courses designed to meet the unique needs of South Asian populations. These new approaches aim to support a more effective and adaptable psychiatry education system. Ultimately, this book represents an effort to document and analyze the landscape of psychiatric education in South Asia. By focusing on the teaching variations, innovations, and regional context, it will provide valuable insights for psychiatric educators, academicians, researchers, and government agencies involved in the continuous improvement of psychiatry teaching and training.

Lucknow, India — Sujita Kumar Kar
Dhaka, Bangladesh — S. M. Yasir Arafat
Puducherry, India — Vikas Menon
Mysuru, India — M. Kishor
Perth, Australia — Mohan Isaac

# Contents

# About the Editors

**Sujita Kumar Kar** is currently working as an Additional Professor of Psychiatry at King George's Medical University, Lucknow, Uttar Pradesh, India. He is the editor-in-chief of the *Indian Journal of Health, Sexuality and Culture*. He is also an editorial board member and reviewer of various national and international journals. He had written 83 book chapters and more than 520 articles in various national and international journals and made 80 presentations at various national and international conferences. He has been included in the global 2% researcher list released by Stanford University in 2021, 2022, 2023, and 2024. His research interests include brain stimulation, neuropsychiatry, and suicide prevention.

**S. M. Yasir Arafat** is currently working as an Associate Consultant of Psychiatry at Bangladesh Specialized Hospital, Dhaka, Bangladesh. He is an Associate Professor of Frontier University Garowe, Somalia, an Associated Fellow of the Bangladesh Academy of Sciences, and a Senior Research Fellow of the Biomedical Research Foundation, Bangladesh. He was affiliated with the University of Bristol, UK, as a Visiting Senior Research Associate (August 2021–2023) and an Honorary Research Fellow with Dnet (October 2023–25).

He completed his MD in Psychiatry from Bangabandhu Sheikh Mujib Medical University, Dhaka, and his MBBS from the Dhaka Medical College, Dhaka, Bangladesh. He also did an MPH in Health Economics and an MBA in Marketing. Dr. Arafat has (co)authored more than 400 peer-reviewed articles and 50 book chapters, and (co)edited more than 15 books with Springer. He has been included in the global 2% researcher list in 2021–23, and 2025. He is an editorial member of more than 10 leading journals in mental health, published by Elsevier, Wiley, Springer, Sage, and Taylor and Francis. His research focused on mental health, suicidal behavior, psychometrics, panic buying, and psycho-sexual disorders.

**Vikas Menon** is currently a Professor of Psychiatry at the Jawaharlal Institute of Postgraduate Medical Education and Research, Puducherry. He completed his postgraduate training in Psychiatry in 2008 from JIPMER. Subsequently, he was awarded the DNB (Psychiatry) degree in 2009. His areas of interest include digital psychiatry, suicidology, and mood disorders. He has published more than 330 peer-reviewed research papers, 20 book chapters in edited volumes, and edited 4 books including the first dedicated book on Dhat syndrome. In 2023, he was awarded the De Leo Fund Award of the International Association for Suicide Prevention in recognition of his outstanding research work on suicidal behaviors carried out in developing countries. He is presently the Deputy Editor of *Indian Journal of Psychiatry*, Chief Associate Editor of the *Indian Journal of Psychological Medicine*, and Editor of the *International Journal of Advanced Medical and Health Research.* He has served on several expert review committees for the Indian Council of Medical Research, the nodal research agency in the country.

**M. Kishor** is currently Head of Department & Professor of Psychiatry, JSS Medical College & Hospital, JSS Academy of Higher Education & Research, Mysuru, Karnataka, India. He did his MBBS from SSMC Tumkur & MD Psychiatry, with University Rank from Bangalore KIMS, Rajiv Gandhi University of Health Sciences, Bengaluru, India. He has published more than 150 peer-reviewed research papers, 18 book chapters in edited volumes, and edited 7 books. He is in speciality editorial board of Indian Journal of Psychiatry, Indian Journal of Psychological Medicine and Digital Journal of Clinical Medicine. He is founder editor of Minds Newsletter, chief coordinator of Indian Teachers of Psychiatry (IToP) and chairperson of Indian Psychiatric Society (IPS) Postgraduate Education.

**Mohan Isaac** is a Clinical Professor of Psychiatry at the Faculty of Medical and Health Sciences, The University of Western Australia, Perth, Australia, and Consultant Psychiatrist, currently in charge of the "Early Interventions in Psychosis" (EIP) Team and the Assertive Community Treatment (ACT) Team at Fremantle Hospital, Fremantle, Australia. He was formerly a Professor of Psychiatry at the UWA (2005–2017) and prior to that Professor and Head of the oldest and largest academic Department of Psychiatry in India at the National Institute of Mental Health and Neurosciences (NIMHANS) in Bangalore. During more than 30 years of his academic and clinical work in India, Mohan was actively involved in the development and implementation of India's National Mental Health Programme (NMHP).His research interests include delivery of mental health services in low-income countries. He is presently involved in a program for "Capacity building for mental health care services, training and research in low- and middle-income Asian countries."Mohan has assisted the World Health Organization (WHO) in various capacities in numerous locations and on numerous occasions, including a stint at the headquarters of WHO in Geneva for about 3 years. Mohan has also assisted various other International Organizations such as the United Nations Relief and Works Agency for Palestinian Refugees (UNRWA), the Asian Development Bank (ADB) Manila, United Mission to Nepal (UMN) Kathmandu, the Royal Netherlands Embassy in India, New Delhi, etc., on matters related to mental health. He works with various non-governmental organizations, particularly in India. He is the immediate past President of the Society for Community Health Awareness Research and Action (2013–2019) and the Medico Pastoral Association (2004–2018), both based in Bangalore, India.

# List of Figures

# List of Tables

# Chapter 1
# Psychiatry Teaching: Global Scene

**Sandeep Grover**

**Abstract** The roots of psychiatry can be traced back to the texts from Ancient India and Greece. However, significant developments in psychiatry occurred from the nineteenth century onward. The emergence of asylums in the nineteenth century led to the development of professional organizations and the starting of training programs for nurses. Clinicians primarily gained their knowledge through hands-on experience in asylums, frequently with the guidance of more experienced medical professionals. Toward the end of the nineteenth century, there was some effort to formulate a curriculum for psychiatry education. Subsequently, psychiatric teaching and training programs have evolved across the globe. However, available data from different surveys suggest a wide variation in the psychiatry teaching and training programs worldwide, with low and middle-income countries lagging behind high-income countries in training and service provisions. The World Psychiatry Association has attempted to formulate the psychiatric curriculum for undergraduate and postgraduate training. Still, these efforts are insufficient to harmonize teaching and training globally. There is a need for more concerted efforts to harmonize psychiatry teaching across the globe.

**Keywords** Teaching · Training · Psychiatry

## 1 Introduction

When one attempts to trace back the history of psychiatry, theories related to mental illness can be seen in texts from Ancient India and Greece. The *Charaka Samhita* can be considered one of the oldest texts related to psychiatry. The history of

S. Grover (✉)
Department of Psychiatry, Post Graduate Institute of Medical Education & Research, Chandigarh, India

Northern Hospital, Melbourne, VIC, Australia



S. K. Kar et al. (eds.), *Teaching and Training in Psychiatry in South Asia*, South Asian Perspectives in Mental Health and Psychology,
https://doi.org/10.1007/978-981-95-1845-6_1

psychiatry in Greek literature can be traced back to Hippocrates, who outlined the physiological basis of mental disorders. Over the centuries, the concept of mental illnesses kept on evolving, and the term "psychiatry" was for the first time used by Johann Christian Reil in 1808, who was a German Physician and Professor at the University of Halle, with the aim of the introduction of a specialty that can focus on the treatment of mind or soul and emphasized the need to treat mental illnesses with the same seriousness as physical conditions (Truong et al., 2020). In terms of the type of treatment for mental disorders, psychiatry has evolved from the use of various inhuman treatments to humane treatments that were initially championed by Pinel, who is considered to be the father of modern psychiatry. In terms of treatment settings, psychiatry as a speciality has evolved from the Asylums to General Hospital Psychiatric Units. Over the years, psychiatry has evolved and developed into various sub-specializations in the subject. The understanding of psychiatry has also changed over the years, and rather than considering it as an isolated speciality of Medicine, it is now well recognized that psychological issues do play a role in etiology, manifestation, treatment seeking, treatment adherence, course, and outcome of almost all diseases. Considering psychiatry's ever-expanding nature and scope, psychiatry is now recognized as an essential subject in the undergraduate medical curriculum. Further, in addition to the traditional postgraduate courses, super-specialization or subspecialisation courses in psychiatry have evolved. When one looks at the history and evolution of psychiatry education, it has run parallel to the history of psychiatry. In this background, this chapter attempts to understand the trends in psychiatry education and training globally. This chapter will primarily focus on the history of psychiatric training and data that has evolved in surveys focusing on psychiatric education and training globally. This chapter does not focus on information collected for a specific country.

## 2 History of Psychiatric Training

Little information is available about psychiatric training and teaching before the establishment of asylums. History can be broadly understood as developments in Europe and the United States. The learning and training in other parts of the world have been broadly guided by development in these parts of the globe.

***History of Psychiatric Teaching and Training in Europe*** Though psychiatry as a branch of Medicine began in the late eighteenth century, it evolved into a specialty only in the mid-nineteenth century. Historically, the development of psychiatry as a medical specialty is mainly attributed to understanding the mind as having active faculties that enabled "mental illnesses," the growing focus on brain and nerve systems instead of humoral concepts of insanity, and the development of asylums. Asylums brought about specialized clinical language and classification systems. Physicians worked as medical superintendents of asylums, and these facilities were soon overcrowded for several reasons. The nineteenth century saw the emergence of these specialized asylums, which were the first to develop training programs for their medical staff. Nurse training schools started in these hospitals to provide good-quality care. Many believe these programs pioneered modern psychiatric residency training. The asylums offered exceptional opportunities to a large, diverse patient population, which enabled the observation, classification, and formation of theories related to mental disorders.

The Association of Medical Officers of Asylums and Hospitals for the Insane, the first national psychiatric organization in the United Kingdom, was established in 1841 and was in line with the culture of mental asylums. In 1865, the Association of Medical Officers of Asylums and Hospitals for the Insane changed its name to the Medico-Psychological Association, which in 1926 was granted a royal charter as the Royal Medico-Psychological Association. The Association's formation also resulted in the publication of a journal in 1853 named *Asylum Journal*, which is now known as the *British Journal of Psychiatry (The Royal College of, The early days, 1841–1865). Similar developments, including the establishment of specialized journals and professional organizations, also occurred in France and Germany. Several attempts were made to categorize the mental illnesses. The following terms, such as schizophrenia, catatonia, manic-depressive insanity, dementia praecox, etc., emerged during this period.*

During this time, phenomenology was emphasized heavily in psychiatry education and training. However, there were no official psychiatric training programs. Psychoanalysis emerged as a result of Sigmund Freud's work in the late nineteenth and the early twentieth centuries, which had a significant influence on psychiatry as a specialty and psychiatric education. The emphasis shifted to psychological explanations and therapeutic interventions by introducing new ideas like the unconscious, transference, and the talking cure through psychoanalysis. There was little official, standardized psychiatric training up until this point. The majority of clinicians with an interest in the topic gained their knowledge through hands-on experience in asylums, frequently with the guidance of more experienced medical professionals. Asylum nurses and attendants also underwent "on-the-job" training, which was occasionally governed by institutional policies and handbooks (Kendler et al., 2022; Nolan, 1991; Freeman, 1996, LE Bonhomme & LE Bras, 2025).

Inhumane treatment of people with mental illness was acknowledged and condemned in the late nineteenth and the early twentieth centuries, and moral treatments emphasizing humane care, minimizing restraints, and providing a therapeutic environment became more prevalent. Even though it was not exactly "education" in the contemporary sense, this method affected how asylum doctors practiced, interacted with, and thought about their patients. It sought to foster moral fortitude and reason via decency, civility, and intentional action. Smaller asylums, more specialized hospitals, outpatient clinics, and, ultimately, community mental health services were all developed as a result. Psychiatric education was inevitably impacted by this change in care settings, necessitating training in various clinical settings and an emphasis on various care models. Formal training programs became more standardized as psychiatry became recognized as a medical specialty. This included certification exams, supervised clinical rotations, and structured curricula. Psychiatric education was progressively incorporated into the core medical curricula of universities and medical schools. As a result, specialized university psychiatry departments were created, encouraging research and more organized academic instruction.

The need for psychiatry to be recognized as a specialty grew as a result of the high prevalence of psychological trauma among soldiers during World Wars I and II. The development of psychopharmacology and other advancements in the United States, starting in the 1950s, impacted the expansion of psychiatry and the instruction and training of psychiatry worldwide (The Royal College of Psychiatrists, 1865–1926; The Royal College of Psychiatrists, 1926–1971). The Royal Medico-Psychological Association received a Supplemental Charter in 1971, transforming into the Royal College of Psychiatrists (Royal College of Psychiatrist, 1971-). This was a significant change, bringing psychiatrists from teaching hospitals and asylum doctors together and reaffirming the College's role in training, education, and professional standards. Teaching, research, and public education were the three primary goals of the Royal College Psychiatrists in the United Kingdom. Since its inception, the Royal College of Psychiatrists has played a key role in creating junior physician training programs, such as the MRCPsych exam, and in setting up training program accreditation and inspection procedures. Additionally, it significantly impacts mental health policy in the United Kingdom, research, and quality improvement. Although the seeds of various subspecialties were sowed during the early part of the twentieth century, College recognized several subspecialties within psychiatry, including child and adolescent psychiatry (CAP), geriatric psychiatry, forensic psychiatry, psychiatry of intellectual disability, and medical psychotherapy (Royal College of Psychiatrist, United Kingdom, 1971-).

***History of Psychiatric Teaching and Training in the United States*** The history of psychiatry teaching in the United States from 1844 to 1944 was reviewed by F G Ebaugh (Ebaugh, 1947). Readers interested in understanding these developments in depth can go through the article. In the following section, this will be discussed briefly. The history of psychiatric teaching can be traced back to Benjamin Rush. In 1812, he published "*Medical Inquiries and Observations upon the Diseases of the Mind*," considered the first American general treatise on mental diseases. The book was based on his 30 years of observation of people with a mental health condition at the Pennsylvania Hospital. This book remained the primary textbook of mental illnesses until the year 1883 when William A. Hammond and C. E. Spitzka published textbooks on insanity, followed by E. C. Mann. It is said that until the 1870s, there were only occasional lectures on mental and neurological diseases in medical colleges (Ebaugh, 1947).

In 1844, Medical Superintendents working in various asylums came together in Philadelphia to form the Association of Medical Superintendents of American Institutions for the Insane (AMSAII). The mission of the Association was to "communicate their experiences to each other, cooperate in collecting statistical information relating to insanity, and assist each other in improving the treatment of the insane." This was later named the American Psychiatric Association (APA). This Association fostered communication among clinicians dedicated to caring for the mentally ill. During this period, Medical Superintendents of asylums were the de facto mental health experts and were responsible for whatever little "education" existed. This often involved practical observation and hands-on experience within the asylum setting rather than formal curricula or lectures in medical schools. The currently known *American Journal of Psychiatry* started in 1844 as the *American Journal of Insanity* (Ebaugh, 1947).

In 1853, Pliny Earle, a physician appointed as a visiting physician to the New York Asylum, delivered his first course of lectures on mental diseases at the College of Physicians and Surgeons. No systematic course was available on mental diseases until 1867 when William A. Hammond was appointed as a professor of nervous and mental diseases at Bellevue Hospital Medical College in New York (Ebaugh, 1947).

Formal teaching positions for mental disorders started emerging in the United States in the 1850s to the 1870s. John E. Tyler was a lecturer on mental disorders at the Harvard Medical School during 1858–1871. A lectureship in mental disease was established at the College of Physicians and Surgeons of New York for E. C. Seguin in 1871. During the same time, Isaac Ray was appointed lecturer on insanity at the Jefferson Medical College of Philadelphia in 1870. The first postgraduate school was established at New York Polyclinic in 1881 and at the Polyclinic in Philadelphia in 1882. At these places, the teaching of postgraduates was limited to outpatient departments of the hospitals, but no systematic teaching was attempted (Ebaugh, 1947).

The lack of psychiatric instruction was formally recognized in 1871 when the AMSAII, at its annual meeting, resolved the following:

1. *"That in view of the frequency of mental disorders among all classes and descriptions of people, and in recognition of the fact that the first care of nearly all these cases necessarily devolves upon physicians engaged in general practice, ...... it is the unanimous opinion of this Association that in every school conferring medical degrees, there should be delivered by competent professors a complete course of lectures on insanity.*
2. *These lectures should be delivered before all the students attending these schools, and no one is allowed to graduate without as thorough an examination on these subjects as in other branches taught in the schools.*
3. *In connection with these lectures, whenever practicable, there should be clinical instructions.........giving the students practical illustrations of the different forms of insanity and the effects of treatment."*

Subsequently, in 1882, the AMSAII and the Prevention of Insanity appointed a committee to draft a circular on psychiatric instruction to be sent to the faculty of every medical school in the country. The commission recommended that all medical schools implement a comprehensive curriculum. However, until the final decade of the nineteenth century, psychiatric practice and teaching was almost entirely confined to the asylums. In 1895, Adolf Meyer established the first pathological laboratory under the interrelation of Clinical Medicine, psychiatry, and pathology. Similar initiatives followed across different institutes. At the beginning of the twentieth century, Adolf Meyer's work led to the evolution of the psychobiological method of approach and the emergence of the subspecialty of Psychosomatic Medicine. J M Mosher established the first psychiatric ward in a General Hospital in 1902, which offered actual therapeutic service, and this led to the emergence of a subspecialty of consultation-liaison psychiatry. At the beginning of the twentieth century, the psychodynamic movement significantly impacted psychiatry teaching. During the same time, the National Committee for Mental Hygiene emerged, which led to psychiatry coming out of the asylums. This movement brought greater attention to mental health and, in turn, to the need for better training of professionals (Ebaugh, 1947) (Table 1.1).

A survey of different medical schools in 1908 showed that there were lectures on mental diseases in most medical schools. However, these were optional, attendance was left to the students, and there was no examination for the subject. In 1914, the Section on Nervous and Mental Diseases of the American Medical Association resolved that there was inadequate psychiatry teaching in a large proportion of American Medical Colleges. The huge number of psychological causalities during World War I highlighted the need to focus on psychiatric education and services in the coming decades. However, psychiatry did not receive much attention during the early twentieth century due to the competing curriculum of the other subjects. However, a 1931 survey undertaken by the Division of Psychiatric Education of the National Committee for Mental Hygiene again brought forth the deficiencies in psychiatry training in the country. This survey resulted in many changes in psychiatric education in the United States. During the late 1920s and the early 1930s, many eminent clinicians of that time recommended the formation of an American Board of Psychiatry and Neurology (ABPN), and several conferences were held on psychiatric education under the direction of the Division of Psychiatric Education of the National Committee for Mental Hygiene. All these developments contributed to the formation of ABPN. This provided a framework for residency training and helped solidify psychiatry's place as a distinct and recognized medical specialty. During the subsequent years, the subspecialty of psychosomatic medicine expanded, which is considered to have provided a significant leap to the recognition of psychiatry. World War II again highlighted the importance of mental health and led to a substantial expansion of mental health services and the formalization of training programs, particularly in the post-war era (Ebaugh, 1947).

After the Second World War, psychiatrists trained in psychoanalysis migrated to the United States, leading to the rise in psychoanalysis in the United States and the formation of the American Psychoanalysis Association (APsaA). In the 1940s, The APsaA urged its members to advocate for the inclusion of psychoanalysis in academic institutions and medical schools. After World War II, during the 1950s, long-term, intensive psychotherapy was emphasized during the postgraduate training. Residents would spend considerable time learning psychoanalytic techniques, interpreting unconscious conflicts, and understanding early childhood experiences as

**Table 1.1** Major psychiatry education developments in the United States (Ebaugh, 1947; Truong et al., 2020)

| Year | Development |
|---|---|
| 1812 | Benjamin Rush published a book titled "*Medical Inquiries and Observations Upon the Diseases of the Mind*," which is considered to be the first American general treatise on the subject of mental diseases |
| 1844 | The Association of Medical Superintendents of American Institutions for the Insane (AMSAII) was founded. It was later named as American Psychiatric Association |
| 1853 | Pliny Earle delivered his first course of lectures on mental diseases at the College of Physicians and Surgeons |
| 1867 | William A. Hammond was appointed as a professor of nervous and mental diseases at Bellevue Hospital Medical College in New York. |
| 1871 | The AMSAII resolved to have instructions/lectures in every medical school |
| 1879 | Construction of an "insane pavilion" at Bellevue Hospital in New York City for observation of patients until proper commitment could be arranged |
| 1882 | The AMSAII and the Prevention of Insanity appointed a committee to draft a circular on psychiatric instruction for every medical school |
| 1895 | Adolf Meyer established the first pathological laboratory in clinical Medicine, psychiatry, and pathology interrelation. Similar initiatives followed across different institutes. |
| 1895 | Establishment in New York City of the Pathological Institute of the New York State Hospitals, which primarily focused on psychiatric Research. Ira Van Gieson was its first director. |
| 1901 | J M Mosher established the first psychiatric ward in a General Hospital in 1902, which offered genuine therapeutic service—led to the emergence of a subspecialty of consultation-liaison psychiatry. |
| 1902 | Adolf Meyer—the evolution of the psychobiological method of approach and emergence of the subspecialty of Psychosomatic Medicine |
| 1909 | Organization of the National Committee for Mental Hygiene |
| 1911 | Formation of American Psychoanalytic Society |
| 1912 | Inclusion of two types of Psychology in the Medical Curriculum, one focusing on normalcy and the second focusing on psychopathology |
| 1934 | Formation of the American Board of Psychiatry and Neurology—aimed to certify standards of training and specialty competence |
| 1952 | Publication of DSM-I |
| 1968 | Publication of DSM-II |
| 1980 | Publication of DSM-III |
| 1987 | Publication of DSM-IIIR |
| 1994 | Publication of DSM-IV |
| 2000 | Publication of DSM-IVTR |
| 2013 | Publication of DSM-5 |
| 2019 | Publication of DSM-5TR |

*DSM* Diagnostic and Statistical Manual of Mental Disorders

root causes of mental illness. In 1946, Mental Health Act was passed, and the National Institute of Mental Health was established in 1949 (Ebaugh, 1947).

During the same time, in 1952, the first Diagnostic and Statistical Manual of Mental Disorders (DSM-I) was published, attempting to standardize psychiatric diagnoses. While still influenced by psychodynamic concepts, it marked an early step toward a more unified diagnostic system. During the same period, there was the introduction of chlorpromazine, which dramatically changed the landscape of mental illness treatment. The introduction of psychotropics led to the emergence of a biomedical model of mental illness and deinstitutionalization. The 1960s also saw the emergence of community mental health centers (CMHCs) that emphasized providing care close to the patient's home (Truong et al., 2020).

Accordingly, psychiatric education and training during the 1950s–1960s started incorporating more neurobiology, pharmacology, and research into brain function. Further, with the CMHCs, there was more focus on outpatient care, crisis intervention, and working with multidisciplinary teams during training. During this period, although there was the emergence of psychopharmacology, psychotherapy remained an essential component of training, with a growing emphasis on shorter-term, more focused therapies. The ABPN and the Accreditation Council for Graduate Medical Education (ACGME) continued to refine and standardize residency training requirements, ensuring consistent competence across programs. From the 1970s onward, there was the emergence of various subspecialties, such as CAP, addiction psychiatry, geriatric psychiatry, and forensic psychiatry, leading to specialized training pathways. Additionally, the period from the 1970s to the 1990s saw multiple revisions of the DSM, the emergence and rise of evidence-based medicine, and the ascendency of biological psychiatry. These developments led to changes in the understanding of mental illness and the inclusion of neurobiology in the form of neurotransmitters, brain circuits, and genetics into the postgraduate curriculum (Geller, 2000; Truong et al., 2020).

Training programs increasingly emphasized critical appraisal of research, empirically supported treatments, and outcomes-based assessment. During the first part of the twenty-first century, the emphasis on neurobiology and psychopharmacology increased. Current psychiatric teaching strongly emphasizes integrated care, where mental health services are co-located or closely coordinated with primary care and other medical specialties. This reflects recognition of the strong link between psychological and physical health. Additionally, current training focuses on recovery-oriented care, empowering patients in their treatment decisions, and focusing on their strengths and goals. Psychiatric education increasingly addresses diversity, equity, and inclusion issues, recognizing the impact of social determinants of health, cultural factors, and disparities in mental healthcare. The COVID-19 pandemic accelerated the adoption of telepsychiatry, and virtual care delivery is becoming a norm. There is also growing interest in and training for digital therapeutics, which use software programs as interventions. Further, more focus on public mental health, prevention, and early intervention is evident in curricula, reflecting a broader societal understanding of mental well-being. Psychotherapy training has evolved, and there is an emphasis on delivering more time-limited and focused interventions.

In 2010, ACGME implemented "Milestones" for residency training in psychiatry and shifted the focus to competency-based education, assessing residents' progression in specific skills and attributes rather than solely relying on time spent in training.

## 3 Evaluation or Surveys of Psychiatry Training Across the Globe

Little information is available about psychiatry training across the globe. The World Psychiatric Association (WPA) has tried to evaluate psychiatry training globally. In one survey from February to July 2001, WPA evaluated the teaching and training in old-age psychiatry across different countries. The survey was sent to 116 WPA member societies from 93 countries, out of which 54 member societies from 48 countries responded to the survey. The survey showed that in only 13% of the countries, old-age psychiatry was recognized as a subspecialty. However, old-age psychiatry services were available in more than four-fifths (83%) of the countries. In countries with old-age psychiatry subspecialty, the curriculum duration ranged between three months to five years (median: two years, data from nine countries). Chairs in Geriatric Medicine existed in 32 participating countries (66%), and chairs in old-age psychiatry existed in 18 countries (38%). Geriatric Medicine and old-age psychiatry were recognized as a subspecialty mainly in European countries, and old-age psychiatry was recognized as a subspecialty in Western Pacific Regions, too. In most countries ($n$ = 30), there were specific learning objectives in old-age psychiatry at the postgraduation level. However, the number of hours dedicated to old-age psychiatry was less than half that of those dedicated to CAP and less than one-tenth of those committed to adult psychiatry. Overall, the perceived need for old-age psychiatry training was reported by 83% of the participating countries. In terms of specific areas, the need for education material was noted most commonly for depression and psychopharmacology, followed by dementia, organization of care, psychotherapy, and psychotic disorders (Camus et al., 2003).

In 2004, the World Health Organization (WHO) and the World Psychiatric Association (WPA) surveyed psychiatric training globally. The questionnaire was initially developed by the mental health professionals associated with the WHO and later modified by those associated with WPA. The questionnaire was circulated in 121 countries through 143 member societies of WPA. The questionnaire was returned from 73 countries and one WHO territory, representing information from 38% of the 192 countries in the world. Another attempt was made to contact the member societies from the countries where information was unavailable to collect the information about the presence or absence of psychiatry training. Overall, information about the presence or absence of psychiatric training was available for 179 countries. The countries were divided into different income categories based on information from the World Bank website in 2005 (Atlas, 2005).

According to the survey, out of the 179 countries for which information was available, 68.2% (122 countries) had psychiatric training programs. Regarding different geographic regions, 94.1% of European countries had psychiatric training programs, whereas this figure was only 47.4% for the African region. Regarding income categories, 55.1% of low-income countries (LIC), 68.5% of lower-middle-income countries (LMIC), 59.5% in high-middle-income countries, and 77.1% of high-income countries (HIC) had psychiatry training facilities (Atlas, 2005).

Regarding the countries where the detailed data was available (73 countries and nd one WHO territory, henceforth mentioned as 74 countries for this chapter), at least one accredited postgraduate diploma course was available in 31 countries, and at least one accredited Master's program was available in 35 countries. An accredited super-specialization course was available in 23 countries, and at least one doctoral course was available in 22 countries. In terms of geographic location, more than half of the European countries had super-specialization courses, whereas none of the countries from the Eastern Mediterranean region had such courses. Similar differences were noted for other courses, too, with more European countries having training programs in the form of Master's courses. The duration of training across different countries varied widely, with the duration of the diploma course in 22 out of 74 countries and the duration of the Master's program in 28 out of 74 countries being 3–4 years. The duration of the super-specialization course in 18 out of the 35 countries in which this was available ranged from 1 to 2 years. The duration of PhD programs in 22 countries varied from 3 to 4 years. In terms of infrastructure, the survey assessed the infrastructure in terms of that related to psychiatry directly (i.e., number of teaching beds, rehabilitation facilities, and psychological testing) and general infrastructure (i.e., biochemical testing, radiology, anesthetist support, library facilities, Biostatistics, ethics committee). Information about the minimum number of beds required for training was available for 45 countries (60.8%) with an average of 136 beds. The average outpatient attendance was a criterion for training centers in 33 (44.6%) countries. The presence of rehabilitation facilities and anesthesia support was a criterion in 40% of the countries. On the other hand, psychological, biochemical, radiological, and neurophysiological testing was a prerequisite in 43%–50% of countries. In terms of other training facilities, data from three-fourths of the countries suggested the presence of open wards, residential facilities, day-care facilities, audiovisual aids, computer facilities, access to electronic databases, and subscriptions to at least five psychiatric journals. Although the information from many countries suggested the presence of rehabilitation and forensic psychiatry services, these were limited to a few centers in those countries. Regarding geographic distribution, most desired facilities in low-income countries were present in most centers in <10% of the countries. In contrast, the entire training infrastructure (except for rehabilitation and forensic psychiatry) was present in most centers in 40%–65% of the higher-middle income countries and HICs. Regarding the workforce, >10 postgraduate teachers were present in 32 countries. A written curriculum was available in 63 countries. In one-third of the countries, rotation in Medicine, Neurology, and multidisciplinary was mandatory in most centers. In only a minority of the countries (19%–27%), training in psychotherapy, national mental health activities, and promoting independence among the trainees was present in most centers. Training skills, including knowledge of psychopathology, diagnostic interviewing, clinical skills, and diagnostic and therapeutic skills, were taught to trainees in most centers in 60% of the countries. Only one-third of the countries were psychotherapy, genetics, basic neurosciences, psychology, research methodology, and public health psychiatry covered in most of the centers. Regarding specific teaching techniques, in 50%–60% of the countries, the most commonly used teaching techniques included case vignettes, case conferences, and seminars. In one-fourth of the countries, the teaching techniques also included self-directed learning and discussion on ethics. The training evaluation was preferably evaluated using oral methods, an ongoing process during training in 39 countries. In contrast, it was used as an assessment method at the end of the training in 46 countries. The teaching, research, and managerial skills were assessed at some point in 55%, 70%, and 40% of the countries, respectively. Research skills were mainly assessed in the written format, such as when submitting a dissertation. In terms of methods recommended by the national bodies, clinical examination (73%) was the most common, followed by essays (66.2%), patient interviews (66.2%), multiple choice questions (63.5%), and dissertations (55.4%). Regarding examiners, in less than half (44.6%) of the countries, the examination was conducted by a combination of internal and external examiners; in one-third (33.8%) of the countries, the examiner panel only included internal examiners. In about one-fifth (20.3%) of the countries, the trainees were evaluated by an independent body, and in another one-fifth (21.6%) of countries, an accrediting body conducted the examination. Super-specialization courses in child psychiatry were available in only 29 countries, whereas de-addiction and forensic training programs were available in 14 and 15 countries, respectively (Atlas, 2005). Regarding inter-country training arrangements, bilateral arrangements were not available in only about half of the countries, and among the countries (28 out of 74) for this was available, the arrangement mostly involved sending trainees from less developed to more developed countries. In only about 15% (11 countries) of countries, there was provision for sending and receiving trainees from other countries. Regarding the number of psychiatrists, 11 countries had <500 psychiatrists residing within the country. However, this survey could not collect information about the quality and uniformity of training. The survey concluded that there is a wide variation in psychiatry training globally, varying across the different centers in a given country. The survey concluded that there is a need for the expansion of psychiatry training across different countries, especially in low-income countries. It was also suggested that developing regional collaborations for psychiatric training could benefit countries with low resources. The survey recommended standardizing the training programs and assessment methods globally. Further, the survey showed limited avenues of advanced training in psychiatry (Atlas, 2005).

In another online survey, in 2017, WPA sent a 15-item self-administered questionnaire in the form of an online survey to 138 Presidents of member societies (44 from HIC and 94 from LMIC as per the 2017 World Bank data) who were representing 118 countries in the WPA. The survey was conducted between September 2016 and February 2017. Fifty-three Presidents representing 47-member societies responded. Regarding regions, 26.4% of responses pertained to Asia, 28.3% to the Americas, 39.6% to Europe, and 5.7% to Africa. The median number of psychiatrists per 100,000 population was seven across the respondent member countries, with a significantly higher number of psychiatrists in HIC than in LMIC. One-fifth of the countries had <1 psychiatrist per 1 lakh population. Overall, there was a low response from the LMIC compared to that from HIC (Ng et al., 2020).

At the postgraduate level, the duration of psychiatry training varied between 1 and 6 years, with a mean duration of 4 years. In about one-third (31%) of countries, the psychiatry training was of ≤3 years, with 10% having training programs for 12–18 months, another 10% having training programs of 19–24 months, and 11% having training programs lasting for 36 months only. Overall, the trainees from LMIC countries spend significantly lower duration in psychiatry training when compared to HIC. Regarding gender, the mean percentage of female trainees was 60%, with no significant difference between LMIC and HIC (Ng et al., 2020). In terms of location of training, about two-fifths (41.8%) of the time was spent in a psychiatry inpatient setting, 26% of the time was spent in the psychiatry outpatient setting, 10.2% was spent in a consultation-liaison psychiatry setting, 6.4% time spent in a primary care clinic setting, and 7.8% time was spent in outreach services in the community (Ng et al., 2020). There was no significant difference in the time spent in different settings during the training period between LMIC and HIC. In terms of time spent in didactic lectures, maximum amount of time was spent on clinical topics (41.9%), followed by psychopharmacology (22.2%), basic sciences (14.8%), psychosocial treatments (12.3%), research methodology (9.5%), psychiatric ethics (6.2%), leadership and administrative topics (5.3%), and other topics such as clinical psychology, philosophy, and history of psychiatry (2.1%). There was no significant difference between LMIC and HIC regarding time spent teaching on different topics. However, it is essential to note that in 41% of the countries, no time was allocated to medical leadership and administration. In terms of training in subspecialty, available information suggested that in 82% of the countries, training in subspecialties was available in various subspecialties apart from the general adult psychiatry, with no significant difference in LMIC and HIC countries in having at least one subspecialty training. Concerning the type of subspecialty, subspecialty training that was available in most countries was that of CAP (71%), followed by addiction psychiatry (60.8%), forensic psychiatry (52.9%), psychotherapy (51%), geriatric psychiatry (41.2%), consultation-liaison psychiatry (39.2%), and neuropsychiatry or perinatal psychiatry (26.1%). When the subspecialty training was compared between HIC and LMIC, the LMIC countries had significantly lower subspecialty training opportunities for CAP, geriatric psychiatry, consultation-liaison psychiatry, and psychotherapy. In about three-fifths (59%) of countries, psychotherapy training was mandatory during psychiatry training, with no significant difference between HIC and LMIC. Among the countries with compulsory psychotherapy training, the median duration of psychotherapy training throughout the training period was 160 hours, with no significant difference between HIC and LMIC. Regarding exposure to training in other medical specialties, 83% of the countries or regions reported that the trainees had a chance of exposure to at least one other medical specialty during the postgraduate training, with no significant difference in the HIC and LMIC. The median number of medical specialties in which rotation was done was two, with a median total duration of training being 6 months (Ng et al., 2020).

Regarding assessment, information from 96% of countries or regions suggested having a mechanism to evaluate trainees' performance. Three-fourth (75%) of the member countries or regions reported having a selection procedure for admission, and 85.4% of countries reported having a mechanism for periodic evaluation of the trainees throughout the training, with no significant difference between the HIC and LMIC countries. There were opportunities in all the member countries for continuing medical education for qualified psychiatrists after the postgraduate psychiatric training (Ng et al., 2020).

## 4 Psychiatry Training at Undergraduate Level Across the Globe

Compared to postgraduate training, less information is available for the undergraduate psychiatry training, and the surveys that have evaluated the postgraduate training had few questions on the undergraduate training. Only occasion surveys have focused explicitly on undergraduate training. The WPA survey that assessed the teaching and training in old-age psychiatry across different countries reported that old-age psychiatry was taught in most countries (92%) at the undergraduate training level (Camus et al., 2003). The 2017 WPA survey showed that at the undergraduate level, only 4% of the time was dedicated to psychiatric education, with no significant difference between HIC and LMIC. Regarding time considered optimal for psychiatry training, participants reported that about 9% of the time should be dedicated to psychiatry during undergraduate training, with no significant difference in response from HIC and LMIC. In terms of the mean percentage of medical graduate students taking up psychiatry at the postgraduate level in the previous 5 years of the survey, the mean was only 3.3%, with significantly lower students from LMIC opting for psychiatry compared to HIC. Further, it was seen that the duration of exposure during undergraduate training had a significant positive correlation with the percentage of students opting for psychiatry at the postgraduate level (Ng et al., 2020).

An online survey was conducted between March and May 2018 by the International Federation of Medical Students' Association (IFMSA), and the WPA that evaluated undergraduate psychiatric training across various countries. The survey explored the inclusion of psychiatry in the undergraduate curriculum, the duration of theory classes, clinical exposure, and assessment methods to determine the knowledge/competencies. The survey was responded to by representatives from 83 countries (66.4% response rate; 66 out of 125 countries). In almost all countries (81 out of 83), psychiatry was mandatory in undergraduate medical education. In two countries, it was an elective subject. The duration of theory classes varied widely across the different countries, with 1 to 15 days in 17 countries, 16 to 30 days in 29 countries, and more than 30 days in 37 countries. In terms of clinical classes, the duration was 1 to 15 days in 29 countries, 16 to 30 days in 28 countries, and more than 30 days in 24 countries. In two countries, there was no provision for clinical classes. Overall, psychiatric education was shorter in Asia and Pacific regions, whereas the duration was longer in America. In terms of evaluation methods, MCQ was the most common method of evaluation of knowledge and competency, with this being the standalone assessment method in 17 countries and being used with another assessment method in 57 countries. The authors concluded that the survey recognizes the need for improvment in psychiatry training at the undergraduate level worldwide (Pinto et al., 2019).

## 5 Impact of Disparity in Psychiatric Training Across the Globe

As evident from the different surveys, there is a vast disparity in psychiatry training globally. Despite the shortage of psychiatrists in LIC and LMIC countries, many psychiatrists from LIC and LMIC move to HIC to pursue their medical careers after their postgraduate studies. However, this immigration process is complex because of the disparity in psychiatry training. Getting their medical degrees and specialized psychiatric training accepted by the developed country's regulatory bodies is a significant challenge. This frequently entails a drawn-out and intricate evaluation procedure, which can be costly, frustrating, and time-consuming. Once accepted to work in developed countries, foreign-trained psychiatrists are still required to pass demanding standardized tests, which may differ significantly from those in their home country regarding format and content.

Furthermore, even after passing exams, they might still need to finish a period of supervised practice, which could last for years, to receive complete registration and start practicing independently. For some, this immigration may entail working exclusively in underserved or needy areas. Many young psychiatrists are unable to migrate to the HIC because of these problems, or if they do, they must complete years of additional training and endure a great deal of stress. In a similar vein, senior psychiatrists are unable to relocate due to equivalency requirements.

## 6 Global Initiatives to Harmonize the Psychiatry Training

Psychiatry as a specialty has evolved over the years, and with the world becoming a global village, there is a need to develop a global uniform curriculum for psychiatry teaching at the undergraduate medical school/college level, at the postgraduate level, and for the subspecialties. There have been some initiatives in this direction. At the beginning of the twenty-first century, WPA, in collaboration with the World Federation for Medical Education, defined the Core Curriculum in Psychiatry. The main educational goal has been "to construct the core elements of a graduate training curriculum in psychiatry in order to ensure high quality of psychiatric services via creation of competent psychiatrists in all areas of the world" (Montenegro, 2002). Later, this Core Curriculum was revised to conform to the ideas of "new medicine," which acknowledges that healing and treatment are insufficient on their own and calls for a greater focus on mental health promotion and mental disorder prevention (Skokauskas et al., 2025). WPA has also developed the *"Institutional Program on the Core Training Curriculum for Psychiatry"* with the educational goal of creating the core elements of a graduate psychiatry training curriculum to ensure good quality of psychiatry services through the creation of competent psychiatrists worldwide (Montenegro, 2002). Unfortunately, these attempts have received little attention at the individual country level to enforce these into training because WPA cannot directly influence the training structure in any given country.

## 7 Conclusions

There is wide variation in psychiatry teaching and training globally, both at the undergraduate and postgraduate levels. In general, the exposure to psychiatry during the undergraduate medical curriculum is more prevalent in HIC than in LMIC and LIC. Further, at the postgraduate level, there is a gap in the level of training across different countries, with, in general, better exposure to the subject in HIC. The current level of efforts to harmonize psychiatry training globally is grossly inadequate.

Psychiatry as a medical specialty has evolved over the centuries, especially in the last three centuries. In the last couple of decades, there has been tremendous growth in the understanding and management of mental illnesses. In recent times, it has been understood that a lack of mental well-being is not only linked to the development of mental disorders but also to a host of chronic physical illnesses. Hence, the subject is receiving wider acceptance and recognition. In this background, there is a need to improve psychiatry training globally, both at the undergraduate and postgraduate levels. Further, there is a need to develop a unified psychiatry course curriculum that can be implemented at the global level. This will not be easy because of the disparity in how medical education is regulated in different countries. Joint efforts of various professional bodies and involving the World Health Organization to achieve harmonization can lead to fruitful results.

## References

Atlas: Psychiatry education and training across the world 2005. World Health Organization, 2005 ISBN: 9241563079.

Camus, V., Katona, C., de Mendonça Lima, C. A., Abdel-Hakam, A. M., Graham, N., Baldwin, R., Tataru, N., & Chiu, E. (2003). World Psychiatric Association section on old age psychiatry. Teaching and training in old age psychiatry: A general survey of the World Psychiatric Association member societies. *International Journal of Geriatric Psychiatry, 18*(8), 694–699. https://doi.org/10.1002/gps.900

Ebaugh, F. G. (1947). The history of psychiatric education in the United States from 1844 to 1944. *Centaur (London, England), 52*(3), 169–178.

Freeman, H. (1996). 250 Jahre englische Psychiatrie [250 years of English psychiatry]. *Fortschritte der Neurologie-Psychiatrie, 64*(8), 320–326. https://doi.org/10.1055/s-2007-996401

Geller, J. L. (2000). The last half-century of psychiatric services as reflected in psychiatric services. *Psychiatric Services, 51*(1), 41–67. https://doi.org/10.1176/ps.51.1.41

Kendler, K. S., Tabb, K., & Wright, J. (2022). The Emergence of Psychiatry: 1650–1850. *The American Journal of Psychiatry, 179*(5), 329–335. https://doi.org/10.1176/appi.ajp.21060614

LE Bonhomme F, LE Bras Anatole. Psychiatric institutions in Europe, nineteenth and twentieth century. Digital Encyclopedia of European History. ISSN 2677-6588, published on 21/10/21, consulted on 29/05/2025. Permalink: https://ehne.fr/en/node/14132

Montenegro, R. (2002). WPA educational programs. *World Psychiatry, 1*(3), 190–191.

Ng, R. M. K., Hermans, M. H. M., Belfort, E., & Bhugra, D. (2020). A worldwide survey on training provisions for psychiatric trainees in WPA member associations. *International Review of Psychiatry, 32*(2), 98–113. https://doi.org/10.1080/09540261.2019.1648241

Nolan, P. W. (1991). The founding of psychiatric nurse training and its aftermath. *The British Journal of Psychiatry, 159*, 46–52. https://doi.org/10.1192/bjp.159.1.46

Pinto da Costa, M., Dima, K., & Ng, R. M. K. (2019). Undergraduate psychiatric education: A snapshot of medical students across the world. *World Psychiatry, 18*(2), 243–244. https://doi.org/10.1002/wps.20642

Skokauskas, N., Chaimowitz, G., El-Gabry, D. A., Fiorillo, A., Lachman, A., Lopez Geist, A., Robertson, P., Yoo, H. J., & Leventhal, B. (2025). The WPA global study on psychiatric training. *World Psychiatry, 24*(1), 147–148. https://doi.org/10.1002/wps.21293

The Royal College of Psychiatrists. The early days (1841–1865). The history of the Royal College of Psychiatrists. https://www.rcpsych.ac.uk/about-us/history%2D%2Dart-and-exhibitions/history/our-history/the-early-days

The Royal College of Psychiatrists. The Medico-Psychological Association (1865–1926). The history of the Royal College of Psychiatrists. https://www.rcpsych.ac.uk/about-us/history%2D%2Dart-and-exhibitions/history/our-history/the-mpa

The Royal College of Psychiatrists. The Royal College of Psychiatrists (1971–). The history of the Royal College of Psychiatrists. https://www.rcpsych.ac.uk/about-us/history%2D%2Dart-and-exhibitions/history/our-history/the-rcpsych

The Royal College of Psychiatrists. The Royal Medico-Psychological Association (1926–1971). The history of the Royal College of Psychiatrists. https://www.rcpsych.ac.uk/about-us/history%2D%2Dart-and-exhibitions/history/our-history/the-rmpa

Truong, A. H., Maguire, G. E., & Maguire, G. A. (2020). A history of psychiatry in the United States of America. *Taiwan Journal Psychiatry, 34*, 59–66. https://doi.org/10.4103/TPSY.TPSY_12_20

# Chapter 2
# Conventional Methods of Psychiatry Teaching in South Asia

**Snehil Gupta , Pooja Shatadal, and Akash Kumar**

**Abstract** Many South Asian countries have adopted competency-based medical education (CBME) for both medical undergraduates (UG) and psychiatry postgraduates (PG). The central theme of CBME is to ensure competency and skill acquisition among the learners and to make the teaching-learning (T-L) experience more engaging and active. Conventional/traditional T-L methods are time-tested approaches to teaching/training, particularly helpful for large groups and resource-limited settings, like South Asia, albeit with some inherent limitations. Lectures, outpatient department (OPD) and bedside teaching, and tutorials are common conventional methods of UG teaching, while case presentations (ward round, grand round, & OPD), case conferences, journal clubs, seminars, thesis writing, and inter-departmental posting are the most used traditional methods in PG training.

Novel T-L methods (simulation, virtual reality, small-group teachings, blended teaching, etc.) have gained prominence, with the introduction of the CBME and during the COVID-19. The relative effectiveness of the novel T-L methods vs. conventional methods (and vice versa) is context dependent, with the suitability of one over the other depending on resources, teachers' expertise, students' motivation, and institutional attitude and policy. In this chapter, we have discussed critical aspects of various conventional T-L methods used in UGs and PGs teaching/training in South Asia and provided future direction.

**Keywords** Conventional · Traditional · Teaching · Learning · Methods · Psychiatry · South Asia

---

S. Gupta (✉)
Department of Psychiatry, All India Institute of Medical Sciences – Bhopal, Bhopal, India

P. Shatadal
Department of Psychiatry, Government Medical College, Surat, Gujarat, India

A. Kumar
Department of Psychiatry, All India Institute of Medical Sciences – Raebareli, Raebareli, India


S. K. Kar et al. (eds.), *Teaching and Training in Psychiatry in South Asia*, South Asian Perspectives in Mental Health and Psychology, https://doi.org/10.1007/978-981-95-1845-6_2

# 1 Introduction

The teaching of medical students (in psychiatry) and the training of psychiatry residents have undergone tremendous change over a couple of decades. South Asia is also not aloof from this development in medical education. Many South Asian countries have, in line with the high-income countries, adopted a competency-based medical education (CBME) curriculum for medical students and postgraduate (PG) psychiatry trainees (Gupta & Menon, 2022; Sahadevan et al., 2021). For instance, India adopted the CBME curriculum for the medical undergraduates in 2018, which was revised in 2024 (National Medical Commission, 2024): likewise, the postgraduate medical education board has released Guidelines for a competency-based postgraduate training program for M.D. in Psychiatry in 2022 (Postgraduate Medical Education Board, National Medical Commission, 2022). The primary goal of the CBME for Indian Medical Graduates (IMG) is to create graduates who can identify and attend to community health needs, including mental health problems, and be able to provide holistic care to patients in a culturally sensitive and empathetic manner (National Medical Commission, 2019). Furthermore, the curriculum has duly recognized and emphasized the importance of students' attitude, medical ethics and communication during patient care (*Attitude, Ethics and Communication (AETCOM) Competencies for the Indian Medical Graduate,* 2018). When it comes to the PG Psychiatry training for the students, the National Medical Commission (NMC, India) provisioned the delivery of a high-quality care to the patients (diagnosis & treatment, preventive care, and develop as a consultant in the health system), research skills, and basic teaching skills (for medical and paramedical students) (Postgraduate Medical Education Board, National Medical Commission, 2022).

For long, traditional or conventional teaching (henceforth, conventional teaching), such as lectures and bedside teaching (for Undergraduates (UGs)) and grand rounds, case discussion, and seminar (for PGs), has been the mainstay of teaching in (Manohari et al., 2013). While such approaches have time-tested efficacy in improving the knowledge, attitude, and skills of the students, they are limited or criticized by the educators and students' body for being less engaging, monotonous, passive, teacher-driven, not accounting unique needs/proficiency of the students, and not being able to teach/train soft skills and clinical skills effectively (Manohari et al., 2013). Furthermore, conventional teaching-learning methods (TL Method) may not effectively impart the competencies among the students, which are required for the students to serve as a primary care physician (medical graduates) or specialist (postgraduates) (Manohari et al., 2013). This becomes particularly critical for psychiatry, where the disease burden is huge, and there is a lack of awareness among patients and the medical fraternity, compounded by the stigma attached to mental illness, limits help-seeking and patients' care (Gupta & Menon, 2022; Manohari et al., 2013; Menon & Kantipudi, 2019).

The novel TL methods, such as small-group teaching (SGT), self-directed learning (SDL), simulated learning, and digital/online-based learning systems, have gained prominence and are more effective in enriching the students' learning experience. Novel TL methods are more engaging, promote active learning, have greater subject's retention and educational outcomes, promoting self-paced or SDL (Gupta & Menon, 2022; Jayaram et al., 2021). A few research studies from the South Asian countries have emerged assessing the perspective of the teachers and students on novel T-L methods, including Internet-based teaching (Gupta & Menon, 2022; Jayaram et al., 2021; Kumar et al., 2024; Verma et al., 2024). Research from Sri Lanka by Rohanachandra et al. (2021), for instance, has evaluated the perspective of the UGs on the child and adolescent psychiatry training (Rohanachandra, 2021). Similarly, a study from Pakistan (Nadeem et al., 2021) analyzed the authors' experience in implementing the online trauma curriculum for medical students (Nadeem et al., 2021). Also, it evaluated the efficacy of such a novel program, involving case-based discussion, flipped classrooms, role-play, and Socratic questioning, on the students' learning. The authors concluded that the curriculum can help with clinical skill development and enhance the participants' knowledge in dealing with trauma survivors.

However, due to a lack of resources (manpower and digital devices) and the teaching skills of the teachers (technical skills in novel TL methods and attitudinal barrier in shifting from teacher-driven learning to student-driven learning), the practical utility of such teaching approaches and their effectiveness are doubtful (Gupta & Menon, 2022; Verma et al., 2024).

The COVID-19 pandemic has exposed the whole education system globally, including in South Asia, to the inherent limitations of the system. Moreover, the perceived need to balance a system where students direct/pace their own learning through online resource materials and shifting to a non-physical classroom platform, with the availability of teachers to guide their learning and being an authentic source of information for quality education (Gupta & Menon, 2022; Kishor, 2021; Kishor et al., 2020; V. P. Singh et al., 2022) (refer to Box 2.1).

More importantly, making psychiatry relevant for the medical colleagues and patients with chronic health problems (and vice versa), it is crucial that our teaching approaches are robust, accurate (learning domain-wise), and in line with the goals and visions of the medical education curriculum (Manohari et al., 2013). Integrated teaching, psychosomatic medicine, early clinical exposure, foundation course with mental health or psychological aspects deeply ingrained in it, attitude ethics, and communication (AETCOM) module, community health visits, and comprehensive assessment are key components for effective psychiatry teaching of our medical graduates (Manohari et al., 2013; Sharma & Chhatwal, 2024). Similarly, for the postgraduates, psychosomatic medicine, psychotherapy rounds, holistic care, research advancement, teaching skills, and community leadership are vital, which need to be imparted through an effective training system (Deshmukh et al., 2022; Manohari et al., 2013; Sawant & De Sousa, 2004).

In this chapter, we intend to provide an overview of the CBME (UG & Psychiatry PG) across the South Asian countries, critically outlining the conventional TL methods in psychiatry teaching. Also, we have highlighted the impact of COVID-19 on our teaching/training practices and how this experience informed us to change/modify our education delivery. Furthermore, we have also compared the effectiveness of the conventional teaching method with the innovative TL approaches. At the end, we have provided the future directions which could inform both the educators and medical students about the potential course of actions.

**Box 2.1 Psychiatry Teaching and Training**

- Psychiatry teaching and training have undergone tremendous changes globally, including in South Asia, with a focus on the CBME
- Traditional/conventional TL methods are time-tested approaches to impart knowledge and skills among the pupils, albeit with some limitations
- However, they can be less engaging, passive, monotonous, and not able to account the unique needs or proficiencies of the students
- Common conventional TL methods for the UGs are lectures, case discussion in the clinical setting, and tutorials
- Psychiatry PG training conventionally involves case discussion in the clinical settings, departmental academic activities, interdepartmental exposures, thesis, attending conferences/ continuous medical education (CMEs), etc.
- COVID-19 pandemic has unraveled the need to innovate in our TL methods, including the conventional teaching

UG Psychiatry Teaching in South Asia: There have been variations in psychiatry teaching in UG curriculum across the South Asian Nations (Arafat et al., 2021). Below, we have provided an overview of Psychiatry as a subject in UG teaching across South Asia:

Bangladesh: As part of the six-year undergraduate degree program, psychiatry has been allocated 20 hours of didactic lectures and a three-week ward posting, but there is no mandatory internship rotation.

India: The latest revision of Competency-Based Medical Education in 2023 allocates 45 hours to psychiatry theory teaching (15 hours lecture, 15 hours SDL, and 15 hours Small Group Discussions [SGDs]) and includes a 2-week posting in the third phase part 1 and 4 weeks in the third phase part 2. A 15-day mandatory psychiatry posting is a part of the Internship. Notably, AIIMS Rishikesh and AIIMS Deoghar (both institutes of national importance) have psychiatry as a separate final year subject; while NMC considers it part of Medicine and allied subjects, wherein, Psychiatry carries 15 marks in the theory exam as part of the medicine paper-2.

Nepal: Duration of psychiatry teaching ranged from 25 to 92 hours in different universities, and a 2-week practical posting is common to all. Most medical schools have a compulsory internship rotation, except one.

Sri Lanka: Psychiatry is given weightage at par with other final year subjects like Medicine, Surgery, and Obstetrics and Gynecology. Psychiatry carries 40–75 hours of theory teaching, compulsory practical posting called clerkship in the fourth and fifth year, and a separate final exam is taken.

# 2 Conventional TL Methods in UG Teaching

## 2.1 *Lecture*

A lecture is a carefully planned oral presentation of facts, organized thoughts, and ideas delivered by a qualified person (Pawar Jayshree & Pawar, 2010). We are all very familiar with lectures as a conventional teaching-learning method. It is the prototype of a large-group teaching method and is still widely utilized. This approach is advantageous in resource-limited settings like South Asian countries. Large portions of the material can be covered by a single faculty member for an entire student body, ranging from 100 to 250 students. It is best suited to introduce and teach cognitive domain competencies. However, it is a teacher-centric method. Its main disadvantages are the passivity of learners, the monotonous one-way flow of information, the lack of consideration for the unique learning needs of individual students, and the limited opportunities for feedback. It is not suitable for teaching psychomotor or affective domains since the softer aspects of professionalism, such as teamwork, critical thinking, and lifelong learning, cannot be taught via lectures. The advent of the Competency-Based Medical Curriculum (CBME) in 2019 has emphasized introducing interactivity into the conventional lecture format. Interactivity ensures more active student involvement. Common interactive strategies suggested include using audio-visual aids, brainstorming, buzz sessions, think-pair-share, posing one-liner questions or multiple-choice questions (MCQs), taking a quiz, etc. (*Competency Based Undergraduate Curriculum for the Indian Medical Graduate*, 2018b). Other useful ways of making lectures more effective are doing set induction by using pictures, a short video clip, a case vignette, etc., at the beginning of the lecture, giving handouts, and summarizing key take-home points at the end.

## 2.2 *Small-Group Teaching*

There is no specific definition for the number of participants in a group that qualifies it as small-group teaching. Rather than the number of participants, there are specific attributes that are emblematic of small-group teaching. These are active participation of group members, working toward a specific task, and reflection. However, roughly 6–12 participants are conventionally considered suitable for small-group teaching (Crosby, 1996). Group discussions, tutorials, seminars, workshops, symposiums, role-play, and panel discussions are a few examples of small-group teaching. Snowballing, fishbowl, circular questioning, narrative or reflective writing for AETCOM, and jigsaw methods are some of the facilitating techniques used in small-group teaching. The advantages of teaching in small groups are that it fosters active learning, deep learning, teamwork, communication skills, and collaboration (Crosby, 1996) The chances of interaction between learners and active participation are much higher in small groups. However, the disadvantages include a lack of motivation from both students and teachers to move away from more conventional teaching styles in favor of small group participation. This approach requires significant pre-planning and resources, such as separate rooms, seating arrangements, and numerous facilitators for effective implementation. Conducting small-group teaching becomes challenging with limited staff available. Psychiatry departments across India vary greatly in faculty numbers, with many college psychiatry departments having only one to three faculty members to fulfill clinical and academic requirements (Kishor et al., 2020). This creates an uphill task for small-group teaching. Practical clinical postings involve teaching psychomotor skills, such as the components of a mental status examination, which are best taught in small group settings. Concepts such as bioethics, communication, and empathy (AETCOM), which constitute the affective domain, also benefit from small-group teaching.

## *2.3 Self-Directed Learning*

Malcolm Knowles, in his pioneering book "*Self-Directed Learning—A Guide for Learners and Teachers*" published in 1975, defined self-directed learning (SDL) as, "a process in which individuals take the initiative, with or without the help of others, in diagnosing their learning needs, formulating learning goals, identifying human and material resources for learning, choosing and implementing appropriate learning strategies, and evaluating, learning outcomes"(Murad & Varkey, 2008). SDL is learner-oriented, on the one hand, while facilitated and monitored by the teacher, on the other hand. SDL does not leave students in their rooms or libraries to study independently. It can be considered a relatively newer method in South Asian countries compared to conventional large-group and small-group teaching. It was introduced as a teaching-learning method in India with the rollout of CBME in 2019 (*Competency Based Undergraduate Curriculum for the Indian Medical Graduate*, 2018b). SDL has been allocated progressively increasing teaching hours from 30 hours in First Professional MBBS to 208 Hours in Third Professional Part II (*Competency Based Medical Curriculum Regulations* 2023, 2023). SDL requires faculty training before it can be effectively implemented. Here, the teacher takes on the role of facilitator. The advantages of SDL are that it fosters and promotes the ability to be a lifelong learner in students, enhances student involvement, and promotes critical thinking and deeper learning (Charokar & Dulloo, 2022). Disadvantages are that it is resource-intensive, requires multiple facilitators to guide and monitor the SDL small groups, learning outcomes are not uniform, and assessment of both process and outcome is difficult. Student motivation is a key factor. They may feel overwhelmed during the process if not adequately supported or oriented toward the SDL process. There is resistance from both students and faculty to SDL methods. Case-Based Learning (CBL) and Problem-Based Learning (PBL) are the two most common examples of SDL-based learning. E-learning Platforms, Learning Management Systems (LMS) are especially useful in conducting SDL. In psychiatry, 15 out of a total of 45 teaching hours have been allocated to SDL (*Competency Based Medical Curriculum Regulations* 2023, 2023)

## 2.4 Clinical Rounds

Clinical rounds include both bedside teaching and OPD-based teaching of UG students. Sir William Osler said, "Medicine is learned by the bedside and not in the classroom." It is a well-known fact that bedside teaching is the cornerstone of teaching clinical skills, communication skills, and affective skills to students. It is a time-tested conventional method of teaching. However, it is being seen that bedside teaching has been slowly dwindling over the years (Ramani & Leinster, 2008). Time constraints, clinical and administrative work demands on the teacher, increasing student strength, lack of physical space in a clinical setting, requirement of multiple skills on the part of the teacher, lack of incentives for teaching, and unpredictable nature of bedside teaching are cited as some of the reasons for its decreasing utilization (Ramani & Leinster, 2008). There are many points a teacher can implement to make bedside teaching a rewarding experience for the students. These are prior preparation, planning and orienting students to the topic at hand. The teacher has to be simultaneously a teacher, clinician, role model, and effective communicator. There could also be resistance from patients for bedside teaching involving privacy, confidentiality, and comfort issues that have to be navigated by the teacher as well. They should encourage student observation, questioning, reflection, and feedback (Ramani, 2003). In psychiatry teaching, full-length history taking and mental status examination (MSE) are too long to be taught in one go at the patient's bedside. However, specific components of history taking and mental status examination can be taken up for ease of teaching. Assessing perceptual abnormalities or delusions, conducting a substance use history, assessment of mood-affect, assessment of thoughts or exploring social circumstances, and the functional impact of illness for individual bedside teaching sessions are some topics to consider (Ruddock, 2021).

## 2.5 DOAP (Demonstration, Observation, Assistance, and Performance)

DOAP is a small-group method for teaching psychomotor skills in practical classes. It allows the student to observe a demonstration, assist the teacher and perform the task either independently or under supervision, but in a simulated environment. Peyton's Four-Step Approach is also a similar technique for teaching psychomotor skills. It has four clearly defined steps—1. The trainer demonstrates the skill in real time without giving instructions or explanatory words ("Demonstration"). 2. The trainer repeats the procedure, this time describing all necessary sub-steps ("Deconstruction"). 3. The trainer performs the skill for a third time, this time following the sub-steps only as described to him by the trainee ("Comprehension"). This step has been identified as the most important step of the Four-Step Approach, as deeper processing mechanisms reflecting what was observed in the first two steps are necessary for the trainees' to be able to give instructions. 4. The trainee performs the skill on his/her own ("Performance") (Skills Training Module for Undergraduate Medical Education Program, 2019, 2019). Peyton's four-step approach is considered effective for teaching psychomotor skills (Giacomino et al., 2020). Pure psychomotor skills that can be taught in this way are few in psychiatry. Guided observation of consultants, followed by a deconstruction of the steps, performance by students on a simulated patient, followed by feedback is a useful approach to teach psychiatry-specific skills. Advantage of DOAP is enhanced skill acquisition, individualized attention and feedback to students, and it helps in the integration of knowledge with skills. However, it is a time-consuming, resource-intensive TL method; it requires adequate prior preparation and is difficult to scale up for large student populations, which are the norm in South Asian countries.

## 2.6 Integrated Teaching

Integration is a learning experience that allows the learner to perceive relationships from blocks of knowledge and develop a unified view of its basis and its application (*Competency Based Undergraduate Curriculum for the Indian Medical Graduate, 2018 Volume II*, 2018a).

Conventional teaching was a study in silos, where each of the UG subjects was taught in a stand-alone fashion. With the advent of CBME, there was a thrust toward the integration and alignment of subjects across the phases of MBBS (Vertical Integration) and between subjects taught in the same phase of MBBS (Horizontal Integration). The purpose of horizontal integration within a phase is to eliminate redundancy and establish interconnectedness. In the earlier phases, the purpose of vertical integration (across phases) is to emphasize the applicative use of the basic science concept taught. In the later phases, its purpose is to utilize and build on prior knowledge and emphasize the foundations of clinical practice (Alignment and Integration Module for Undergraduate Medical Education Program, 2019, 2019). Temporal coordination, sharing, correlation, and nesting are the strategies used (Harden, 2000).

Psychiatry is vertically integrated with Pharmacology, Forensic Medicine, and Community Medicine, while it is horizontally integrated with General Medicine and Pediatrics. About 20% of the entire portion is integrated and aligned when formulating timetable (*Competency Based Undergraduate Curriculum for the Indian Medical Graduate, 2018 Volume II*, 2018a).

Advantages of integrated teaching are it fosters holistic understanding, reduction of repetitions and redundancies, more relevance to clinical practice and improves interdisciplinary collaboration. Disadvantages are logistical considerations, time constraints, and faculty resistance, as they may have other compelling commitments; cooperation from different departments is difficult, and if not adequately planned, it can be overwhelming for the learners.

**Box 2.2 Conventional Teaching-Learning Methods in UG**

1. Lecture: Teacher-centric, cost-effective for LGT in resource-limited settings, and suits cognitive learning. However, it limits interaction, ignores individual needs, and is ineffective for teaching psychomotor or affective skills.
2. Small-Group Teaching (SGT): Group discussions, tutorials, seminars, workshops, symposiums, role-play, and panel discussions; promotes active learning, teamwork, and communication. However, requires significant planning, resources, and motivation to move away from didactic settings.
3. Self-Directed Learning (SDL): Promotes lifelong learning, critical thinking, and student engagement but is resource-intensive, and requires student motivation. CBL, PBL, and LMS platforms support SDL.
4. Clinical Rounds: A cornerstone for clinical, and AETCOM, is a time-tested method. However, it is declining due to time constraints, teachers' engagement in multiple competing roles, administrative burdens, privacy and space issues.
5. DOAP (Demonstration, Observation, Assistance, and Performance): Pure psychomotor skills to be imparted through DOAP are limited in psychiatry. It promotes skill acquisition and offers individualized feedback. However, it is time-consuming, resource-intensive, and difficult to implement in a large student groups.
6. Integrated Teaching—Integrated teaching promotes holistic understanding, reduces redundancies, and enhances clinical relevance and interdisciplinary collaboration. However, it faces challenges like time constraints, faculty resistance, logistical issues, and may overwhelm learners if not well-planned.

CBL—Case-based learning, PBL–Problem-based learning, LGT—Large group teaching, LMS—Learning management system

## 3 Conventional T-L Methods in Psychiatry Postgraduate (PG) Teaching

Overview—PG teaching and training in psychiatry aim to produce specialists capable of delivering clinical care in diverse clinical settings across the country. These specialty trainees are expected to provide clinical care, teach medical undergraduates and paramedical staff, contribute to research, and lead mental health-related awareness programs and community projects (Postgraduate Medical Education

Board, National medical commission, 2022). PG psychiatry training across the globe shares some common TL methods. However, differences exist in course duration, stages of clinical exposure, and exit criteria from training programs across the nations (Sartorius, 2009), including in South Asian countries (Kallivayalil & Enara, 2021) (refer to Box 2.3).

Below, we have provided a country-wise overview of psychiatry PG training:

- Afghanistan: There is no separate postgraduate course in psychiatry.
- Bangladesh: Postgraduate psychiatry training began with shorter courses like the Diploma in Psychological Medicine and Master of Philosophy, which were later discontinued. These were replaced by longer programs such as the MD-, Fellow of Bangladesh College of Physicians and Surgeons (FCPS)-, and Member of the College of Physicians and Surgeons (MCPS) in psychiatry. The FCPS now lasts five years with both entrance and exit exams, while the MCPS is a one-year psychiatry training course without an entrance exam. The MD in Psychiatry, introduced in 2010, includes two phases with separate exams: Phase A (two years) covers general and liaison psychiatry; Phase B (three years) focuses on adult and subspecialty psychiatry. A similar five-year MD in Child and Adolescent Psychiatry began in 2016, with Phase B dedicated to child-specific topics (Arafat, 2020; *Bangladesh Association of Psychiatry – Courses*, n.d.).
- Bhutan—A 4-year MD Psychiatry program was initiated in 2018. However, details of it is not available in the public domain.
- India: Offers a 3-year MD or DNB program, with final assessments comprising theory exams, practical examinations, and mandatory thesis/dissertation submission (Postgraduate Medical Education Board, National medical commission, 2022). Over the years, there have been many revisions in postgraduate training in psychiatry in India (*Advances in Psychiatry Training and Faculty Development in India – Venkata Lakshmi Narasimha, Satish Suhas, M Kishor, Advait Dixit, Pratima Murthy,* 2024). Significant variations can be found across institutions, comparing central institutes or institutes of National Importance (INIs) and state-level institutes, autonomous institutes and state-governed colleges, General Hospital Psychiatric Units (GHPUs) and mental health institutions, and newly established departments and well-established ones. Variations are also observed based on the type of program, such as Doctor of Medicine (MD) versus Diplomate of National Board (DNB) (*Advances in Psychiatry Training and Faculty Development in India – Venkata Lakshmi Narasimha, Satish Suhas, M Kishor, Advait Dixit, Pratima Murthy,* 2024; S. Singh & Singh, 2022).

State colleges and some central universities follow the NMC-mandated curriculum, which is largely fixed. In contrast, INIs like the All India Institute of Medical Sciences (AIIMS) and the National Institute of Mental Health and Neuro Sciences, Bengaluru (NIMHANS) are free to innovate or develop their own curricula and training programs. Even among INIs, such as various AIIMSs which have been established by the Government, although the core curriculum may be similar, differences do exist based on internal policies and institute infrastructure or priorities. Likewise, state-level institutions vary in rural/community postings, district postings, and service bond requirements (Grover et al., 2018; *Resource Material | Indian Psychiatric Society*, n.d.). Some authors have contended that there is a need for greater uniformity in PG training and greater dialogue between the NMC, INIs, and professional bodies like the Indian Psychiatric Society (IPS) (*Advances in Psychiatry Training and Faculty Development in India - Venkata Lakshmi Narasimha, Satish Suhas, M Kishor, Advait Dixit, Pratima Murthy,* 2024; Grover et al., 2018).

- Maldives: There are no dedicated postgraduate courses in psychiatry in the Maldives.
- Nepal: Offers a 3-year postgraduate program. However, there is a lack of uniformity in curriculum design and evaluation processes (Rai et al., 2021).
- Pakistan: Follows the Fellowship of the College of Physicians and Surgeons (FCPS) in the Psychiatry system, with two parts to the examination. After clearing Part I, candidates have to undergo four years of structured training, including mandatory workshops and minimum case requirements in adult psychiatry, psychotherapy, etc., to qualify for the Part II examination. The total duration of FCPS is about 4 years, and the assessment method is Task Oriented Assessment of Clinical Skills (TOACS), which is a modified version of Objective Structured Clinical Examination (OSCE) (Isaac et al., 2018)
- Sri Lanka: Has a 5-year MD Psychiatry program, which includes training in general adult psychiatry and brief exposure to subspecialties, followed by two years of senior registrar training (Gambheera & Williams, 2010). This contrasts with India, where a Senior Residency (SR)-ship in psychiatry is for three years and can only be pursued following completion the MD course (three years)

In South Asian countries, training faces several challenges, including a low psychiatrist-to-patient ratio, long working hours, inadequate infrastructure, and insufficient or outdated training for educators (Gambheera & Williams, 2010). Research is another area of concern, often hindered by limited funding and resources, resulting in basic or poor-quality research output. These issues have been widely highlighted in the literature, emphasizing the need to strengthen research training and support. Postgraduate training in the region tends to concentrate more on clinical service delivery, often at the expense of a more holistic educational approach (Sharan et al., 2009). In recent years, efforts have been made to improve skill acquisition and promote research involvement (*Advances in Psychiatry Training and Faculty Development in India – Venkata Lakshmi Narasimha, Satish Suhas, M Kishor, Advait Dixit, Pratima Murthy,* 2024; Pal et al., 2024; Postgraduate Medical Education Board, National medical commission, 2022).

**Box 2.3 Salient Points on the PG Psychiatry Training in South Asia**

- PG psychiatry training in South Asian countries faces several challenges, primarily due to the limited number of psychiatrist educators
- TL methods across these nations remain similar; however, differences exist in terms of course duration and exit examinations
- The differences in teaching and training are also attributed to institutional policies, available resources, exposure to subspecialties, and institutional priorities
- Training programs predominantly emphasize clinical exposure, while the research orientation and related SDL are limited

In Table 2.1, we have provided a list of commonly used TL methods during psychiatry postgraduate training across institutes (the list is inclusive rather than being exhaustive).

## *3.1 Lectures*

The Postgraduate psychiatry teaching and training primarily focus on developing critical thinking and encouraging reflective learning among students. Learning typically occurs in clinical settings, beginning with observation and gradually progressing to independent performance, in line with Miller's pyramid of clinical competence (Kishor, 2024). Therefore, Lectures play a limited role in postgraduate teaching due to their inherently passive nature. However, with certain modifications—such as incorporating interactive elements, demonstrations, or role-plays—lectures can be transformed into a more engaging and active learning experience (Postgraduate Medical Education Board, National medical commission, 2022).

## *3.2 Bedside Teaching and Ward Rounds*

A major component of postgraduate psychiatry teaching is bedside teaching and ward rounds, which have long been foundational methods in clinical training. These approaches facilitate simultaneous learning of clinical skills and theoretical concepts (Chandran et al., 2019). Although time-tested and effective, they have to navigate through certain challenges, especially in high-turnover settings, where time constraints can impede in-depth assessment and discussion (Ramani, 2008). Additionally, such teaching is often restricted to inpatient cases, potentially limiting the diversity of clinical exposure.

**Table 2.1** Conventional methods of psychiatry post graduate teaching and training

| Teaching methods | Principle | Advantage | Disadvantage |
|---|---|---|---|
| 1. Lecture | • Can be didactic or interactive<br>• Focuses on quick knowledge acquisition | • Useful for quick sensitization and providing information on specific topics<br>• Can be beneficial in the initial phase of training | • Inadequate in promoting critical thinking and cognitive engagement (Schmidt et al., 2015)<br>• Passive mode of teaching<br>• Not suitable for PG training; to be used sparingly (Postgraduate Medical Education Board, National Medical Commission, 2022) |
| 2. Ward rounds/ bedside teaching | • Most common clinical T-L method<br>• Promotes practical aspects of learning related to clinical care | • Primary training method embedded in routine clinical care<br>• Important for learning communication, documentation, teamwork work, and group dynamics<br>• Provides clinical competency and confidence to students; feedback received during the process is cornerstone to learning (Jenkins et al., 2007) | • Ethical concerns regarding discussions in front of patients and families<br>• Students may hesitate to express or accept errors<br>• Teachers may avoid direct feedback to the trainee or the teachers may not accept his or her own shortcomings in front of patients<br>• Can only be used for those patients requiring inpatient care.<br>• Short hospital stays and high patient load can restrict teaching time. |
| 3. Grand rounds | • It consists of case presentation by a trainee and discussion among the treatment team<br>• Includes eliciting, demonstration of clinical findings, including MSE, psychopathology, management, coupled with discussing relevant theory (Chandran et al., 2019) | • Can provide ample time and space for discussion, identify students' limitations, and focus on developing clinical skills among trainees<br>• Enhance case presentation skills<br>• Opportunity for inculcating a team spirit among participants | • Time-consuming and requires collective availability<br>• May create anxiety in trainees due to workload pressures, fear of scrutiny, and interruptions (e.g., CL calls, emergency cases, disruption by ward patients, or other immediate or urgent issues)<br>• Can get restricted to specific clinical area (e.g., addiction psychiatry, interventional neuropsychiatry, forensic psychiatry) based on the interest or expertise of the facilitators |

(continued)

**Table 2.1** (continued)

| Teaching methods | Principle | Advantage | Disadvantage |
|---|---|---|---|
| 4. OPD case discussion | • Supervised case discussions, treatment planning, and follow-ups<br>• Brief psychological interventions, treatment plans, and psychoeducation sessions | • Exposure to a wide range of commonly encountered psychiatric disorders<br>• Learning the art of time-bound workups, presentations, learning psychological (including psychoeducational) skills<br>• Opportunity to follow-up on worked-up cases on a long-term basis<br>• Opportunity to observe effects of medication, dose titration, learning strategies to deal with compliance issues and managing minor side effects on OPD basis | • Time constraints due to high OPD footfall and limited staff<br>• Some patients may not agree to stay in the facility for an extended period for a detailed assessment or may want to directly consult with senior doctor instead<br>• If adequate supervision and discussion time are not given to the trainees, their learning can be superficial and a trainee may feel overwhelmed |
| 5. Subspecialties psychiatry training(Addiction, Child & Adolescent psychiatry, Geriatric psychiatry, CLP, Sleep medicine, Psychosomatic medicine, Emergency psychiatry, Neuromodulation, Community psychiatry, etc.) | • Rotational postings for PGs in various subspecialties | • Provides a platform to refine their skills and learn intricacies of subpopulation or specific interventions<br>• Students get exposed to various subspecialties which stimulate them to pursue their own interest and create a niche for themselves in future, including pursuing a higher training<br>• Can help to place student in a position to excel in subspecialty and on cutting-edge research and clinics of particular subspecialty | • Many institutes lack access to all subspecialties<br>• Research shows only about 70% on centers across India had deaddiction and child guidance clinics (Grover et al., 2018) (*Resource Material \| Indian Psychiatric Society*, n.d.)<br>• There is a lack of exposure across residency program especially to child and adolescent-, geriatric-, rTMS, rehabilitation-, forensic-psychiatry, CLP, community psychiatry, etc. (Grover et al., 2018) (*Resource Material \| Indian Psychiatric Society*, n.d.)<br>• Some of these subspecialties may not have well-defined boundaries in psychiatry<br>• Some of these are only available in reputed institutes which offer dedicated services to PWMI<br>• Unequal exposure can create bias in choosing treatment modality. E.g. in institutes where exposure to psychotherapy is minimal or lacking, residents may tend to rely more heavily on pharmacotherapy and may even develop a dismissive attitude toward psychological interventions (Kakunje et al., 2019; S. Singh & Singh, 2022)<br>• Institutes with DM/PDF may limit MD student exposure (*Advances in Psychiatry Training and Faculty Development in India – Venkata Lakshmi Narasimha, Satish Suhas, M Kishor, Advait Dixit, Pratima Murthy,* 2024)<br>• Logistical challenges in accommodating all clinical rotations in a time-bound curriculum |

| | | | |
|---|---|---|---|
| 6. Departmental academic activities/presentations | • Case conference—Case presentation in front of the department with focus on areas like difficulty in management, diagnostic clarification, demonstration of psychopathology, etc. | • Interactive forums for skill building and discussion<br>• Promotes clinical skills and critical thinking<br>• Platform for discussion and getting feedback on cases and their management<br>• Apprise candidates on current practices, clinical practice guidelines, and recent updates | • Often, there is a challenge for faculty to include regular academics during clinical hours<br>• Faculty/resident burnout may reduce quality of discussion<br>• There may be resistance to informal formats (e.g., movie/book review) in some institutes |
| | • Journal club—Learning selecting article from a journal, understanding the methodology, statistics, results, discussion, etc., and presenting one's own critical appraisal of the research paper | • Familiarize students with latest research and innovation, different methodologies, learning to critically evaluate a paper and draw inference using their understanding and continually improving it | |
| | • Seminar—Learning a given topic from basic concepts to recent advances after going through text books, recent articles, online search, and making a presentation in a group | • Promotes in-depth and critical understanding of a topic<br>• Acquiring the art of literature review, making presentations, and discussing a topic in a group, receive feedback & respond to the audience's queries<br>• Opportunity to participate and lead in collective learning | |
| | • Movie club and Book review—selecting a movie or book relevant to psychiatry and discussions based on the idea, content and pattern of depiction and understanding of psychiatry in society | • Understanding the view of prevalent society toward mental illness and PWMI and their caregivers, the challenges and stigma associated with them | |
| | • Guest lectures—Inviting a field expert from other institute for delivering a lecture of discussion on a topic of expertise. | • Exposure to latest advances, and practical aspects of the topic, getting to know, clarify their doubts and may draw inspiration from the expert | |
| | • Debate and Quiz—Based on different topics of psychiatry | • Provide a competitive environment to excel and do better<br>• Provide a positive reinforcement for learning | |

(continued)

**Table 2.1** (continued)

| Teaching methods | Principle | Advantage | Disadvantage |
| --- | --- | --- | --- |
| 7. Dissertation/thesis and publications | • Compulsory and one of the essential requirements for award of the final degree (Postgraduate Medical Education Board, National Medical Commission, 2022) | • Familiarize student with basic research skills, like choosing a topic, planning methodology, statistics, literature review, protocol writing, data collection, analysis, and paper writing<br>• Launchpad for future research and academic pursuits | • Balancing clinical work with research is challenging, especially in poorly motivated student<br>• Lack of incentives or resources can be prominent hurdles<br>• If not guided properly, the research endeavor can be overwhelming for the candidate, can result into indulgence in plagiarism, may lead to poor quality of research work/publication, hence demotivating the students to further participate in such activities |
| 8. Psychotherapy forum | • Discussions on basic principles of psychology, psychotherapy, and case-based learning of psychological intervention<br>• Involve psychiatrist, psychologist, PG students, etc. | • Encourages learning psychological interventions<br>• Promotes a holistic approach to patient care (Grover et al., 2018) | • Time constraints.<br>• Shortage of clinical psychologists<br>• Can be overburdening for the psychiatry teachers<br>• Lack of training and skills among the psychiatry educators can be a bottleneck (S. Singh & Singh, 2022) |
| 9. Interdepartmental activities | • Collaboration with departments like neurology, pharmacology, forensic medicine, medicine, psychology | • Ensures exposure of specific cases and comorbid cases<br>• Exposures of basic skills of examinations and patients' evaluation<br>• Enhances communication and collaborative care skills | • May be challenging to accommodate in the course duration<br>• Coordination with the relevant department, including ensuring their availability, can be challenging<br>• Sometimes PGs may serve as proxy psychiatrists in the posted department instead of receiving training in the posted department |
| 10. Inter-institute clinical postings | • To promote comprehensive learning, mainly in those aspects for which resources is sub-optimal in the parent institute (e.g., a trainees working in a GHPU can benefit with posting in dedicated mental health institutes; likewise the latter can establish link with the former to improve CL psychiatry training of their PG trainees.) | • Promotes exposure of different types of cases and management strategies as per available resources<br>• May broaden the point of view of assessment and managing the cases and overcoming any inherent shortcomings of the parent institute, such as a lack of subspecialties psychiatry services especially in GHPUs, or lack of CLP cases in dedicated psychiatry institutes | • Not all institutes have policy and enough resources to send their PG trainees to different institute<br>• Host institutes may face accommodation/training constraints<br>• No national policy ensuring such postings |

| | | | |
|---|---|---|---|
| 11. DRP (district residency program) | • Posting PGs to nearby district hospitals for community exposure | • Improves access to specialist care in underserved areas<br>• Raises awareness about mental health in rural populations<br>• Help residents understand the manifestations of various psychiatric conditions, different common mental health conditions in the community, and challenges in management | • Poor implementation and variable practice of DRP often lead to time and resource inefficiency |
| 12. CME/Conferences | • PG students are required to attend at least two CME programs in 3 years by the course guidelines by NMC<br>• Also required to present a minimum number of one poster, one paper at national/state conference, and one research paper presentation with publication (Postgraduate Medical Education Board, National Medical Commission, 2022) | • Help the students to develop skills of presenting their research findings, compete for different awards<br>• Provide opportunity for attending workshops/ symposiums to enhance their learning, widen their perspective, getting exposure to the advancement in the field, network, and stay updated<br>• Enhance their interaction with experts from different national and international institutes thus inspiring them to excel in their fields | • PG students usually do not get any institute funding or financial support for attending or presenting their work<br>• In small or new department, it may affect clinical services in the institute |

*CIP* Central Institute of Psychiatry, Ranchi, *CLP* Consultation liaison psychiatry, *CME* Continuing Medical Education, *DM* Doctorate of Medicine, *GHPU* General Hospital Psychiatry Unit, *IHBAS* Institute of Human Behaviour and Allied Sciences, *IPS* Indian Psychiatric Society, *MD* Doctor of Medicine, *MSE* Mental state examination, *NIMHANS* National Institute of Mental Health and Neuro Sciences, *NMC* National Medical Commission, *OPD* Outpatient department, *PDF* Post doctoral fellowship, *PWMI* Person with Mental Illness, *rTMS* Repetitive transcranial magnetic stimulation

## 3.3 Grand Rounds

It can be considered an extension of ward rounds, involving the full clinical team and featuring more detailed case presentations and discussions. These sessions offer the advantage of direct assessment and feedback on student performance, promote collective learning, and aid in treatment planning and addressing clinical challenges. They also help boost confidence and decision-making skills within the team (Ramani & Leinster, 2008).

## 3.4 Clinical Discussion in the Outpatient Department (OPD)

Routine OPDs provide opportunities to learn from short cases and those typically managed without admission. OPDs also allow students to practice time-bound clinical assessments and management, thereby improving their clinical efficiency. Subspecialty OPD postings, such as those in addiction medicine or child and adolescent psychiatry, expose students to complex and specialized cases and help them learn treatment strategies, such as psychological assessment, psychosocial interventions, beyond routine care (Ramani & Leinster, 2008).

## 3.5 Departmental Academic Activities

They serve as a platform where clinical work, theoretical learning, and research converge. Case conferences by focusing on specific aspects—such as psychopathology or management difficulties—sharpen students' presentation and communication skills. Journal clubs and seminars enhance understanding of research methodology, statistics, and critical appraisal. To break routine monotony while encouraging learning from diverse sources, methods such as movie clubs, book reviews, guest lectures, debates, and quizzes are also incorporated. Hands-on research training occurs primarily through dissertations and publications. Despite challenges like busy schedules and limited funding, dissertation work ensures that students at least gain basic familiarity with research concepts, forming a foundation for future academic work (Chandran et al., 2019).

## 3.6 Psychotherapy Forum and Focused Groups

Postgraduate training often emphasizes clinical service due to the limited availability of community-based psychiatric care. However, many established institutes—and some newer ones provide exposure to psychology and psychotherapy through dedicated forums, serving as an introduction to further learning and skill development. However, training in psychotherapy remains limited in South Asian countries (Grover et al., 2018; Hanwella, 2012).

### 3.7 *Intramural Interdepartmental Postings*

During the PG training, students are also posted in other departments, such as neurology and general medicine, to enhance their understanding of comorbid conditions and interdisciplinary management. In some instances, students are sent to other institutions to gain exposure to different settings—for example, from GHPUs to specialized mental health institutes, and vice versa. Subspecialty clinic rotations further broaden clinical experience. Similarly, posting in community programs like district residency programs (DRPs) has the potential to provide service to service deprived area and on the same time familiarize the students to needs of the community. Continuing Medical Education (CME) programs and academic conferences are essential for staying updated on recent advances, networking with experts from other institutions or countries, and fostering future collaborations among participants (Chandran et al., 2019) (refer to Box 2.4).

**Box 2.4 Key Features of the CBME with Regard to PG Psychiatry Training**

- CBME has been adopted in several institutions, promoting a learner-centered, outcome-focused, and skills-driven approach to medical education, in contrast to the conventional knowledge-based, time-bound model
- Didactic lectures are less recommended; clinical teaching is mainly delivered through ward rounds, OPDs, subspecialty postings, and case conferences
- Research and academic enrichment are supported through thesis work, publications, CMEs, journal clubs, seminars, and interactive formats such as guest lectures, movie clubs, book reviews, debates, and quizzes
- Trainees are also exposed to varied clinical settings beyond their parent department/institution through interdepartmental and inter-institutional collaborations, e.g., DRP

## 4 After the Introduction of CBME

The NMC of India, for instance, has introduced the CBME framework in 2019, marking a significant shift from traditional, time-bound, and knowledge-based training to a more learner-centric, outcome-oriented, and skills-driven approach.

This paradigm shift has also been reflected in the updated MD Psychiatry curriculum released by the NMC in 2022 (Postgraduate Medical Education Board, National medical commission, 2022). Under the CBME framework, psychiatry training now emphasizes clearly defined learning outcomes across three core domains: the cognitive domain (knowledge acquisition), the affective domain (attitudes and professionalism), and the psychomotor domain (clinical and procedural skills). Each domain is aligned with specific competencies and learning objectives that are observable and measurable. A key component of CBME is the emphasis on both formative (ongoing) and summative (final) assessments. Many institutions have already integrated these principles into their postgraduate psychiatry training programs. Formative assessments serve not only as evaluation tools but also promotes learning, enabling continuous improvement through regular, structured feedback from supervising faculty. The guideline also focuses on teaching skills, research mindset, leadership role in the community mental health, communication with the relevant disciplines, and teamwork.

## 5 COVID-19 Pandemic and Shift in Conventional Psychiatry Teaching and Training

A cross-sectional study from India on the COVID-19's impact on the postgraduate teaching-learning-evaluation (TLE), including innovative TL methods adopted, involving 77 psychiatry teachers, showed that the conventional methods of teaching (case discussion, case vignette based training, demonstration, JCs, resource access, and live-streaming), though delivered in a simulated or enriched with audio-visual aids, can ensure effective training of the students. In contrast, Massive Open Online Courses (MOOCs), Objective Structured Long Examination Record (OSLER), and online Objective Structured Clinical Examination (OSCE) might not be handy for the PGs. The online teaching approach, though effective, needs to be tailored, coupled with ensuring participation of the teachers to ensure the experiential learning of the PG trainees (Deshmukh et al., 2022).

Notably, another multi-center cross-sectional survey involving medical students (n = 877) on healthcare students' perspective on the lecture as TL method during the COVID-19 pandemic revealed that the students perceived the lecture and organized learning delivered by teachers as indispensable for UG teaching and cannot be replaced by online teaching (Singh et al., 2022). However, the participants highlighted that the lecture's success heavily depends on the quality of teachers (delivery, communication skills, soft skills, and role modeling). Furthermore, they opined that to make lectures engaging and effective, audio-visual aids must be incorporated into them, particularly by those teachers who may not be very effective in lecture delivery. The potential solution put forth by the participants to overcome the current limitations in the educational system was having more teachers onboard, an effective lesson plan, setting induction, summarization at the end, and seeking students' feedback to improve.

The COVID-19 pandemic informed us that our teaching approach needs to be more flexible (blended), innovative, with scope for students to self-determine their learning (high touch or low touch—based on the relative involvement of teachers during the learning process, with high touch approach requiring greater teachers' involvement and utilized for the complex concepts; short courses—credit or non-credit based). Furthermore, having a peer group, just-in-time learning, and teachers' availability can ensure effective learning in psychiatry for both medical UGs & Psychiatry PGs (Jayaram et al., 2021).

## 6 Evidence on the Effectiveness of the Conventional Teaching Methods Vs. Novel Methods

Research has shown mixed results for the effectiveness of innovative learning methods over conventional teaching methods. This variations in the research findings can be attributed to research methodology, student participants, study period (COVID-19 vs. non-COVID; pre-CBME vs. post-CBME), and mode of delivery of the teaching.

For instance, global research, one by McParland et al. (2004) from London involving medical UGs indicates that the problem-based learning vs. conventional teaching methods lead to greater performance in the examination (MCQ-based and viva), have a more versatile learning style (including deep learning and strategic learning), promote SDL, and improve clinical performance (McParland et al., 2004).

Similarly, research dated back to the 1970s from the USA showed better performance of university students regarding objective test scores, clinical skills, and proficiency in patient management enrolled in the psychiatric learning system versus conventional teaching. The latter was a self-instrumental system, incorporating self-paced, programmed text- and audio-visual content delivery (psychopathology, MSE, signs/symptoms in psychiatry) module (Randels et al., 1976).

Although robust comparative research from India is lacking in terms of learning effectiveness and students' satisfaction with the conventional teaching vs. innovative teaching-learning methods, a few available studies have shown mixed results of latter TL methods vs. the innovative teaching methods.

A scoping review on the research funded by the Minds trust-IToP found that two comparative studies, one on the effectiveness of online-based teaching (of psychopharmacology) and another on skill acquisition of the interns following the CBME vs. the conventional teaching program had negative results (Verma et al., 2024).

The review also pointed out the potential utility of the innovative TL methods in medical education and their equal or greater efficacy over conventional teaching. For instance, a mixed-method study by Ruben et al. showed that role-play-based learning and simulation-based learning were the preferred innovative TL methods by the medical undergraduates and teachers (Ruben et al., 2022). Similarly, a comparative research by Guruprasad (2024) on the outcome of teaching cum learning related to suicide-risk assessment using mobile app versus conventional teaching for medical students using semi-structured questionnaire found that mobile-app-based teaching vs. the conventional teaching method was better comprehended by participants. Moreover, the implementation of the mobile-app-based suicide risk-assessment session was not inferior to the conventional method (Verma et al., 2024).

Notably, a cross-sectional study from Haryana, India, exploring the perspective of the medical students on the competency-based curriculum showed that students did not consistently prefer various innovative teaching methods as part of the competency-based curriculum (Sharma & Chhatwal, 2024). Particularly, SDL, reflective writing, small-group teaching, and log-book-based assessment were less favorably perceived by the students. In contrast, early clinical exposure, community health visits, AETCOM, foundation course, integrated teaching, and formative assessment, a tool to promote learning, were rated high by the majority of the study participants. It must be emphasized that participants, as well as the authors, identified the crucial role of the teacher in effectively conducting SGT/SDL/reflective writing sessions. The authors also recommended that the SGT/SDL mandated by the competency-based curriculum require faculty training and proper orientation of the students and teachers using this active TL method.

Another study from the Mumbai, India, though before the implementation of the CBME, involving 160 interns revealed that majority of the students felt that conventional teaching method for the theory, such as lecture helped them learn the subject matter in a better way; however, one fourth felt that lecture was a waste of time. The limitation of the lecture could be overcome by incorporating the A-V aids. The participants also reported that for the practical skills, case demonstration and bedside teaching were the preferred modes over ward rounds. These findings indicate that conventional TL methods are still preferred by the students, which may indicate that UGs still want a passive method of teacher-driven learning versus active, self-directed learning (Sawant & De Sousa, 2004).

**Box 2.5 Conventional Teaching Methods Vs. Novel T-L Methods Comparison and Evidence**

- Conventional or traditional TL methods with adequate utilization of A-V aids can ensure the effective teaching of the medical students.
- Teacher's quality, effective lesson plan, discussion with fellow educators, and feedback from the students are essential for the success of the conventional teaching.
- The comparative effectiveness of the novel TL methods over conventional teaching and vice versa is context dependent (domains of learning, resources, students' motivation, and learning environment).
- Though research globally shows superiority of the novel TL methods over conventional teaching methods, literature from India and South Asian countries have mixed results and varied students' perspective.

# 7 Future Direction

In this chapter, we have highlighted the scope of the conventional teaching methods both for the medical students and PG psychiatry trainees in enhancing their learning in the era of the CBME (Boxes 2.6, 2.7). As mentioned above, the utility of the conventional teaching methods depends greatly on the content to be taught, the setting where T-L is taking place, the available resources, the teaching skills of the teachers, and the motivation for learning among the students. It must be emphasized that the lately institutional teaching-learning environment is significantly getting impacted by the prevailing private coaching, which is often app-based, crisp, and aiming to pass the examinations or crack the competitive exams. Therefore, whether conventional or innovative, the effectiveness of the teaching methods will be confounded by the students' involvement in private coaching (Banerjee, 2020).

However, to effectively use the time-tested conventional teaching methods in both medical UG and PG psychiatry training, the medical teachers need to undergo medical education technology training and prioritize teaching over other activities (administrative, clinical care, or research). The latter is not an easy task given the quantum of work entrusted to the faculty members, particularly in public-run hospitals, and the disproportionately high faculty–student ratio. Below, we have provided some future directions that can enrich the teaching and learning experience of both the students and teachers.

**Box 2.6 Future Direction for Improving the Effectiveness of the Conventional T-L Methods in Psychiatry for the Medical UGs**

*Making the session interesting and engaging*

- The conventional teaching (lecture, bedside teaching, etc.) must engage students using role-plays, demonstration, A-V aids, PBL, and group discussions.
- Effective set induction, session plan, and succinct learning objectives will streamline the session flow and make the session effective.
- Allowing quizzes, summarization, and key take-home points at the end, and seeking feedback from the students can have long-term implications.

*Faculty training in TL methods*

- Faculty training in the CBME, including use of the various T-L methods and robust assessment methods to test students' learning can have a lasting effect.
- Peer faculty support and lesson plan discussion can improve teaching quality.

(continued)

**Box 2.6 (continued)**

*Faculty training in digital technology (A-V aids)*

- With the advent of technology and students' active involvement in it, faculty need to be trained in using various learning management systems (Google Classroom, Moodle, etc.)
- The teaching can be enhanced by engaging the students through in-class questions using Slido, VoxVote, etc.
- Using catchy and succinct graphics/slides/video/simulation can enrich students' learning experience.

*Blended teaching (simulation, role-play, and online teaching blended with the physical classroom-based teaching)*

- *The era of student-driven, preference of self-paced learning, coupled with limited teaching hours in psychiatry, the educators can blend the classroom teaching with the virtual/online lectures or providing resource materials.*
- *The high touch and low touch TL methods for difficult and easier topic, respectively, can help stakeholders' utilizing time and resources* effectively.

*Integrated teaching*

- For make psychiatry teaching relevant for the students, it has to be seamlessly integrated with other subjects throughout the medical course.
- The communication, soft-skills, and ethical aspects that psychiatry can teach can be integrated with the humanities or behavioral sciences in the foundation years and with AETCOM module throughout the course.
- Psychiatry can also be effectively integrated with the vertically (pharmacology, forensic medicine) and horizontally integrated (community medicine, internal medicine, sleep medicine, psycho-sexual medicine, etc.) with other subjects.

*Robust assessment of the competencies*

- The assessment of psychiatry in part-2 section B of medicine needs to be done by the psychiatrist, including setting the question paper.
- The formative assessment should also focus on the key learning domains if the psychiatry is delivered through lectures (e.g., Short answer questions, MCQs) or clinical teaching (e.g., OSCEs).

*Faculty development program and imparting teaching skills among the psychiatry residents*

- The conventional teaching's (lectures, bedside teaching, demonstration) effectiveness can be ensured by taking onboard more academic teachers.

(continued)

**Box 2.6 (continued)**

- The psychiatry residents, either under supervision (microteaching) or independently (at a later stage) must be involved in students' teaching.
- Resident (mostly senior residents) training in medical education can bridge the existing gaps in medical students' teaching in psychiatry.
- Residents are also more tech-savvy and aware of the learning styles and needs of the students.

*Feedback of the stakeholder and course correction*

- A bidirectional feedback system, after each T-L encounter will help teachers to understand the strengths and limitations of their teaching skills.
- Moreover, students will feel counted and validated for their inputs when it comes to providing feedback and getting it implemented.

**Box 2.7 Future Direction for Improving Effectiveness of the Conventional T-L Methods in Psychiatry for the Psychiatry PGs**

*Regular formal teaching sessions for the PGs by the faculty members and senior residents*

- Active learning through role-plays, demonstration, A-V clips, live-interview with PWMI can improve basic knowledge and clinical skills of the PG trainees.
- Group discussions, PBL, and focussed case discussions involving senior residents and psychiatry faculty can keep the residents motivated in learning.

*Faculty training in T-L methods*

- Training of faculty and senior residents in medical education technology will improve their teaching skills, including effective time and resource utilization.
- Senior PG trainees can be encouraged to teach their junior colleagues and medical students to learn teaching skills and consolidate their learning.

*Faculty training in digital technology (A-V aids)*

- Like for UG teaching, PG teaching also requires faculty members to be well-versed with the digital tools frequently used in medical education.
- A command on the digital technology can also equip faculty members in ensuring continuity of teaching during the uncertain periods (e.g., COVID-19).

(continued)

**Box 2.7 (continued)**

*Blended teaching (simulation, role-play, and online teaching blended with the physical classroom-based teaching)*

- PG teaching requires greater degree of practical and professional skills, blended teaching methods can help realize this.
- Multimodal teaching methods (simulation, role-play, skill-labs, and interaction with a real patient in a controlled environment) can enrich PGs learning experience and make the conventional teaching methods more effective.

*Integrated teaching*

- Multidisciplinary ward rounds or academic activities will make psychiatry relevant to other disciplines and ensure holistic patient care.
- Psychosomatic clinics, CL psychiatry, grand rounds, community-, emergency- psychiatry are effective integrated teaching approaches for the PG trainees.
- Integrated teaching help residents learn the wider aspects of patient care and management.

*Robust assessment of the competencies*

- Effective assessment through OSCEs, Viva, and case presentation, preferably involving multiple assessors—both as a part of formative and summative assessments—is vital for residents training.

*Feedback from the stakeholders and course correction*

- A bidirectional feedback involving residents and teachers can help enriching the learning experience of the student.
- This will also provide students with the inputs on their learning needs, learning styles, strengths, limitations, and future course of action.
- Feedback also informs the teachers on their teaching methods and content delivery, which thus can be utilized to improve one's teaching skills.

*Psychotherapy forum*

- Psychosocial interventions are key to psychiatric treatment, and students must learn the art of counseling/psychotherapy to develop as a better specialist.
- Regular psychotherapy rounds involving CPs, PSW, psychiatrists, and peer residents are vital in enriching the learning of the psychiatry trainees.

A-V: Audio-visual, CPs: Clinical psychologists, OSCEs: Objective structured clinical examination, PBL: Problem-based learning, PWMI: Persons with mental illness, PSW: Psychiatry social workers, SRs: Senior residents

# 8 Conclusion

South Asian nations have increasingly adopted CBME, with a focus on competency and novel T-L methods to enrich students' learning experience. The COVID-19 pandemic has unraveled the significance of blended teaching methods and effective incorporation of digital technology in various conventional T-L methods. Conventional teaching methods, particularly in UGs, may not be holistic in teaching psychomotor and AETCOM domains. Lectures, clinical case discussions, and tutorials are commonly used conventional T-L methods for UGs; while clinical case discussions, seminars, case conferences, dissertations, and CMEs are major conventional T-L methods in PG training. However, there are variations in training programs and relative importance given to various aspects of psychiatry (including subspecialties) in South Asian countries. Each conventional T-L method has its own advantages and limitations; therefore, they should be utilized based on the context and available resources. The comparative analysis of the effectiveness of conventional teaching/training methods vs. novel T-L methods has shown mixed results and varied students' perspectives. Teachers' characteristics and students' level of motivation are key determinants of the success of the conventional T-L methods. Future research must aim to explore the effective blending of conventional teaching methods with technology and other novel T-L approaches to make the former teaching patterns relevant and effective.

# References

Alignment and Integration Module for Undergraduate Medical Education Program, 2019. (2019). Medical Council of India.

Arafat, S. M. Y. (2020). The current status of psychiatric education in Bangladesh. *Asian Journal of Psychiatry, 52*, 102108. https://doi.org/10.1016/j.ajp.2020.102108

Arafat, S. M. Y., Kar, S. K., Sharma, P., Marahatta, K., & Baminiwatta, A. K. A. B. (2021). A comparative analysis of psychiatry curriculum at undergraduate level of Bangladesh, India, Nepal, and Sri Lanka. *Indian Journal of Psychiatry, 63*(2), 184–188. https://doi.org/10.4103/psychiatry.IndianJPsychiatry_615_20

Attitude, Ethics and Communication (AETCOM) Competencies for the Indian Medical Graduate, 2018. (n.d.). Retrieved April 21, 2025, from https://www.nmc.org.in/wp-content/uploads/2020/01/AETCOM_book.pdf

Banerjee, A. (2020). Coaching Classes… Competency-Based Curriculum… Bed of Procrustes… Deck Chairs on the Titanic. *Medical Journal of Dr. D.Y. Patil Vidyapeeth, 13*(1), 1. https://doi.org/10.4103/mjdrdypu.mjdrdypu_292_19

Bangladesh Association of Psychiatry—Courses. (n.d.). Retrieved May 18, 2025, from https://bapbd.org/education_course.php

Chandran, S., Isaac, M., Mysore, A., Sreedaran, P., Manohari, S., Kumar, K., George, S., Menon, V., Shamasundar, C., Behere, R., Kumar, A., Eiman, N., Murthy, P., Dere, S., Deshpande, S., Tripathi, A., Kakunje, A., Shah, N., Bharathi, G., & Manohar Rao, K. (2019). *Perspectives in psychiatry training* (1st ed.).

Charokar, K., & Dulloo, P. (2022). Self-directed learning theory to practice: A footstep towards the path of being a life-long learner. *Journal of Advances in Medical Education & Professionalism, 10*(3), 135–144. https://doi.org/10.30476/JAMP.2022.94833.1609

Competency Based Medical Curriculum Regulations 2023. (2023, August 1). National Medical Council.

Competency based Undergraduate curriculum for the Indian Medical Graduate, 2018 Volume II (Vol. 1–Vol II). (2018a). Medical Council of India.

Competency based Undergraduate curriculum for the Indian Medical Graduate (Vol. 1). (2018b). Medical Council of India.

Crosby, J. (1996). AMEE Medical Education Guide No. 8. Learning in small groups. *Medical Teacher, 18*(3), 189–202. https://doi.org/10.3109/01421599609034160

Deshmukh, D., Patil, A. V., Deore, R., & Bhise, M. C. (2022). Impact of COVID-19 pandemic on postgraduate psychiatry teaching-learning and evaluation in India: A Nationwide Survey. *Indian Journal of Psychological Medicine, 44*(5), 479–484. https://doi.org/10.1177/02537176221114439

Gambheera, H., & Williams, S. (2010). Shared challenges in psychiatric research in India and Sri Lanka. *Indian Journal of Psychiatry, 52*(Suppl 1), S80–S82. https://doi.org/10.4103/0019-5545.69217

Giacomino, K., Caliesch, R., & Sattelmayer, K. M. (2020). The effectiveness of the Peyton's 4-step teaching approach on skill acquisition of procedures in health professions education: A systematic review and meta-analysis with integrated meta-regression. *PeerJ, 8*, e10129. https://doi.org/10.7717/peerj.10129

Grover, S., Sahoo, S., Srinivas, B., Tripathi, A., & Avasthi, A. (2018). Evaluation of psychiatry training in India: A survey of young psychiatrists under the aegis of research, education, and training foundation of Indian Psychiatric Society. *Indian Journal of Psychiatry, 60*(4), 445–460. https://doi.org/10.4103/psychiatry.IndianJPsychiatry_334_18

Gupta, S., & Menon, V. (2022). Psychiatry training for medical students: A global perspective and implications for India's competency-based medical education curriculum. *Indian Journal of Psychiatry, 64*(3), 240. https://doi.org/10.4103/indianjpsychiatry.indianjpsychiatry_187_22

Hanwella, R. (2012). Postgraduate training in psychotherapy in Sri Lanka: The need for a systematic approach. *Sri Lanka Journal of Psychiatry, 2*(2), 49. https://doi.org/10.4038/sljpsyc.v2i2.4039

Harden, R. M. (2000). The integration ladder: A tool for curriculum planning and evaluation. *Medical Education, 34*(7), 551–557. https://doi.org/10.1046/j.1365-2923.2000.00697.x

Isaac, M., Ahmed, H. U., Chaturvedi, S. K., Hopwood, M. J., Javeed, A., Kanba, S., Mufti, A. A., Maramis, A., Samaniego, R. M., Udomratn, P., Yanling, H., Zainal, N. Z., & Sartorius, N. (2018). Postgraduate training in psychiatry in Asia. *Current Opinion in Psychiatry, 31*(5). https://doi.org/10.1097/YCO.0000000000000444

Jayaram, M., Shields, G., & Buisman-Pijlman, F. (2021). Novel methods of teaching psychiatry to medical and postgraduate students. *Current Opinion in Psychiatry, 34*(5), 491–496. https://doi.org/10.1097/YCO.0000000000000725

Jenkins, C., Page, C., Hewamana, S., & Brigley, S. (2007). Techniques for effective bedside teaching. *British Journal of Hospital Medicine, 68*(Sup9), M150–M153. https://doi.org/10.12968/hmed.2007.68.Sup9.27182

Kakunje, A., Punnoose, V. P., Ponnusamy, K. P., Mysore, A. V., & Daniel, S. J. (2019). Revisiting Postgraduate (PG) psychiatry training in India. *Indian Journal of Psychological Medicine, 41*(4), 380–387. https://doi.org/10.4103/IJPSYM.IJPSYM_15_19

Kallivayalil, R. A., & Enara, A. (2021). Education and training in psychiatry in South Asian countries. Asia-Pacific. *Psychiatry, 13*(4), Article 4. https://doi.org/10.1111/appy.12494

Kishor, M. (2021). What to teach and how to teach medical students in the middle of COVID-19? Guidance for teachers in psychiatry. *Indian Journal of Psychological Medicine, 43*(4), 357–359. https://doi.org/10.1177/02537176211023886

Kishor, M. (2024). Psychiatry training in competency-based medical education: What to teach? How to teach? *Indian Journal of Psychological Medicine, 46*(2), 101–102. https://doi.org/10.1177/02537176241237962

Kishor, M., Menon, V., Vinay, H., Bhise, M., Isaac, M., Chandran, S., Kumar, A., Nebhinani, N., Gupta, R., Dere, S., Kakunje, A., Bharathi, G., Ashok, M., & Nischal, A. (2020). COVID-19 pandemic highlights the need to reconsider psychiatry training of Indian medical graduate. *International Journal of Health and Allied Sciences, 9*(5), 104–104.

Kumar, A., Gupta, S., Jain, J., Ghosh, S., Basera, D., Pakhre, A., & Modak, T. (2024). Perceived learning and feedback of students following the competency-based clinical rotation in psychiatry: A retrospective review from tertiary-care teaching Institute in Central India. *Indian Journal of Psychological Medicine, 46*, 429–438. https://doi.org/10.1177/02537176241277518

Manohari, S. M., Johnson, P. R., & Galgali, R. B. (2013). How to teach psychiatry to medical undergraduates in India?: A model. *Indian Journal of Psychological Medicine, 35*(1), 23–28. https://doi.org/10.4103/0253-7176.112196

McParland, M., Noble, L. M., & Livingston, G. (2004). The effectiveness of problem-based learning compared to traditional teaching in undergraduate psychiatry. *Medical Education, 38*(8), 859–867. https://doi.org/10.1111/j.1365-2929.2004.01818.x

Menon, J., & Kantipudi, S. J. (2019). Crossroads in postgraduate psychiatry training in India. *Indian Journal of Mental Health and Neurosciences, 2*(2), Article 2. https://doi.org/10.32746/ijmhns.2019.v2.i2.40

Murad, M. H., & Varkey, P. (2008). Self-directed learning in health professions education. *Annals of the Academy of Medicine, Singapore, 37*(7), 580–590.

Nadeem, T., Asad, N., Hamid, S. N., Gul, B., & Aftab, R. (2021). Experiences from implementing an Lessons from teaching psychiatry trainees at a tertiary care hospital in Karachi, Pakistan. *Asian Journal of Psychiatry, 65*, 102865. https://doi.org/10.1016/j.ajp.2021.102865

Narasimha, V. L., Satish Suhas, M. Kishor, A. D., Murthy, P. (2024). *Advances in psychiatry training and faculty development in India*. Retrieved April 15, 2025, from https://journals.sagepub.com/doi/10.1177/02537176241284348?int.sj-abstract.similar-articles.1

National Medical Commission. (2019). National Medical Commission-competency-based medical education curriculum for the Indian Medical Graduates. www.nmc.org.in/wp-content/uploads/2020/01/UG-Curriculum-Vol-II.pdf

National Medical Commission. (2024). Guidelines for Competency Based Medical Education (CBME) Curriculum; 2024. National Medical Commission.. https://www.nmc.org.in/MCIRest/open/getDocument

Pal, A., Parmar, A., Nath, S., Chawla, N., Gupta, S., Vinay, H. R., & Kishor, M. (2024). Survey of Felt Needs Among Teachers of Psychiatry in Institutes of National Importance (INI) to improve the quality of undergraduate and postgraduate training. *Indian Journal of Psychological Medicine, 46*(5), 439–444. https://doi.org/10.1177/02537176241273919

Pawar Jayshree G, & Pawar GS. (2010). *A Good Lecture Class and Delivery, 19*, 31–32.

Postgraduate Medical Education Board, National medical commission. (2022, August). Guidelines for competency based postgraduate training programme for M.D. in Psychiatry. National medical commission. https://www.nmc.org.in/wp-content/uploads/2019/09/MD-Psychiatry.pdf

Prasad, C. G., Jotibannad, D. Y., Kilagi, A. K., NHY, R. (2024). A comparative study of outcome of teaching related to suicide risk assessment using mobile app versus conventional teaching for undergraduate medical students. *Natl J Physiol Pharm Pharmacol, 14*, 1869–1869. https://doi.org/10.5455/njppp.2024.14.04155202407042024

Rai, Y., Gurung, D., & Gautam, K. (2021). Insight and challenges: Mental health services in Nepal. *BJPsych International, 18*(2), E5. https://doi.org/10.1192/bji.2020.58

Ramani, S. (2003). Twelve tips to improve bedside teaching. *Medical Teacher, 25*(2), 112–115. https://doi.org/10.1080/0142159031000092463

Ramani, S. (2008). Twelve tips for excellent physical examination teaching. *Medical Teacher, 30*(9–10), 851–856. https://doi.org/10.1080/01421590802206747

Ramani, S., & Leinster, S. (2008). AMEE Guide no. 34: Teaching in the clinical environment. *Medical Teacher, 30*(4), 347–364. https://doi.org/10.1080/01421590802061613

Randels, P. M., Kilpatrick, D. G., McCurdy, L., & Saunders, P. J. (1976). Comparison of the psychiatry learning system and traditional teaching of psychiatry. *Journal of Medical Education, 51*(09), 751–757. https://doi.org/10.1097/00001888-197609000-00006

Resource Material | Indian Psychiatric Society. (n.d.). Retrieved April 15, 2025, from https://indianpsychiatricsociety.org/resource-material/

Rohanachandra, Y. M. (2021). Child and adolescent psychiatry teaching in medical undergraduates in a Lower Middle-Income Country (LMIC) – Perspectives from Sri Lanka. *Asian Journal of Psychiatry, 61*, 102674. https://doi.org/10.1016/j.ajp.2021.102674

Ruben, J.-P., Shah, H., Sreedaran, P., Chandran, S., Selvam, S., & Kurpad, S. S. (2022). Effective and innovative teaching methods in psychiatry for the medical undergraduates in South India: An exploratory study of teachers' and students' perspectives. *Indian Journal of Psychiatry, 64*(6), 545. https://doi.org/10.4103/indianjpsychiatry.indianjpsychiatry_954_21

Ruddock, K. (2021). Bedside teaching: An invaluable tool in undergraduate medical education. *BJPsych Open, 7*, S154. https://doi.org/10.1192/bjo.2021.431

Sahadevan, S., Kurian, N., Mani, A. M., Kishor, M. R., & Menon, V. (2021). Implementing competency-based medical education curriculum in undergraduate psychiatric training in India: Opportunities and challenges. *Asia-Pacific Psychiatry, 13*(4), e12491. https://doi.org/10.1111/appy.12491

Sartorius, N. (2009). Training psychiatrists for the future. *Asia-Pacific Psychiatry, 1*(3), 111–115. https://doi.org/10.1111/j.1758-5872.2009.00038.x

Sawant, N., & De Sousa, A. (2004). Attitudes of medical graduates to psychiatry and their evaluation of the teaching learning methods. *Indian Journal of Psychological Medicine, 26*(3), 52–58. https://doi.org/10.1177/0975156420040307

Schmidt, H. G., Wagener, S. L., Smeets, G. A. C. M., Keemink, L. M., & van der Molen, H. T. (2015). On the use and misuse of lectures in higher education. *Health Professions Education, 1*(1), 12–18. https://doi.org/10.1016/j.hpe.2015.11.010

Sharan, P., Gallo, C., Gureje, O., Lamberte, E., Mari, J. J., Mazzotti, G., Patel, V., Swartz, L., Olifson, S., Levav, I., de Francisco, A., Saxena, S., & World Health Organization-Global Forum for Health Research – Mental Health Research Mapping Project Group. (2009). Mental health research priorities in low- and middle-income countries of Africa, Asia, Latin America and the Caribbean. *The British Journal of Psychiatry: the Journal of Mental Science, 195*(4), 354–363. https://doi.org/10.1192/bjp.bp.108.050187

Sharma, S., & Chhatwal, J. (2024). Perspectives of undergraduate medical students regarding competency-based curriculum. *The National Medical Journal of India, 36*(6), 379–383. https://doi.org/10.25259/NMJI_461_2022

Singh, S., & Singh, D. V. (2022). Post Graduate Psychiatric Education in India—Current practice and future directives. *Indian Journal of Clinical Psychiatry, 2*(02), Article 02.

Singh, V. P., Ramakrishna, A., Sinha, N., Khandelwal, B., Joseph, N., & Barua, P. (2022). Perception of health care students towards lectures as a teaching and learning method in the COVID era—A multicentric cross-sectional study from India. *F1000Research, 11*, 665. https://doi.org/10.12688/f1000research.110100.2

Skills Training Module for Undergraduate Medical Education program, 2019. (2019). Medical Council of India.

Verma, N., Gupta, S., & Shatadal, P. (2024). Research in psychiatry medical education through "MUST Enrich Grant": A scoping review. *Indian Journal of Psychological Medicine, 46*, 382–390. https://doi.org/10.1177/02537176241265742

# Chapter 3
# Principles of Learning and Psychiatry Teaching

**Arghya Pal, Bandita Abhijita, and Vikas Menon**

**Abstract** Psychiatry education is largely underrepresented in the extant medical curriculum. It is essential to adopt the adult andragogical learning principles into psychiatry education. Experience-based, self-directed, problem-focused learning approaches can potentially facilitate interest and motivate students. In addition, well-structured specific learning objectives aligned with competencies laid down by the national medical curriculum can enhance knowledge acquisition. Integration of innovative teaching-learning methods and appropriate use of media can tap effectively into the psychomotor, cognitive, and affective domains of learning. Despite considerable advances, challenges exist in the form of limited resources, inadequacies and inequities in infrastructure and technology, structural issues, and regulatory challenges. Addressing these gaps through curricular reforms and improved teaching methodologies can enhance psychiatry education, ultimately improving mental health care and patient outcomes.

**Keywords** Adult learning · Psychiatry education · Competencies · Specific learning objectives · Teaching-learning methods

A. Pal
Department of Psychiatry, All India Institute of Medical Sciences, Kalyani, West Bengal, India

B. Abhijita (✉) · V. Menon
Department of Psychiatry, Jawaharlal Institute of Postgraduate Medical Education and Research (JIPMER), Puducherry, Pondicherry, India



S. K. Kar et al. (eds.), *Teaching and Training in Psychiatry in South Asia*, South Asian Perspectives in Mental Health and Psychology, https://doi.org/10.1007/978-981-95-1845-6_3

# 1 Introduction

Mental illnesses are one of the leading causes of global disease burden (Ferrari, 2022). Despite this, psychiatry education is a neglected domain in medical curricula, leading to poor knowledge and negative attitudes among undergraduates. That psychiatry should be a major part of the medical curricula is agreed upon by the World Psychiatric Association (Kallivayalil & Enara, 2020). Psychiatry emphasizes the unity of body and mind, which is essential in all medical practices. Some of the skills learnt in psychiatry, such as building patient relationships, assessing mental state, and delivering bad news, are crucial for all doctors. Also, psychiatric disorders are common across medical settings, with around one-third of patients visiting general medical settings having associated psychiatric issues (van Niekerk et al., 2022). Thus, all medical students require a foundational understanding of psychiatry to provide comprehensive care.

# 2 Principles of Learning

Learning as we know it today is derived from early efforts of teaching young children knowledge and skills such as reading, writing, and arithmetic, which was largely directed by teachers. Such a form of learning is known as 'pedagogy' ('ped'—child, 'agogos'—leading). It was only in the 1920s that adult learning 'andragogy' ('andr'—man) was discussed (Glicken, 2004). The term 'andragogy' was introduced by Alexander Kapp and popularized by Malcolm Knowles. Table 3.1

**Table 3.1** Key differences between andragogy and pedagogy

| | Andragogy | Pedagogy |
|---|---|---|
| Learner's role | Self-directed, responsible for their learning | Dependent on the teacher for guidance and instruction |
| Motivation | Internal (e.g., career growth, personal development) | External (e.g., grades, rewards) |
| Experience | Builds on prior knowledge and experiences | Limited prior experience, relies on new knowledge |
| Teacher's role | Facilitator, guide, and resource provider | Authority figure, instructor, and knowledge provider |
| Curriculum structure | Flexible, customized based on learners' needs | Structured, predetermined by educational standards |
| Learning approach | Problem-based, practical, and immediately applicable | Subject-based, theoretical, and knowledge-focused |
| Reason for learning | Learners seek relevance to real-life applications | Learning is often mandatory and preparation for future life |
| Assessment methods | Self-assessment, reflective learning, and application-based evaluation | Formal assessments, tests, and teacher-driven evaluations |

highlights the key differences between andragogical and pedagogical forms of learning (Mukhalalati & Taylor, 2019).

## 3 Foundations of Adult Learning

### *3.1 Relevance*

Adults are relevance-driven learners who need a clear purpose for acquiring new knowledge. Learning is most effective when it directly applies to their work or daily responsibilities. To ensure engagement, instructors should establish clear learning objectives before starting any course. Additionally, theories and concepts should be presented in a context that is familiar and meaningful to participants. One effective approach is to allow learners to select projects aligned with their own interests, making the learning process more practical and personalized.

### *3.2 Self-Concept*

Adult learning is largely self-driven, where adults take charge of planning, managing, and evaluating their own learning. This humanistic approach supports learner-based personalized learning, with educators serving as facilitators rather than instructors.

### *3.3 Experience*

The most effective learning is from shared experience; learners learn from each other, and the trainer often learns from the learners. They can learn through concrete experience, observation, and active experimentation. Case studies, therefore, are an effective way of teaching (Subedi & Pandey, 2021).

### *3.4 Orientation to Learn*

Children shift from subject-based learning to problem-based learning as they grow. This brings in the importance of scenario-based learning, wherein they are allowed to solve problems in a realistic risk-free situation. This also allows greater participation and retention of the learners. It is important to choose a relevant, cost-effective scenario with minimal distractions and the right medium.

### 3.5 *Motivation to Learn*

At a younger age, often the motivation to learn lies in the external world, be it teachers or parents. However, adults are primarily driven by internal motivation such as improving their skills, getting a job or promotion, or maintaining a balanced professional life. It is important for the trainer to identify the motivators that can shape the learning process (Cook & Artino, 2016).

## 4 Factors Affecting Learning

### 4.1 *Physiological Factors*

Several physiological factors can significantly affect learning, including: stress hormones (like cortisol), sleep quality, nutrition, hydration, sensory perception, physical activity, and overall health conditions like chronic pain or illness, which can all impact cognitive function and learning ability.

### 4.2 *Psychological Factors*

Psychological factors that are internal to the learner are, often, the major factors affecting learning (Chen et al., 2023). These include:

- *Intelligence*: Intelligence refers to the ability of problem-solving, reasoning, critical thinking, regulating emotions, moral understanding, and environmental adaptation. In other words, intelligence is closely linked to a student's learning capacity, with better learning seen in those possessing higher intelligence as compared to those with lower intelligence levels.
- *Motivation*: Motivation drives learning behaviour. It can be intrinsic (learning for personal satisfaction) or extrinsic (learning for rewards). A combination of different motivation-enhancing techniques, such as providing incentives, sharing success stories, holding exams, etc., should be used by educators to facilitate learning.
- *Readiness to Learn*: Learning is effective only when the learner has the will to learn. To make him/her ready, the educator can adopt various motivating strategies and address other physiological, psychological, and environmental barriers effectively.
- *Emotions*: It is presumed that positive emotions such as happiness enhance learning, while negative emotions such as fear and sadness can be a hindrance.

### *4.3 Environmental Factors*

Learning is also shaped by external influences such as family environment, peer influence, cultural norms, socioeconomic status, and social expectations. The teaching environment also plays a crucial role in shaping learning experiences. A positive and inclusive institutional environment fosters better learning. The availability of physical infrastructure such as libraries, laboratories, and classrooms affects learning efficiency. Lastly, the availability of well-trained teachers using effective teaching methods can significantly improve adult learning outcomes.

### *4.4 Teaching-Learning Process-Related Factors*

The use of appropriate teaching-learning methods, as discussed later in the chapter, can facilitate learning in today's media-driven world. Media can be in the form of print or non-print media. Print media such as texts, articles, or magazines are often used as learning aids. Adults prefer modern electronic media such as audio-visual aids, artificial intelligence techniques, flipcharts, films, and role-plays. These not only motivate the learners but also encourage active participation in the teaching-learning process.

## 5 Framing Educational Objectives in Psychiatry

Active andragogical learning is widely adopted within medical education. When we talk about learning in medical curriculum, especially psychiatry, it is crucial to understand the key differences between objectives, competencies, and entrustable professional activities (EPA) (ten Cate & Schumacher, 2022) (Fig. 3.1).

## 6 Introduction to Specific Learning Objectives: Components, Benefits, and Linking with Competencies

A well-designed learning objective should be Specific, Measurable, Attainable, Relevant, and Time-bound (SMART) (Chatterjee & Corral, 2017). A specific learning objective (SLO) has the following benefits; it offers both the learner and educator a clear roadmap. It helps in designing fair evaluation tools. It also offers graded learning from simple to complex concepts. To sum up, SLOs improve learners' engagement and increase participation and self-directed learning.

For instance, an SLO in psychiatry would be: '*By the end of the lecture, the student will be able to list five causes of delirium in medical and surgical settings*'.

**Objectives**

- Objectives are defined as the intended knowledge, skills, or attitudes a learner should acquire by the end of a teaching session or curriculum
- Specific and measurable

**Competencies**

- Competencies describe broader capabilities that integrate multiple objectives and skills
- Underlying abilities
- In psychiatry, competencies may include patient-centered care, professionalism and communication.

**EPA**

- EPAs are the real-world tasks or responsibilities that learners must be able to perform independently before progressing to the next level
- Observable and assessable clinical activities
- e.g. Conducting a psychiatric interview

**Fig. 3.1** Objectives vs. competencies vs. entrustable professional activities (EPA)

It is important that SLOs are aligned with competencies to achieve broader educational goals.

For example,

- SLO: List the common side effects of selective serotonin reuptake inhibitor antidepressants.
- Competency: Select an appropriate first-line antidepressant for a patient with major depressive disorder.
- EPA: Initiating and monitoring antidepressant medication for a patient with major depressive disorder.

Benjamin Bloom and colleagues divided SLOs into three broad domains—cognitive, affective, and psychomotor (Sewagegn, 2020). The cognitive domain represents intellectual skills; affective domain represents attitudes, feelings; and psychomotor domain represents skills/performance.

Examples of SLOs in Psychiatry

i. *Cognitive Domain*

   For the cognitive/knowledge domain, information is available in textbooks and is mostly rote knowledge.

   Example—'*By the end of the lecture session, the student will be able to enlist diagnostic criteria of major depressive disorder as per ICD-11*'.

ii. *Psychomotor Domain*

   This domain focuses on the development of practical and procedural skills.

   This needs clinical demonstration by the teacher in addition to the knowledge.

   Example—'*By the end of the training module, the student will be able to administer a long-acting injection of antipsychotic to a patient with schizophrenia*'.

   Other examples:

- Eliciting extrapyramidal symptoms in a patient on antipsychotics.

iii. *Affective Domain*

This domain includes empathy, communication, and professional skills.

Example—'*By the end of the clinical posting, the student will be able to demonstrate active listening when interacting with a patient suffering from depressive disorder*'.

Other examples include:

- Breaking bad news.
- Obtaining informed consent for modified electroconvulsive therapy from a family member.

# 7 Teaching-Learning Methodologies in Psychiatry

Teaching in the setting of a medical college is challenging yet a rewarding proposition. These issues become more prominent for a subject like psychiatry, because of its relatively unique status in the curriculum. As an example, in the undergraduate curriculum, where psychiatry has very limited representation in the summative assessment, the general drive among students to study psychiatry may be feeble. On the other hand, in a postgraduate setting, where students would have selected psychiatry as their subject of choice, the level of interest will be high. The teaching-learning methods in either of these situations will be different. The following subsection intends to provide a snapshot of the various options for teaching-learning methods available to a psychiatry teacher.

## *7.1 Large Group Teaching*

Large group teaching (LGT) is a mode of imparting knowledge simultaneously to a large group, often considered to indicate a group bigger than 30 students. There are various ways of imparting large group teaching but lecture remains the most popular as well as time-tested method of LGT. LGT remains a very effective way when the teacher–student ratio is very skewed; hence, it is a very cost-effective way of teaching. The various common modes of LGT have been illustrated in Fig. 3.2.

LGT has been subjected to intensive criticism from educationists, to the extent that some have even pondered whether they are outdated. However, the alternative viewpoint regarding this matter posits that LGT is essential and relevant, but there needs to be proper preparation for the method to be effectively implemented (Cantillon, 2003). Figure 3.3 discusses the key features of LGT in an attempt to demonstrate the scope of this teaching method in the curriculum.

While preparing for LGT, the preparation of the teacher is governed by a few important factors. They may include the purpose of the class, the target population, objectives to be covered, the teaching media and audio-visual aids to be used, and availability of these media and aids. The answers to the above question may be

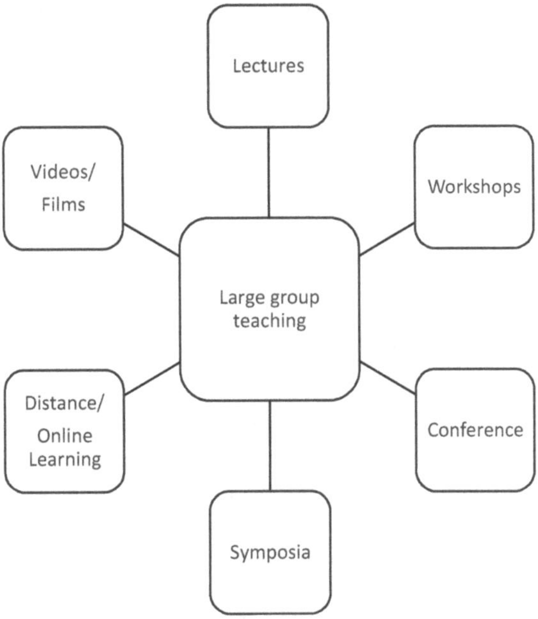


**Fig. 3.2** Large group teaching methods

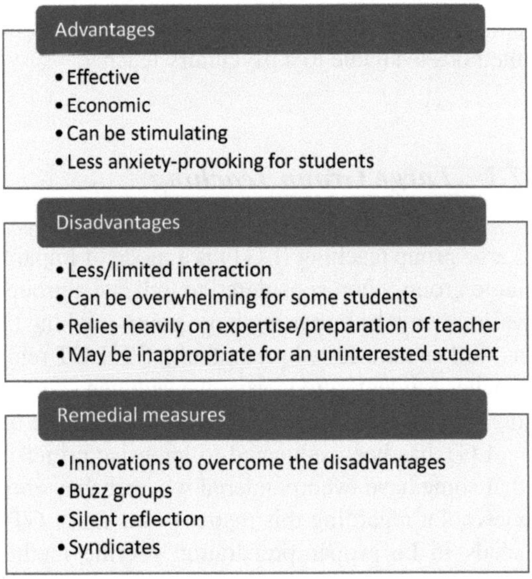


**Fig. 3.3** Features of large group teaching

helpful in designing the plan for LGT. All facilitators must prepare a lesson plan that addresses the aforementioned considerations in preparing for an LGT session.

Over the recent years, there have been numerous innovations made to retain the learners' interest in an LGT-like lecture. Examples of some of these strategies include buzz groups, silent reflection, and three minutes each way. Buzz groups are small groups (about 3–5) created within the large group, who are given specific subtopics or related activities to discuss ('buzz') for a short time (typically, a minute or two at most). Following this, the group presents the salient points to the larger group.

Another technique, referred to as 'silent reflection' is designed to involve the quieter students who are given a few minutes to reflect on an issue and then present it to the class. Three minutes each way is another method of involving the students and is often useful if the class is restless or finding it difficult to maintain silence. In this technique, each student is asked to communicate on a specific topic with a classmate on each side for three minutes. Subsequently, selected representatives may be asked to speak on that topic. It is often a very effective way to break the ice if the large group is largely unknown to each other.

## 7.2 *Small Group Teaching*

Small group teaching (SGT) typically involves teaching to a more limited group of students (around 2–10) with, generally, a higher level of interaction between the teachers and students. In general, such classes are less didactic in nature, and the teacher often acts as a facilitator, thus shifting the focus of interaction from lecturer-centred to student-centred mode (Biggs, 1989). These kinds of teaching activities are particularly useful for facilitating competencies in the affective and psychomotor domain that are essential in psychiatry. The various kinds of SGT include tutorials, seminars, workshops, debates, student-led groups, etc. The key attributes of SGT have been depicted in Fig. 3.4.

In SGT, there are multiple innovations to increase student participation as well. Though detailed discussion about this topic is out of the scope of this chapter, some of the examples of innovations include cross-over and fishbowl techniques. Cross-over involves distributing the small group into subgroups where each subgroup is

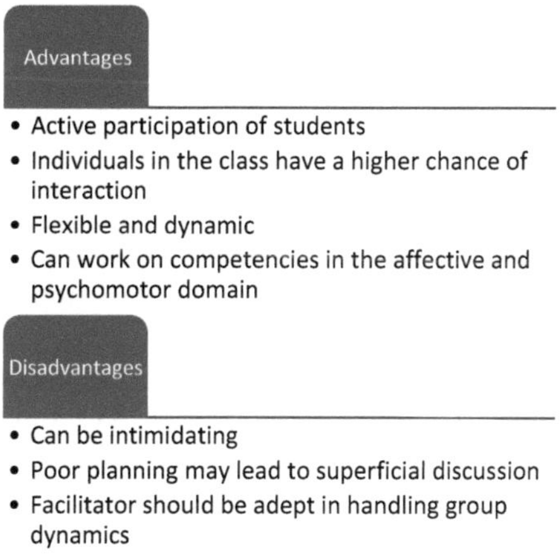


**Fig. 3.4** Features of small group teaching

given a subtopic to discuss. In the second phase, each member of the subgroup is redistributed into new subgroups, which will be comprised of one member who has studied each subtopic; thus, in the reconstituted subgroup, the whole topic can be discussed. The fishbowl technique involves splitting the small group into two circles. The inner circle will be actively deliberating on a given topic and the outer circle will be involved in actively listening to and documenting the discussion (Jaques, 2003).

## 8 Innovations in Teaching-Learning Methods

Over the last couple of decades, the field of psychiatry education has seen various newer teaching-learning methods that have been effectively used in this context. Of note, all these methods represent ways to promote active learning. Some of these innovations are depicted below:

### *8.1 Flipped Classroom*

Flipped classroom is a teaching method that reverses the traditional approach of students first receiving a lecture in the classroom and proceeding home for assignments or further reading. In flipped classroom, the student comes prepared to the classroom, having gone through resource material provided in advance either by the teacher or made available through other sources; thus, time in the class can be used for activities that promote higher-order thinking. There is a growing body of positive evidence for flipped classrooms in various aspects of psychiatry education (Sarvarizadeh et al., 2024). Some of the key aspects that can be addressed by this method include language issues and cultural barriers in psychiatry teaching.

### *8.2 Problem-Based Learning*

The premise of problem-based learning (PBL) is to enable the students to engage in active learning by using real-world problems or clinical situation. The approach is typically group work on a problem that reflects a real-world clinical situation and is commonly open-ended so that the complexities and ramifications of the choices can be demonstrated. PBL has been widely used and found to be effective in teaching psychiatry and its various subdomains across settings and types of students (Iwatsuki et al., 2021; Shad et al., 2023). For example, PBL can be a useful tool when teaching a group of students who have shown inclination to clinical exposure but adequate patients are not immediately available. It can also be a useful tool to foster teamwork and break the monotony of bedside clinics. PBL is also helpful to foster higher-order thinking by carefully choosing the problem and modulating the discussion.

### *8.3 Role-Plays and Simulations*

In psychiatry, irrespective of undergraduate or postgraduate curriculum, several skills that need to be taught are in the affective and psychomotor domain. In competencies pertaining to domains like psychotherapy, it might be very difficult to delineate between the affective and psychomotor domains of learning. Role-plays and simulations may be effective tools in dealing with such skills. These experiential teaching methods are based on direct observation of the verbal and non-verbal behaviours of the teachers/actors/clients. It may also be customized where the students take up assigned roles as individuals or as members of a group to hone a particular skill (King et al., 2014).

### *8.4 Self-Directed Learning and E-Learning*

Over the last decades, especially since the advent of the coronavirus pandemic, there has been a shift in learners' preferences. As people became more adept with online media and the reach of this media became apparent, self-directed learning through online media has gained considerable traction globally. Self-directed learning is a method where the learning topics, methods, and outcomes are determined by the choice of the learners; in other words, the decisions pertaining to planning and evaluation are their responsibility (Lai et al., 2022).

### *8.5 Integrated (Interdisciplinary) Learning*

Interdisciplinary learning allows students to examine a fundamental problem from various viewpoints of different disciplines. This approach helps students not only to understand a problem in a comprehensive manner but also enables them to appreciate the various connections that exist in the knowledge base and become aware of the ambiguity of the topic (Shahar, 2021). It can be horizontal integration, when the disciplines that are taught simultaneously in an academic year are integrated (e.g. psychiatry and medicine) or vertical integration, when subjects that are taught in different years are integrated (e.g. pharmacology and psychiatry).

## 9 Principles of Choosing a Teaching-Learning Method

Many factors need to be considered by a teacher when the teaching-learning method is being selected. These factors can be grossly divided into learning objectives (whether cognitive, affective, or psychomotor domains); learning styles (profile of the students); learning environment (small group or large group); learning feedback (ways of evaluation) and learning outcome (the level of clinical competence that the student has to demonstrate). Figure 3.5 demonstrates a few common factors that might affect the choice of the teaching-learning method. Figure 3.6 illustrates a practical situation of how the teaching-learning method may change for the same learning objective based on the profile of the students.

## 10 Innovations in Teaching-Learning in Psychiatry

Over the last decade, and with the advent of the pandemic, teaching-learning methods have seen numerous changes. A number of factors have precipitated these innovations. The physical distancing that was mandated during the pandemic situation created hindrances in educational endeavours in psychiatry training. Several innovations that used the enormous reach of the Internet became the need of the hour, and even after the resolution of the pandemic, the appeal of digital learning platforms has continued (Shan et al., 2023). Some of the important innovations in this regard have been discussed in the subsequent section.

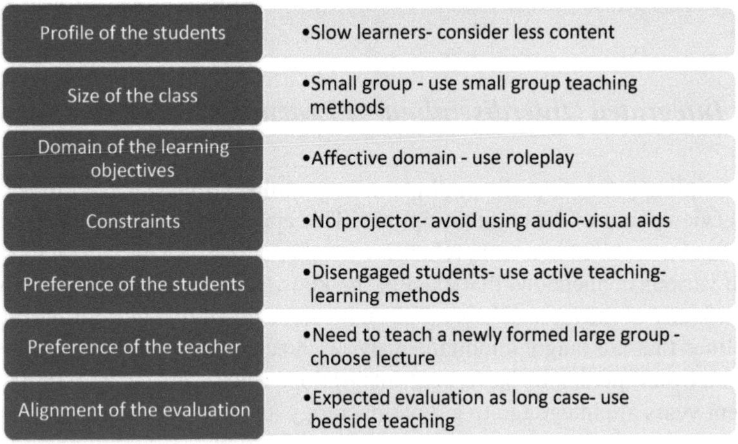


*Note: Excerpts on the right column denote common examples encountered in clinical teaching in psychiatry*

**Fig. 3.5** Factors governing the choice of teaching-learning methods

| Learning Objective- Management of depression | Class | Teaching- Learning Method |
|---|---|---|
| | Undergraduate | Lecture, tutorial |
| | Undergraduate (Elective posting) | Self directed learning, Case-based learning |
| | Postgraduate | Seminar, Problem-based learning |

**Fig. 3.6** Choice of teaching-learning methods based on the profile of the students

## *10.1 Digital Learning*

Digital learning is the process of using technology in any form for the purpose of learning. Digital learning in some form was adopted by most universities in the pandemic times, but digital learning was in vogue much earlier. This mode of teaching-learning allows ease of access as it is self-paced and flexible. Additionally, it has unmatched reach and demands modest infrastructure, time-saving, and cost-effective. This mode of teaching is also very popular when the experts or teachers of the topic are limited or when there is a lack of uniform training curriculum; thus, the technique has become quite popular in the training of the evolving subdomains of psychiatry (Bairy et al., 2019). However, such a mode requires appropriate training of faculty and familiarization of the platform intended to be used for the teaching-learning activities (Orsolini et al., 2021).

## *10.2 Artificial Intelligence in Psychiatry Teaching*

Artificial intelligence (AI) refers to technology that allows computers to mimic human learning and decision-making. It has been used in diagnostics and also in the development of therapeutic interventions in psychiatry (Ray et al., 2022). However, there is a paucity of information on the use of AI in psychiatry in the context of psychiatry education. However, in the field of medical education, there has been extensive use of AI (Gordon et al., 2024; Narayanan et al., 2023). A review on this topic found that AI has been used in the fields like recruitment, admissions, teaching, assessment, clinical reasoning, and automation of log entries. Hence, AI may hold similar promise in the field of psychiatry education.

### *10.3 Virtual Reality in Psychiatry Teaching*

Virtual reality (VR) is the technology of recreating an immersive real-world situation using a computer-generated algorithm that can be experienced in real-time. It has been widely used in the field of medical education. It has been used in the process of recreating clinical scenarios, depicting surgical anatomy and anatomical orientation of structures, and also in surgical training, amongst various other uses (Gan et al., 2023; Jiang et al., 2022; Mergen et al., 2024). In the field of psychiatry, it has been used with encouraging results in the training of psychopathology and psychotherapy (Pedersen & Musaeus, 2023). It has been also used in mental health research in creating quasi-clinical experimental situations (Lee et al., 2024). This technology has been able to recreate clinical situations and also can be used in creating Objective Structured Clinical Exam situations. The field holds great promise in transforming psychiatry education to a more engaging and immersive style.

## 11 Challenges in Teaching-Learning in Psychiatry

Teaching psychiatry is fraught with unique challenges. Challenges like the need to teach psychopathology in a manner that reflects the complexities arising out of the intertwining of phenomenology and socio-cultural and religious attributes. Choosing an appropriate teaching-learning method for such a complex subject can be a challenging proposition and leaves a lot of scope for innovation (Gupta & Khurana, 2015; Masson, 2011).

On the other hand, a lot of challenges have arisen in the new age of digital revolution. It has to be acknowledged that the field of mental health has been associated with significant stigma. As psychiatry educators, it is our responsibility to address this issue so that the medical students of tomorrow can effectively advocate against stigma and discrimination. In order to train them, the affective domain of learning has to be reinforced. Similarly, fields like psycho-pharmacology and neuro-stimulation have seen considerable evolution in the recent past. These fields require rigorous training in the psychomotor domain of the students, which should be kept in mind while designing the curriculum (Fiorillo et al., 2013).

Finally, one of the most unique needs of a psychiatry faculty is to impart training in psychotherapy. Training in psychotherapy needs skills that fall in the cognitive, psychomotor, and affective domains. Thus, there is a need to choose the teaching-learning methods that address all these domains. However, it also needs to be mentioned that though training needs are substantial, the availability of trained experts is limited, and those inclined towards teaching are even more infrequent. Thus, there is a need for upskilling teachers of psychiatry in this regard, so that mental health services can be augmented in the clinical and community setting (Al-Uzri, 2022).

## 12 Conclusion

Psychiatry is a unique subject in the medical curriculum in various ways. It is one of those subjects where the need for learning objectives in the affective domain is very important. However, in many undergraduate curricula, not enough emphasis has been given to psychiatry, resulting in the students' dwindling interest. In this regard, we want to emphasize that teachers of psychiatry should be aware of the various principles of learning and should also be able to appreciate the situations where either of the principles can be best implemented. As teachers, we also need to be aware of the various factors that can influence the student's learning experience and how that can be further improvised. Psychiatry educators should also be able to frame well-designed specific learning objectives, and further the teaching-learning methods should be well-aligned with the SLOs. Finally, the teaching-learning methods in psychiatry have seen much evolution in the recent past. Yet, there remains a palpable need for further innovation and research in this field, particularly given the advent of newer techniques and disruptive technology.

## References


Al-Uzri, M. (2022). Education and training in psychiatry: Challenges and consequences of the last two years, future perspectives and actions needed. *European Psychiatry, 65*(Suppl 1), S10. https://doi.org/10.1192/J.EURPSY.2022.51

Bairy, B. K., Ganesh, A., Govindraj, D., & Chand, P. K. (2019). Role of digital learning in addiction psychiatry. *Digital Psychiatry, 2*(1), 25–33. https://doi.org/10.1080/2575517X.2019.1622983

Biggs, J. B. (1989). Approaches to the enhancement of tertiary teaching. *Higher Education Research and Development, 8*(1), 7–25. https://doi.org/10.1080/0729436890080102

Cantillon, P. (2003). Teaching large groups. *BMJ, 326*(7386), 437. https://doi.org/10.1136/BMJ.326.7386.437

ten Cate, O., & Schumacher, D. J. (2022). Entrustable professional activities versus competencies and skills: Exploring why different concepts are often conflated. *Advances in Health Sciences Education, 27*(2), 491–499. https://doi.org/10.1007/S10459-022-10098-7

Chatterjee, D., & Corral, J. (2017). How to write well-defined learning objectives. *The Journal of Education in Perioperative Medicine: JEPM, 19*(4), E610. https://doi.org/10.46374/volxix-issue4-chatterjee

Chen, D. P., Chang, S. W., Burgess, A., Tang, B., Tsao, K. C., Shen, C. R., & Chang, P. Y. (2023). Exploration of the external and internal factors that affected learning effectiveness for the students: A questionnaire survey. *BMC Medical Education, 23*(1), 49. https://doi.org/10.1186/S12909-023-04035-4

Cook, D. A., & Artino, A. R. (2016). Motivation to learn: An overview of contemporary theories. *Medical Education, 50*(10), 997. https://doi.org/10.1111/MEDU.13074

Ferrari, A. (2022). Global, regional, and national burden of 12 mental disorders in 204 countries and territories, 1990–2019: A systematic analysis for the Global Burden of Disease Study 2019. *The Lancet Psychiatry, 9*(2), 137–150. https://doi.org/10.1016/S2215-0366(21)00395-3

Fiorillo, A., Malik, A., Luciano, M., Del Vecchio, V., Sampogna, G., Del Gaudio, L., Rojnic Kuzman, M., Jovanovic, N., Nawka, A., & Volpe, U. (2013). Challenges for trainees in psychiatry and early career psychiatrists. *International Review of Psychiatry, 25*(4), 431–437. https://doi.org/10.3109/09540261.2013.812960

Gan, W., Mok, T. N., Chen, J., She, G., Zha, Z., Wang, H., Li, H., Li, J., & Zheng, X. (2023). Researching the application of virtual reality in medical education: One-year follow-up of a randomized trial. *BMC Medical Education, 23*(1), 1–12. https://doi.org/10.1186/S12909-022-03992-6

Glicken, A. D. (2004). Becoming an effective teacher: Applied principles of adult learning. *Journal of Veterinary Medical Education, 31*(3), 268–272. https://doi.org/10.3138/jvme.31.3.268

Gordon, M., Daniel, M., Ajiboye, A., Uraiby, H., Xu, N. Y., Bartlett, R., Hanson, J., Haas, M., Spadafore, M., Grafton-Clarke, C., Gasiea, R. Y., Michie, C., Corral, J., Kwan, B., Dolmans, D., & Thammasitboon, S. (2024). A scoping review of artificial intelligence in medical education: BEME Guide No. 84. *Medical Teacher, 46*(4), 446–470. https://doi.org/10.1080/0142159X.2024.2314198

Gupta, R., & Khurana, H. (2015). Challenges in undergraduate psychiatric training in India. *Developments in Psychiatry in India: Clinical, Research and Policy Perspectives* (pp. 593–610). https://doi.org/10.1007/978-81-322-1674-2_31

Iwatsuki, J., Kondo, T., Takahashi, N., Takami, H., Nishigori, H., Bustos-Villalobos, I., Aleksic, B., Kasuya, H., Ban, N., Yagi, T., & Skokauskas, N. (2021). Problem-based learning in child and adolescent psychiatry: A perspective from Japan. *Advances in Medical Education and Practice, 12*, 1329–1335. https://doi.org/10.2147/AMEP.S333958

Jaques, D. (2003). Teaching small groups. *BMJ, 326*(7387), 492–494. https://doi.org/10.1136/BMJ.326.7387.492

Jiang, H., Vimalesvaran, S., Wang, J. K., Lim, K. B., Mogali, S. R., & Car, L. T. (2022). Virtual reality in medical students' education: Scoping review. *JMIR Medical Education, 8*(1), e34860. https://doi.org/10.2196/34860

Kallivayalil, R. A., & Enara, A. (2020). Undergraduate education in psychiatry in India. *Global Psychiatry, 3*(1), 9–16. https://doi.org/10.2478/GP-2020-0006

King, J., Hill, K., & Gleason, A. (2014). All the world's a stage: Evaluating psychiatry role-play based learning for medical students. *Australasian Psychiatry: Bulletin of Royal Australian and New Zealand College of Psychiatrists, 23*(1), 76–79. https://doi.org/10.1177/1039856214563846

Lai, Y., Saab, N., & Admiraal, W. (2022). University students' use of mobile technology in self-directed language learning: Using the integrative model of behavior prediction. *Computers & Education, 179*, 104413. https://doi.org/10.1016/J.COMPEDU.2021.104413

Lee, M., Kim, S. K., Go, Y., Jeong, H., & Lee, Y. (2024). Positioning virtual reality as means of clinical experience in mental health nursing education: A quasi-experimental study. *Applied Nursing Research, 77*, 151800. https://doi.org/10.1016/J.APNR.2024.151800

Masson, N. (2011). Undergraduate psychiatry education: the challenges ahead: Commentary on… Teaching Medical Undergraduates. *Advances in Psychiatric Treatment, 17*(2), 110–113. https://doi.org/10.1192/APT.BP.110.008169

Mergen, M., Graf, N., & Meyerheim, M. (2024). Reviewing the current state of virtual reality integration in medical education – A scoping review. *BMC Medical Education, 24*(1), 1–25. https://doi.org/10.1186/S12909-024-05777-5

Mukhalalati, B. A., & Taylor, A. (2019). Adult learning theories in context: A quick guide for healthcare professional educators. *Journal of Medical Education and Curricular Development, 6*, 23821205198403З. https://doi.org/10.1177/2382120519840332

Narayanan, S., Ramakrishnan, R., Durairaj, E., & Das, A. (2023). Artificial intelligence revolutionizing the field of medical education. *Cureus, 15*(11), e49604. https://doi.org/10.7759/CUREUS.49604

van Niekerk, M., Walker, J., Hobbs, H., Magill, N., Toynbee, M., Steward, B., Harriss, E., & Sharpe, M. (2022). The prevalence of psychiatric disorders in general hospital inpatients: A systematic umbrella review. *Journal of the Academy of Consultation-Liaison Psychiatry, 63*(6), 567–578. https://doi.org/10.1016/J.JACLP.2022.04.004

Orsolini, L., Jatchavala, C., Noor, I. M., Ransing, R., Satake, Y., Shoib, S., Shah, B., Ullah, I., & Volpe, U. (2021). Training and education in digital psychiatry: A perspective from Asia-Pacific region. *Asia-Pacific Psychiatry, 13*(4), e12501. https://doi.org/10.1111/APPY.12501

Pedersen, K., & Musaeus, P. (2023). A phenomenological approach to virtual reality in psychiatry education. *Frontiers in Virtual Reality, 4*, 1259263. https://doi.org/10.3389/FRVIR.2023.1259263/BIBTEX

Ray, A., Bhardwaj, A., Malik, Y. K., Singh, S., & Gupta, R. (2022). Artificial intelligence and psychiatry: An overview. *Asian Journal of Psychiatry, 70*, 103021. https://doi.org/10.1016/J.AJP.2022.103021

Sarvarizadeh, M., Miri, S., Darban, F., & Farokhzadian, J. (2024). Innovative cultural care training: The impact of flipped classroom methods on critical cultural competencies in psychiatric nursing: A quasi-experimental study. *BMC Nursing, 23*(1), 1–12. https://doi.org/10.1186/S12912-024-02001-Z

Sewagegn, A. A. (2020). Learning objective and assessment linkage: Its contribution to meaningful students learning. *Universal Journal of Educational Research, 8*(11), 5044–5052. https://doi.org/10.13189/ujer.2020.081104

Shad, M. U., Onwuameze, O., Sioson, K., Khan, A. H., Khalid, K., & Glick, I. (2023). Problem-based learning in psychopharmacology. *Academic Psychiatry, 47*(1), 111–112. https://doi.org/10.1007/S40596-022-01661-W

Shahar, G. (2021). Interdisciplinarity and integration: An introduction to the special issue on psychopathology in medical settings. *Journal of Clinical Psychology in Medical Settings, 28*(1), 1–5. https://doi.org/10.1007/S10880-020-09752-2

Shan, Y., Zhou, X., Qi, W., Liu, X., & Huang, C. (2023). Innovations in teaching during the COVID-19 pandemic: Comparisons of the impacts of different teaching approaches in psychiatric nursing on undergraduate nursing students. *BMC Medical Education, 23*(1), 1–12. https://doi.org/10.1186/S12909-023-04819-8

Subedi, P., & Pandey, M. (2021). Applying adult learning theories in improving medical education in Nepal: View of medical students. *JNMA: Journal of the Nepal Medical Association, 59*(234), 210. https://doi.org/10.31729/JNMA.5292

# Chapter 4
# Teaching and Training in Psychiatry in Afghanistan

**Mohammad Akbar Paiman**

**Abstract** Decades of violence, displacement, and economic instability have significantly increased mental health burdens. Forced displacement disrupts family and community structures, compounding psychological distress. Refugees and internally displaced persons face additional challenges, including unemployment, social isolation, and lack of access to mental health services. Culturally, Afghanistan's tribal and kinship-based society influences mental health perceptions and psychiatric education. In Kabul, several universities, including Kabul University, Kabul Medical University, and private institutions such as Khatam Al-Nabieen University, offer undergraduate and graduate courses in psychology and psychiatry. Kabul Medical University is the main institution offering structured training in psychiatry. Provincial universities, such as Herat University, Nangarhar University, Balkh University, Kandahar University, Bamyan University, and Kunduz University, also offer psychology and psychiatry training. These institutions typically follow curricula similar to Kabul's universities but with notable limitations due to fewer resources, trained faculty, and clinical facilities. The core curriculum generally includes courses in general psychology, abnormal psychology, mental health assessment, counseling, and community-based mental health practices. Provincial universities rely significantly on partnerships with local and international organizations to facilitate practical experiences and internships, enabling students to engage with real-world cases.

**Keywords** Conflict · Displacement · Mental health · Psychiatric education · Stigma · Community-based · Trauma · Psychosocial support

---

M. A. Paiman (✉)
World Health Organization, Abuja, Nigeria



S. K. Kar et al. (eds.), *Teaching and Training in Psychiatry in South Asia*, South Asian Perspectives in Mental Health and Psychology,
https://doi.org/10.1007/978-981-95-1845-6_4

## 1 Historical Background

Afghanistan is located between Central and South Asia, with a rich yet turbulent history shaped by its geographical significance as a cultural and trade nexus (Yar et al., 2023). Repeated invasions, wars, and regime changes have significantly influenced its social, cultural, and healthcare structures, including the provision of mental health services (Rasool et al., 2024). During the Silk Road times, this country served as a key center for trade and cultural exchange (Rasool et al., 2024). The emergence of Afghanistan as a modern nation-state in the eighteenth century unified fragmented regions, but persistent instability due to tribal divisions and external interference has continued to affect its governance and development (Jalali, 2021). The nineteenth and twentieth centuries were marked by colonial interests, particularly the British-Afghan wars, followed by modernization efforts in the 1920s, which were later disrupted by political unrest (Saikal, 2004). The Soviet invasion (1979–1989), ensuing civil war, Taliban rule (1996–2001), and two decades of conflict after the U.S.-led intervention (2001–2021) severely weakened Afghanistan's health infrastructure, exacerbating mental health disorders such as trauma, depression, and anxiety. Following the withdrawal of international forces and the collapse of the Afghan government, the Taliban's return in 2021 further restricted health and human rights, particularly for women and vulnerable populations (Saikal, 2004; Alemi et al., 2023). Decades of violence, displacement, and economic instability have significantly increased mental health burdens. Studies estimate that almost half of the displaced Afghans suffer from Post-Traumatic Stress Disorder (PTSD), depression, or anxiety, especially among those directly exposed to violence (Alemi et al., 2023). Forced displacement disrupts family and community structures, compounding psychological distress. Refugees and internally displaced persons (IDPs) face additional challenges, including unemployment, social isolation, and lack of access to mental health services (Alemi et al., 2023). The recent mass expulsion of refugees from Pakistan, Iran, and even some European countries further deteriorated the situation. Culturally, Afghanistan's tribal and kinship-based society influences mental health perceptions. Mental illness remains stigmatized, often perceived as a moral or spiritual weakness, delaying professional treatment (Mustafaeva, 2015). Gender disparities further shape mental health outcomes—women are disproportionately affected due to gender-based violence, forced marriages, and restricted autonomy (Mustafaeva, 2015). The bans on women's education and employment have exacerbated psychological distress, violated fundamental human rights, and further limited access to care (Shoib et al., 2024). Just before 2021, The Human Development Index (HDI) of Afghanistan was 0.51. Afghanistan is having a rank of 169 (out of 189 nations) in the domains of education, life expectancy, and overall living standards. Since the regime change in 2021, conditions for women, girls, religious, and other minorities have deteriorated, and the economy has been struggling due to market disruptions and freezing of reserves of the Afghanistan central bank by the United States (US) and the sanctions imposed on Afghanistan by the international community. Afghanistan is once again an isolated country, and the de facto authorities are not formally recognized as a government by the world. Millions have been pushed into extreme poverty, with an estimated 55% of the population now in urgent need of humanitarian assistance while many of the healthcare gains achieved over the past two decades are also at risk of being lost (Alemi et al., 2023).

## 2 Development of Psychiatry in Afghanistan

The development of psychiatric care in Afghanistan has been slow, shaped by traditional beliefs, religious interpretations, and limited institutional support. Historically, mental illnesses were attributed to supernatural causes, such as Jinn possession, with treatment sought from religious scholars and traditional healers (Mustafaeva, 2015; Alemi et al., 2023). Islamic theology framed mental suffering as a divine test, which, while fostering community support, also contributed to stigma and delayed medical interventions (Rasool et al., 2024).

In 1985, the government began developing community-based mental health services by creating a Department of Mental Health (DMH) within the Ministry of Health and by launching four community mental health centers in Kabul. However, in 1992, these facilities were looted after the fall of the Soviet-backed government. The ensuing years of civil war and the Taliban regime severely disrupted Afghanistan's newly established mental health system (Rahimi & Azimi, 2012; van de Put, 2002). A significant advance occurred in 1999 with the initiation of a three-month diploma course in basic psychiatric practice to train 20 medical practitioners; however, this program was unsustainable due to ongoing insecurity (Rahimi & Azimi, 2012). By 2002, mental healthcare facilities employed only two psychiatrists and a limited number of doctors with minimal training. In the early 2000s, the Afghan Government and donor communities decided to rebuild the healthcare system through non-governmental organizations (NGOs) (Alemi et al., 2023). In Nangarhar province, HealthNet TPO integrated mental health services into basic healthcare, targeting conditions such as depression, anxiety, psychosis, and epilepsy. This initiative resulted in an increase in the utilization of mental health services from less than 0.5% to about 5% of all healthcare consultations (Oriya & Alekozai, 2022). Between 2005 and 2008, the program expanded to six additional provinces, registering over 125,000 mental health consultations. These consultations primarily addressed depression (66.6%), followed by anxiety (14.9%), epilepsy (9.5%), psychosis (4.3%), intellectual disabilities (1.2%), substance use disorders (0.7%), and unexplained somatic complaints (2.8%). The publication of the Basic Package of Health Services (BPHS) in 2003 marked a significant milestone in the reconstruction of Afghanistan's health system, as it defined the minimum services available at primary health centers, including the management of mental health issues. In 2005, the appointment of a national coordinator for mental health in primary healthcare led to the establishment of a mental health unit within the Ministry of Health (Alemi et al., 2023; Ventevogel et al., 2007). Afghanistan has undergone a significant transformation in mental health service delivery, moving from a hospital-centric approach to a more integrated model within primary healthcare. This transition included substantial training initiatives: by 2018, non-governmental organizations (NGOs) had facilitated short-term mental health training for approximately 1000 physicians and over 1200 nurses and midwives, utilizing curricula developed by the Ministry of Public Health. The WHO's Mental Health Gap Action Programme (mhGAP) was also implemented, beginning in three provinces in 2013 and followed by a national-level training of trainers in 2022 (WHO, 2016). A major milestone in this transformation was the mandated inclusion of psychosocial counselors in comprehensive health centers, aligned with the 2009 revision of the Basic Package of Health Services (BPHS). NGOs such as IPSO and HealthNet TPO helped standardize the training process, eventually establishing formal diploma programs at the Ghazanfar Institute of Health Sciences (Alemi et al., 2023). By 2019, roughly 750 psychosocial counselors had been absorbed into the national health workforce, and by 2021, the Ghazanfar Institute had graduated 190 counselors through a two-year program. Public universities also began offering programs in counseling psychology, and Kabul University opened a Model Counseling Center in 2018, which remained operational even after the 2021 political transition. Before 2004, Afghanistan's secondary mental healthcare system was limited to one national psychiatric hospital in Kabul and a few psychiatric wards in provincial hospitals. The increased prioritization of mental health led to the development of specialized psychiatric wards in several regional and provincial hospitals, although many continued to face challenges such as inadequate staffing and poor infrastructure. The National Mental Health Strategy (2019–2023) set an ambitious goal to provide mental health services across all district and provincial hospitals, including the establishment of regional mental health wards and psychiatry residency programs. Despite progress, the system continues to suffer from significant limitations in financing, human resources, infrastructure, and information management (Table 4.1) (Alemi et al., 2023). Between 2017 and 2022, around two million mental health consultations were recorded annually, making up approximately 4% of total primary care visits. Nevertheless, reports of insufficient staffing, substandard care, and reliance on pharmacological treatment—often without adequate supervision—persist. Afghanistan's response to substance use disorders has also been insufficient, with only 104 treatment centers serving about 30,000 clients annually, despite estimates suggesting 2.5 million people suffer from substance use disorders. Relapse rates remain high, and services such as opioid agonist therapy are limited and politically sensitive, with several facilities shutting down after the 2021 regime change (Alemi et al., 2023; WHO, 2016).

Following the fall of the Taliban in 2001, numerous international agencies introduced community-based psychosocial support programs inspired by socioecological models that valued traditional practices, cultural norms, and local support systems. These initiatives emphasized strengthening families' and communities' resilience rather than relying solely on clinical services. For example, the cultural practice of storytelling among Afghan women was utilized as a therapeutic tool (de Berry, 2004; Mannell et al., 2018). Programs were developed collaboratively with

**Table 4.1** SWOT analysis of psychiatry teaching and training in Afghanistan

| SWOT analysis | Description and key points |
|---|---|
| Strengths | Established psychiatry education programs in Kabul and some provinces. The existence of structured curricula including general psychiatry, clinical rotations, and internships at Kabul Medical University. Integration of mental health into primary healthcare via BPHS and mhGAP. International collaborations and NGO support for training and program development. |
| Weaknesses | Insufficient qualified psychiatric professionals (only a handful of psychiatrists). Limited practical clinical training and insufficient resources in provincial universities. Low quality of research and dissertations heavily dependent on translated materials. Gender-based restrictions severely limiting female participation in medical education. |
| Opportunities | Potential to strengthen mental healthcare by leveraging existing community-based psychosocial programs. Expansion of training initiatives through international and local partnerships. Integration of psychiatry training with broader primary healthcare education. |
| Threats | Political instability and recent regime changes have drastically impacted access and quality. Ongoing security issues affecting service provision. Stigma related to mental health and cultural beliefs delaying professional care. Economic decline and reduced international funding after 2021. |

local stakeholders and often involved training schoolteachers and community members in psychosocial support techniques. Many of these efforts contributed to formal social work education, influencing national standards through the National Skills Development Program (Kostelny, 2006). Previous experiences working with Afghan refugees in Pakistan informed several of these efforts. For instance, teacher training programs initiated in refugee camps by the International Rescue Committee were later replicated inside Afghanistan. Other organizations, like War Child Holland and HealthNet TPO, focused on building safe spaces for children and restoring community trust through participatory planning and culturally sensitive approaches to issues such as gender-based violence (Ventevogel et al., 2006). Evaluations of these community-based interventions, though limited, have demonstrated encouraging outcomes. For example, activities led by international NGOs across 150 Afghan villages helped create child-centered spaces and community-led child protection committees, which improved school attendance, child safety, and social integration while reducing aggressive behavior (Snider & Triplehorn, 2003). A comparative study showed that interventions targeting water and sanitation had broader psychosocial benefits than stand-alone mental health programs. Innovative self-help approaches like the "Focusing" technique—a body-centered mindfulness practice adapted to Afghan culture—were introduced to promote emotional awareness and healing outside clinical environments (Loughry et al., 2005). These techniques, drawing from Persian and Afghan poetry, were integrated into training for educators and NGO staff. Between 2002 and 2008, the American Friends Service Committee (AFSC), in partnership with Kabul University and local organizations, trained dozens of interns and thousands of teachers in psychosocial methods (Omidian & Lawrence, 2007). Evaluations showed that these programs were well-received across various literacy levels. Donors like USAID and the EU supported such initiatives until funding was disrupted in 2021. Overall, these efforts highlight the importance of culturally grounded, community-driven approaches in addressing Afghanistan's complex mental health needs (Alemi et al., 2023).

## 2.1 *Teaching and Training in Psychology and Psychiatry in Afghanistan's Universities*

There is an urgent need for fundamental reforms in the collective mindset of Afghan society regarding the critical importance of education, particularly female education, which has been banned for the past four years (Table 4.2). This deeply rooted issue stems from a combination of rigid interpretations of religious values, traditional Afghan cultural norms, and the prevailing attitudes held by a significant portion of the population. A striking contradiction is evident: while many young Afghan men express a desire to marry educated women, they simultaneously restrict their own sisters and female relatives from attending school. This mindset must be actively and systematically challenged at all levels—within households, across

**Table 4.2** Gap identification in psychiatric training and suggested solutions in Afghanistan

| Gaps identified in psychiatric training | Suggestions to bridge the gaps |
|---|---|
| Insufficient clinical training opportunities | Strengthen partnerships between universities, NGOs, and international organizations to enhance practical internships and clinical rotations. Expand psychiatry wards in regional and provincial hospitals to support practical training. |
| Limited quality of research and original data | Establish structured mentorship and support systems for research, emphasizing original studies relevant to Afghanistan's context. Promote research integrity through rigorous evaluation processes and training in research methodologies. |
| Severe shortage of qualified psychiatric staff | Accelerate and expand training programs, including residency programs in psychiatry, especially in provincial areas. Implement continuous professional development initiatives using remote and hybrid training models to overcome geographical barriers. |
| Restrictions on female education | Advocate internationally and domestically for policies to lift restrictions on women's education. Develop targeted distance-learning programs specifically designed to safely include and empower female students in healthcare education. |
| Cultural stigma delays treatment | Launch community awareness and mental health education campaigns that address cultural and religious misconceptions. Engage religious and community leaders in advocacy to promote acceptance of mental health care. |
| Limited financial resources and infrastructure | Increase investment and international collaboration to secure sustainable financing for psychiatric education and healthcare infrastructure. Advocate for prioritizing mental health services within national and international humanitarian budgets. |

communities, and at district, provincial, national, and international platforms. The opposition to education must be addressed not only as a social issue but as a critical barrier to national development and prosperity. Sustainable progress in Afghanistan will require bold efforts to dismantle discriminatory attitudes and practices and to promote education as a universal right for all, regardless of gender (Najam et al., 2024).

Teaching and training in psychology and psychiatry at Afghanistan's universities are critical areas of academic and healthcare development, particularly given the country's prolonged exposure to conflict and resulting widespread mental health issues (Alemi et al., 2023). The curriculum, pathways to specialization, and availability of professional literature significantly influence the country's capability to address mental health needs (Table 4.1) (Kovess-Masfety et al., 2021). With high levels of trauma, stress-related disorders, depression, anxiety, and PTSD prevalent among the population, there is a critical need for well-trained professionals in psychology and psychiatry. Kabul and various provincial universities have established curricula aimed at addressing these pressing mental health issues, although resources and infrastructure remain limited (Alemi et al., 2023). Psychology and psychiatry education in Afghanistan primarily takes place within the faculties of medicine and psychology departments at major universities. Undergraduate psychology programs typically last four years, providing foundational knowledge in various psychological theories, methodologies, counseling techniques, developmental psychology, abnormal psychology, clinical psychology, and social psychology. Courses cover essential psychological concepts, history, major theoretical approaches, and fundamental research methods. Students are also introduced to counseling skills, including effective communication, assessment techniques, basic psychotherapy, and ethics in psychological practice (Alemi et al., 2023).

## 2.2 *Curriculum for Psychology and Psychiatry in Kabul Universities*

In Kabul, several universities, including Kabul University, Kabul Medical University (KMU), and private institutions such as Khatam Al-Nabieen University, offer undergraduate and graduate courses in psychology and psychiatry. Kabul Medical University is the main institution offering structured training in psychiatry (Missmahl et al., 2012). Medical students at KMU begin their exposure to psychiatry during their third and fourth years through introductory courses. The curriculum typically includes general psychiatry, child and adolescent psychiatry, forensic psychiatry, clinical psychology, psychotherapy, counseling techniques, psychopharmacology, and neuropsychiatry. Students participate in theoretical classes, clinical rotations, and internships, primarily at mental health hospitals such as Kabul Mental Health Hospital (Ali Abad) (Missmahl et al., 2012). Clinical training is central to KMU's psychiatry program, providing students direct interaction with patients under supervision, allowing them to develop essential diagnostic and therapeutic skills. The university collaborates closely with international organizations such as the World Health Organization (WHO) and international NGOs to ensure updated methodologies and treatment approaches (WHO, 2016). At Kabul University's Department of Psychology, students undertake comprehensive undergraduate programs. The curriculum covers foundational topics such as developmental psychology, educational psychology, clinical psychology, social psychology, cognitive-behavioral therapy, psychological assessments, psychometric testing, and various research methods. Practical training is encouraged through supervised internships in schools, hospitals, rehabilitation centers, and community mental health programs, enhancing students' hands-on experiences (Alemi et al., 2023).

### *2.3 Curriculum in Provincial Universities*

Provincial universities, such as Herat University, Nangarhar University, Balkh University, Kandahar University, Bamyan University, and Kunduz University, also offer psychology and psychiatry training. These institutions typically follow curricula similar to Kabul's universities but with notable limitations due to fewer resources, trained faculty, and clinical facilities. The core curriculum generally includes courses in general psychology, abnormal psychology, mental health assessment, counseling, and community-based mental health practices. Provincial universities rely significantly on partnerships with local and international organizations to facilitate practical experiences and internships, enabling students to engage with real-world cases (Missmahl et al., 2012).

## 3 Specialization Process in Psychiatry

Medical education with a specialization in psychiatry follows a distinct path. Initially, students pursue a medical degree (MD), which typically requires seven years, including clinical rotations in various specialties, of which psychiatry is one component for a limited time. During their undergraduate medical training, students are introduced to core psychiatric concepts, psychiatric assessment methods, common psychiatric disorders, psychopharmacology, basic psychotherapies, and ethical and legal issues in psychiatry. Residency programs (specialization, *Takhassus*) usually last three to four years (Missmahl et al., 2012). Trainees rotate through various psychiatric sub-specialties, including adult psychiatry, child psychiatry, geriatric psychiatry, addiction psychiatry, forensic psychiatry, and emergency psychiatry. The training is designed to provide residents with both theoretical knowledge and extensive practical exposure through clinical rotations, patient evaluations, and supervised clinical interventions (Missmahl et al., 2012). Residency programs in psychiatry in Afghanistan typically include a research component, requiring residents to complete a thesis or research project aimed at contributing to the understanding of psychiatric conditions prevalent in the country. However, based on the author's experience, the quality of these final dissertations is generally low. Many projects rely heavily on translated materials, often sourced from Iranian textbooks, rather than original research or locally relevant data. Furthermore, the widespread presence of advertisements in Kabul and other provinces offering dissertation writing services for students reflects deeper concerns about the quality of education and research integrity in the country. Upon successful completion of the residency training and passing the required national examination administered by the Ministry of Public Health (MoPH) and the Afghanistan Medical Council (AMC), graduates become certified psychiatrists (Alemi et al., 2023) (Tables 4.1 and 4.2).

## 4 Conclusion

Decades of prolonged conflict and persistent political instability in Afghanistan have had a devastating impact on the mental well-being of its people. These challenges have contributed to a high prevalence of mental health disorders across all age groups. On one hand, continuous violence and insecurity have exposed individuals to trauma, loss, and chronic stress. On the other hand, the destruction of traditional social support systems—including extended family networks, community cohesion, and cultural safety nets—has left individuals, particularly women and children, highly vulnerable. Education, a fundamental human right enshrined in international law, has been heavily politicized and manipulated in Afghanistan. Schools and educational institutions have not only suffered from systemic neglect but have also been deliberately targeted during periods of unrest. In many instances, schools—especially those for girls—have been burned or bombed. More alarmingly, there have been documented cases where female students were attacked with acid to deter them from pursuing education. This targeted violence and ideological repression have led to widespread fear, especially among families who might otherwise support their daughters' education. As a result, literacy rates remain critically low—particularly among women—and the overall quality of education at both school and university levels has been significantly compromised. The breakdown of the education sector not only stifles intellectual and social development but also limits the country's long-term prospects for peace, stability, and recovery.

The teaching and training of psychiatry in Afghanistan is deeply affected by the broader challenges facing the country's fragmented education system. Since the reduction of international support and the mass departure of skilled professionals following the political shift on 15 August 2021, many of the advancements achieved over the past two decades are now at serious risk of being reversed. Notably, over the last four years, no female students have graduated from high school or university, and no female medical graduates have been permitted to sit for the Afghanistan Medical Council (AMC) exit examination, which is a prerequisite for obtaining a license to practice medicine in the country. This alarming situation underscores the urgent need to depoliticize and reform Afghanistan's education system, with particular attention to medical education. Strengthening the foundational elements of education—such as access, quality, equity, and academic freedom—is essential for improving graduate-level teaching and training. This includes revitalizing the field of psychiatry education, which is vital for addressing the growing burden of mental health disorders in the population. Without immediate and sustained efforts, the country risks further deterioration in human capital, public health, and social stability.

## References

Alemi, Q., Panter-Brick, C., Oriya, S., Ahmady, M., Alimi, A. Q., Faiz, H., Hakim, N., Hashemi, S. A. S., Manaly, M. A., & Naseri, R. (2023). Afghan mental health and psychosocial well-being: Thematic review of four decades of research and interventions. *BJPsych Open, 9*, e125. https://doi.org/10.1192/bjo.2023.502

de Berry, J. (2004). Community psychosocial support in Afghanistan. *Intervention Journal of Mental Health and Psychosocial Support in Conflict Affected Areas, 2*, 143–151.

Jalali, A. A. (2021). *Afghanistan: A Military History from the Ancient Empires to the Great Game*. University Press of Kansas.

Kostelny, K. (2006). A culture-based, integrative approach. *A world turned upside down: Social ecological approaches to children in war zones* (pp. 19–38).

Kovess-Masfety, V., Karam, E., Keyes, K., Sabawoon, A., & Sarwari, B. A. (2021). Access to care for mental health problems in Afghanistan: A national challenge. *International Journal of Health Policy and Management, 11*, 1442. https://doi.org/10.34172/ijhpm.2021.46

Loughry, M., Macmullin, C., Eyber, C., Ababe, B., Ager, A., Kostelny, K., & Wessells, M. 2005. Assessing Afghan children's psychosocial well-being: A multimodal study of intervention outcomes. *Unpublished report,* CCF, Oxford University, Queen Margaret University. *http://www.forcedmigration. org*.

Mannell, J., Ahmad, L., & Ahmad, A. (2018). Narrative storytelling as mental health support for women experiencing gender-based violence in Afghanistan. *Social Science & Medicine, 214*, 91–98. https://doi.org/10.1016/j.socscimed.2018.08.011

Missmahl, I., Kluge, U., Bromand, Z., & Heinz, A. (2012). Teaching psychiatry and establishing psychosocial services–lessons from Afghanistan. *European Psychiatry, 27*, S76–S80. https://doi.org/10.1016/S0924-9338(12)75712-7

Mustafaeva, S. (2015). *The cultural shaping of depression: A qualitative investigation into Afghan women's perspectives on depression*. The University of Regina (Canada).

Najam, R., Patrinos, H. A., & Kattan, R. B. (2024). *The mis-education of women in Afghanistan*. The World Bank Group Policy Research Working Paper.

Omidian, P., & Lawrence, N. J. (2007). A community based approach to focusing: The Islam and Focusing Project of Afghanistan. *The Folio,* 152.

Oriya, S., & Alekozai, T. (2022). The impact of persons with mental health problems on family members and their coping strategies in Afghanistan. *Intervention Journal of Mental Health and Psychosocial Support in Conflict Affected Areas, 20*, 28–35. https://doi.org/10.4103/intv.intv_13_21

Rahimi, Y. A., & Azimi, S. (2012). War and the crisis of mental health in Afghanistan. *International Psychiatry, 9*, 55–57.

Rasool, G., Mukhtarova, K., & Jan, B. N. (2024). The role of Afghanistan in Central Asia: Risks and future prospects overview. *International Relations & International Law Journal/Seriâ Meždunarodnye Otnošeniâ & Meždunarodnoe Pravo, 106.*

Saikal, A. (2004). *Modern Afghanistan: A history of struggle and survival.* Bloomsbury Publishing.
Shoib, S., Hussaini, S.S., Nazari, S.K., Saeed, F. (2024). Mental Healthcare in Afghanistan. In: Arafat, S.M.Y., Kar, S.K. (eds) Access to Mental Health Care in South Asia. Springer, Singapore. https://doi.org/10.1007/978-981-99-9153-2_2
Snider, L., & Triplehorn, C. (2003). *Assessment of CCF's emergency entry program into Afghanistan: Its impact on child well-being and protection.* Christian Children's Fund.
Van de Put, W. (2002). Addressing mental health in Afghanistan. *The Lancet, 360*, s41–s42.
Ventevogel, P., Azimi, S., Jalal, S., & Kortmann, F. (2007). Mental health care reform in Afghanistan. *Journal of Ayub Medical College Abbottabad, 14.*
Ventevogel, P., Van Huuksloot, M., & Kortmann, F. 2006. Mental health in the aftermath of a complex emergency: The case of Afghanistan. *Advances in psychological and social support after disasters* (pp. 83–93).
WHO. (2016). mhGAP intervention guide for mental, neurological and substance use disorders in non-specialized health settings: mental health Gap Action Programme (mhGAP). *mhGAP intervention guide for mental, neurological and substance use disorders in non-specialized health settings: mental health Gap Action Programme (mhGAP).*
Yar, F. G. M., Zahid, S., & Miakhil, J. M. (2023). Afghanistan's geopolitical and geo-economic significance in regional connectivity and development. *Journal of Political and Legal Sovereignty, 1*, 78–86.

# Chapter 5
# Psychiatry Teaching, Training, and Research in Bangladesh

**S. M. Yasir Arafat**

**Abstract** Bangladesh gained independence at the end of 1971, and over the last 50 years, teaching, training, and research in mental health have remained underdeveloped. The first undergraduate medical curriculum was developed in 1988. Before that, there was a syllabus based on the existing colonial medical education system. Teaching and training in psychiatry are grossly neglected in the undergraduate level curriculum in Bangladesh, with 20 hours of lecture and four weeks of clinical ward placement. The *Diploma in Psychological Medicine* was the first postgraduate degree in Bangladesh, started in 1975, which was stopped later. The *Master of Philosophy* (MPhil) course in psychiatry was initiated in 1995, but was stopped later. A fellowship (*Fellow of Bangladesh College of Physicians and Surgeons [FCPS]*) was opened in 1979, and it is continuing. There is a membership (*Member of the College of Physicians and Surgeons [MCPS]*) program with a shorter duration. In 1995, the *Doctor of Medicine* (MD) in psychiatry was opened, which was revamped as "Residency Program" in 2010. There are two academic journals with a scope in mental health in Bangladesh. This chapter highlights the teaching, training, and research in mental health in Bangladesh.

**Keywords** Psychiatry · Curriculum · Teaching · Training · Mental health · Mental health research

## 1 Introduction

Bangladesh was a part of the Indian subcontinent that was ruled by the British till 1947. Then it was under Pakistan as East Pakistan till 16 December 1971. After liberation, Bangladesh made enormous progress in health, per capita income of the country, and socioeconomic status. Recently, the country has moved to the lower

S. M. Y. Arafat (✉)
Department of Psychiatry, Bangladesh Specialized Hospital Limited, Dhaka, Bangladesh



S. K. Kar et al. (eds.), *Teaching and Training in Psychiatry in South Asia*, South Asian Perspectives in Mental Health and Psychology,
https://doi.org/10.1007/978-981-95-1845-6_5

middle income from the low-income group. Historically, mental health services were started during the British period in Dhaka as an asylum in 1815, which was demolished, and the hospital mental services were established in 1957 in Pabna (Arafat, 2024a). During the Pakistan period, the hospital services for mental health disorders were inadequate in Bangladesh (East Pakistan of that time) based on the needs and burden of mental disorders (Morning News, 1970). After the liberation, the mental health service was extended gradually all over the country. However, as an academic entity, psychiatry has been considered as a neglected branch of medicine (Hasan et al., 2021). This chapter aims to highlight the academic teaching, training, and publishing in psychiatry in Bangladesh based on available evidence, personal experience, and expert opinion.

## 2 Academic Psychiatry Education in Bangladesh

### *2.1 Psychiatry in Undergraduate Curriculum*

There was no formal undergraduate medical curriculum in Bangladesh till 1988. The *Bangladesh Medical and Dental Council (BMDC)* had a syllabus for medical colleges to be followed in medical education (Majumder, 2003). Before that, there was a typical colonial medical education system with traditional lecture-based, teacher-dominant, discipline-focused, examination-driven, and hospital-ccntric. After the first formal medical curriculum, there were important developments for ensuring the medical education system in the country during the 1990s (Majumder, 2003). Since the early days of curriculum development, psychiatry has been considered a tiny part and small branch of medicine at the graduation level (Hasan et al., 2021). After graduation, there are specialized degrees mandatory for becoming a psychiatrist.

The BMDC released the latest undergraduate medical curriculum [*Bachelor of Medicine, Bachelor of Surgery (MBBS)*] in 2021 (BMDC, 2021). It needs at least five academic years and an additional one year of internship after passing out MBBS. The five academic years are divided into four phases. Anatomy, Physiology, and Biochemistry are taught in the first phase with a duration of one and a half years and a professional exam. Forensic Medicine and Community Medicine are taught in the second phase, with a duration of one year and a professional exam. Pathology, Microbiology, and Pharmacology are taught in the third phase with a duration of one year and a professional exam. Medicine and allied subjects, Surgery and allied subjects, and gynecology are taught in the fourth phase with a duration of one and a half years and the final professional exam. These four phases were also noted in 2012 curriculum (BMDC, 2012). However, there were three phases (phase 1: 1.5 years; phase 2: 2 years; and phase 3: 1.5 years) with the same duration and three professional exams in 2002 curriculum (BMDC, 2002). Psychiatry has been taught as an allied subject of Medicine. The latest curriculum contains twenty hours for lectures which is divided into two hours in the second phase and the rest eighteen hours are in the phase four (BMDC, 2021; Arafat, 2024b). Additionally, there are four weeks allocation for the clinical ward placement divided into third and fourth phase for two weeks each (Arafat, 2024b; BMDC, 2021). There was difference with the curriculum of 2012 where the twenty hours lectures was allocated in the fourth phase only and there was a placement at clinical ward with a duration of 3 weeks in the fourth phase (Arafat, 2024b; BMDC, 2012; Roy & Arafat, 2018; Hasan et al., 2021). The curriculum of 2002 allocated the twenty hours of lecture classes divided into third (second phase) and fourth year (early third phase, i.e. final phase) for ten hours each and a place of four weeks in the clinical ward during the fourth year (Arafat, 2024b; BMDC, 2002). Overall, psychiatry has an allocation of twenty hours of lectures and four weeks of clinical ward placement at MBBS level in Bangladesh. The time duration was reduced in 2012 curriculum when compared to the 2002 curriculum in clinical placement, which raised criticism among mental health professionals, urging additional time allocation (Table 5.1). The allocated duration is lowest when compared to the other three South Asian neighboring countries, i.e. India, Nepal, and Sri Lanka (Arafat et al., 2021). Psychiatry has been considered as a major discipline at the graduation level in Sri Lanka with the highest course duration in the curriculum, Nepal has various durations in different universities, whilst has already started a competency-based medical curriculum (Arafat et al., 2021). One study found that about 85% of 307 physicians considered that there should have more emphasis on Psychiatry in the curriculum (Hasan et al., 2021).

Important topics are highlighted in the latest (2021) curriculum, i.e. evolution of psychiatry and classification of disorders, importance of communication in physician–patient relationship, behavioral perspectives of learning, memory, intelligence, personality constructs, phenomenology, examination of mental state, delirium, dementia, neurodevelopmental disorders with special focus on autism, sexual dysfunctions, biological management of psychiatric disorders, substance abuse and emerging behavioral addictions, psychoses, mood disorders (mania and depression), suicidal behavior, non-suicidal self-injury, emergencies in psychiatry, generalized anxiety disorder (GAD), phobia, obsessive-compulsive disorder (OCD), and panic disorder, somatoform disorders, stress related disorders, movement disorders, seizure disorder, eating disorders, sleep disorders, and women's reproductive psychiatric disorders.

Having patients admitted in the hospital is necessary for clinical placements during the ward rotations. However, out of 37 public medical colleges, indoor facilities

**Table 5.1** Psychiatry time duration in different curricula

| Variable | 2021 | 2012 | 2002 |
|---|---|---|---|
| Total phases | 4 (1.5, 1, 1, & 1.5 years) | 4 (1.5, 1, 1, & 1.5 years) | 3 (1.5, 2, & 1.5 years) |
| Lecture | 20 hours (2 hours in phase 2 and 18 hours in phase 4) | 20 hours (phase 4) | 20 hours in fourth year |
| Clinical ward placement | 4 weeks (2 weeks in third and fourth phase) | 3 weeks (fourth phase) | 4 weeks in fourth year |

are available in only ten medical colleges. Among the 67 private medical colleges, indoor facilities are available in only four institutes (Government of the People's Republic of Bangladesh, 2022).

## 2.2 *Specialist Courses in Psychiatry in Bangladesh*

To become a psychiatrist in Bangladesh, one has to complete at least one of the available BMDC-recognized degrees. With the course of time the duration of degrees has been changed, some degrees have been discontinued, some started and are continuing.

### 2.2.1 Fellow of Bangladesh College of Physicians and Surgeons (FCPS)

A fellowship in psychiatry in Bangladesh was launched in 1979 at the *Bangladesh College of Physicians and Surgeons* (BCPS) (Arafat et al., 2020). There is an entry exam to be enrolled in the program, and then a training period with a dissertation, followed by an exit exam. However, there is no bar in case of the number of participants and the number of qualifying students in both entry and exit exams. Till 2019, a four-year duration of training was needed to sit in the exit exam. The training duration has been increased from four to five years to qualify for the exit exam (Arafat, 2020). A new fellowship (FCPS in *Child and Adolescent Psychiatry*) has been started in January 2022 (BCPS, 2021).

### 2.2.2 Doctor of Medicine (MD)

This course was started at the Bangladesh Medical University (BMU) [former *Bangabandhu Sheikh Mujib Medical University (BSMMU)]* in 1995 and was discontinued for some time. Eventually, in 2010, a new curriculum, i.e., MD Residency, was launched with a duration of five years in two phases (A and B). Phase A continues for the initial two years, followed by a mandatory completion exam and then Phase B continues for the next three years with completion of a clinical exam and a thesis. Gradually, the extent of this program has been extended on the basis of the subjects as well as new institutions. Currently, the MD in Psychiatry course is available at the BMU, the *National Institute of Mental Health (NIMH)*, Dhaka, and *MAG Osmani Medical College*, Sylhet. The seats are limited, and the entry exam is highly competitive. An MD in child and adolescent psychiatry was started at BMU in 2016 (Arafat, 2024b).

### 2.2.3 Member of the College of Physicians and Surgeons (MCPS)

The BCPS also offers shorter duration membership programs, namely *Member of the College of Physicians and Surgeons (MCPS)* in different subjects (Arafat, 2020; Arafat et al., 2020). For MCPS, no entry exam is needed, and the seats are not limited. However, the participants must pass at least four years after completing graduation with clinical training of a certain duration from BCPS-certified institutions (Arafat, 2020). In 2022, BCPS made some changes to the criteria of the MCPS exam. The gap between the MCPS exam and the completion of graduation increased from four to five years. Additionally, the required clinical training period has been increased from one to two years (BCPS, 2022). An MCPS in *Child and Adolescent Psychiatry* is yet to be started. A membership qualification enables a person to see patients as a psychiatrist and a consultant. However, it does not help in achieving academic promotions like professorship (Arafat, 2024b).

### 2.2.4 Master of Philosophy (MPhil)

The MPhil in psychiatry was launched in 1995 when the DPM was discontinued. The duration of this degree was three years. The MPhil course was continued under the BMU and the *Sylhet MAG Osmani Medical College*. There were some entry criteria to sit for an entry exam for the degree, and the number of seats was limited based on the institution. Eventually, this course was discontinued, and the launch of longer courses was attempted (Karim et al., 2006; Mullick, 2007).

### 2.2.5 Diploma in Psychological Medicine (DPM)

It was the first degree started in Bangladesh to recognize psychiatrists in 1975 at the BMU, which was named as *Institute of Postgraduate Medicine and Research* (IPGMR). It was started by *Professor Dr. A K M Nazimuddowla Chowdhury,* who completed DPM from England in 1958 (Chowdhury et al., 2024). This diploma course was discontinued in 1995 (Arafat et al., 2020).

## *2.3 Mental Health and Psychiatric Nursing*

The *National Institute of Advanced Nursing Education and Research (NIANER)* is the pioneer organization of mental health nursing in Bangladesh. It initiated the master's level (MSc) courses in mental health nursing in the country (Arafat, 2019, 2024b). The MSc in mental health course was started in 2013 to enhance the academic milieu, ensure skilled human resources, and improve mental health services (Arafat, 2019). The NIANER launched a separate MS in mental health and psychiatric nursing program in BSMMU in July 2016. *Advanced Mental Health and*

*Psychiatric Nursing*, *Advanced Mental Health Nursing Intervention*, *Advanced Psychiatric Nursing Practicum for People with Mental Disorders*, and *Advanced Mental Health Nursing Practicum for Vulnerable Populations* are the available courses in the curriculum. Later in July 2022, BMU launched a separate MSc mental health and psychiatric nursing program. In 2024, a Diploma in Psychiatric Nursing with one duration course has been started at NIMH, Dhaka, with an allocation of 20 seats.

At private sector, several institutions have been attempting to open the courses. The *Universal Nursing College*, Dhaka, launched the MSc in mental health and psychiatric nursing program in July 2022 (Universal Nursing College, 2024). The *Enam Nursing College* is another private institution that opened MSc in *Mental Health & Psychiatric Nursing* program recently (Enam Nursing College, 2024). The *SAIC Nursing College* and the *International Nursing College* have been offering the courses.

## 3 Research Systems in Psychiatry in Bangladesh

Mental health research has been an underdeveloped agenda in Bangladesh. Fortunately, some interest has been noted since the COVID-19 pandemic. Research is merely considered in policy making, institutional recognition, academic promotions and benefits (Arafat, 2024b). It was noted in the WHO-ATLAS data (2020) that only 35 peer-reviewed papers were published in mental health subject in Bangladesh (World Health Organization, 2022). The *Scimago Journal Rank* (SJR) under Subject area – Medicine; followed by Subject Category – Psychiatry and Mental Health (https://www.scimagojr.com/) revealed that Bangladesh held 59th position with 569 documents and 53 h-index from 1996 to 2023. Among the South Asian countries, Bangladesh holds the third position after India (15th) and Pakistan (47th). Additionally, it is prudential to consider that a good proportion of articles do not reach Scimago-listed journals as none of the local mental health journals is listed and writing quality and quality of research also restrict the papers from reaching well-indexed journals. Several challenges have been discussed in Bangladesh attributing to the status quo such as scarcity of role model in psychiatry research, extreme political influence in academic appointment and promotion, lack of motivation of clinicians in research, inadequate funds in mental health research, lack of supervision and research facilities, and authorship misconduct (Arafat et al., 2022a). Bangladesh needs immediate attention to mental health research to change the status, influence the policy level implications, developing human resource and other facilities in the country.

## *3.1 Psychiatry Journals in Bangladesh*

### 3.1.1 Bangladesh Journal of Psychiatry (BJP)

*Bangladesh Journal of Psychiatry* (BJP) is the officially affiliated journal of the *Bangladesh Association of Psychiatrists* (BAP). It publishes paper in the open-access model, two issues in a year (January and July). The latest online accessible issue was Vol 37 Issue 2 (2023) (till 27 October 2024). It is free of charge for publication for authors. Also, there is no subscription charge for the journal.

### 3.1.2 Archives of NIMH (AN)

The Archives of NIMH (AN) is a newer open-access psychiatry journal. It was launched in 2018. Like the BJP, it also releases two issues in a year. It publishes articles without charging fees from the authors. Also, there are no subscription charges.

Both of the journals are available in Bangladesh Journals Online (BanglaJOL). However, the journals are yet to be included in DOAJ, PubMed, PMC, Embase, and Web of Science (Arafat, 2024b; Arafat et al., 2022a). The journals do not launch any special or thematic issues, and do not have an online submission and peer review platform.

One study assessed the gender distribution of psychiatry journals in South Asia (Arafat et al., 2022b). Reanalysis of the data after extracting the editorial board members of two mental health journals in Bangladesh revealed that about three-fourths of the total board members were males, editor-in-chief of both journals were males (Fig. 5.1, Arafat, 2024b). The proportion of the total male editors was lower when compared to the South Asia (73 vs. 78%) (Arafat et al., 2022b). Additionally, 96% of the editorial positions were occupied by psychiatrists (Arafat, 2024b).

Table 5.2 revealed that BJP published 5 papers per issue with 3 original articles, whereas AS published more than 8 papers per issue with more than five original articles. AN published review articles, whereas BJP published original articles and case reports.

## 4 Conclusions

The academic psychiatry teaching, training, and research have received inadequate attention in Bangladesh. A little attention has been paid to psychiatry in the undergraduate medical curriculum. Therefore, general practitioners face challenges during clinical practice with mental health symptoms. Bangladesh needs immediate attention to academic psychiatry teaching, training, and the curriculum to meet the pace of demand as the economy is expanding rapidly, and the awareness about

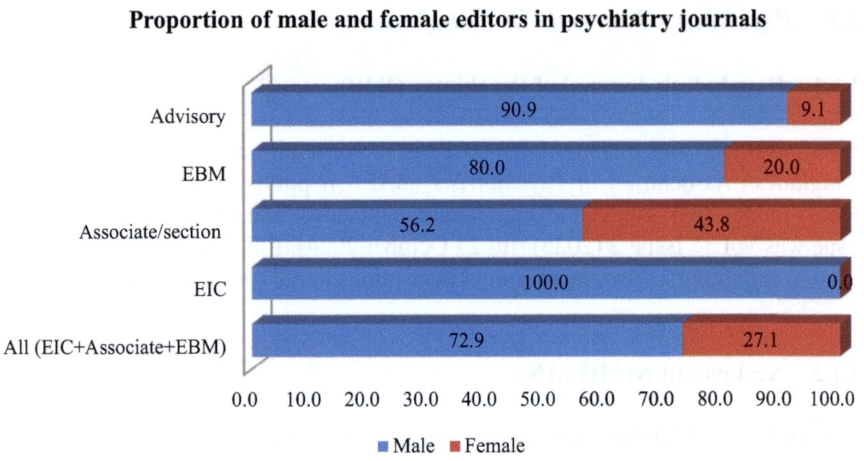


**Fig. 5.1** Gender distribution of editors in mental health journals in Bangladesh (Adapted from Arafat, 2024b). EIC—Editor-in-Chief; EBM—Editorial Board Member

**Table 5.2** Distribution of papers published in two mental health journals in Bangladesh

| Volume | Volume (Issue) | Original | Review | Case report | Editorial | Total |
|---|---|---|---|---|---|---|
| *Archives of NIMH* (AN) | | | | | | |
| 2023 | 6 (1) | 6 | | 1 | 1 | 8 |
| 2023 | 6 (2) | 7 | | 1 | 1 | 9 |
| 2022 | 5 (1) | 6 | | | 1 | 7 |
| 2022 | 5 (2) | 7 | | 1 | 1 | 9 |
| 2021 | 4 (1) | 6 | 1 | 1 | 1 | 9 |
| 2021 | 4 (2) | 6 | 1 | 1 | 1 | 9 |
| 2020 | 3 (1) | 5 | 1 | 1 | 1 | 8 |
| 2020 | 3 (2) | 7 | 1 | 1 | 1 | 10 |
| 2019 | 2 (1) | 4 | 1 | 1 | | 6 |
| 2019 | 2 (2) | 4 | 1 | 1 | 1 | 7 |
| *Bangladesh Journal of Psychiatry* (BJP) | | | | | | |
| 2023 | 37 (1) | 3 | | 2 | | 5 |
| 2023 | 37 (2) | 3 | | 2 | | 5 |
| 2022 | 36 (1) | 3 | | 2 | | 5 |
| 2022 | 36 (2) | 3 | | 2 | | 5 |
| 2021 | 35 (1) | 3 | | 2 | | 5 |
| 2021 | 35 (2) | 3 | | 2 | | 5 |
| 2020 | 34 (1) | 3 | | 1 | 1 | 5 |
| 2020 | 34 (2) | 3 | | 2 | | 5 |
| 2019 | 33 (1) | 3 | | 2 | | 5 |
| 2019 | 33 (2) | 3 | | 2 | | 5 |

psychiatric disorders and treatment has been increasing day by day. Additionally, the country needs attention to mental health research to develop culture-appropriate interventions for psychiatric disorders as culture plays significant role in presentation and treatment of psychiatric disorders.

## References

Arafat, S. M. Y. (2019). History of psychiatry in Bangladesh. *Asian Journal of Psychiatry, 46*, 11–12. https://doi.org/10.1016/j.ajp.2019.09.024

Arafat, S. M. Y. (2020). The current status of psychiatric education in Bangladesh. *Asian Journal of Psychiatry, 52*, 102108. https://doi.org/10.1016/j.ajp.2020.102108

Arafat, S. M. Y. (2024a). Mental health services in Bangladesh. In S. M. Y. Arafat (Ed.), *Mental health in Bangladesh*. Springer. https://doi.org/10.1007/978-981-97-0610-5_3

Arafat, S. M. Y. (2024b). Psychiatric education and research system in Bangladesh. In S. M. Y. Arafat (Ed.), *Mental health in Bangladesh*. Springer. https://doi.org/10.1007/978-981-97-0610-5_12

Arafat, S. M. Y., Mullick, M. S. I., & Islam, H. (2020). Development of psychiatric services in Bangladesh. *Asian Journal of Psychiatry, 47*, 101870. https://doi.org/10.1016/j.ajp.2019.101870

Arafat, S. M. Y., Kar, S. K., Sharma, P., Marahatta, K., & Baminiwatta, A. K. A. B. (2021). A comparative analysis of psychiatry curriculum at undergraduate level of Bangladesh, India, Nepal, and Sri Lanka. *Indian Journal of Psychiatry, 63*(2), 184–188. https://doi.org/10.4103/psychiatry.IndianJPsychiatry_615_20

Arafat, S. Y., Ali, S. A. E. Z., Saleem, T., Banerjee, D., Singh, R., Baminiwatta, A., & Shoib, S. (2022a). Academic psychiatry journals in South Asian countries: Most from India, none from Afghanistan, Bhutan and the Maldives. *Global Psychiatry Archives, 5*(1), 1–9. https://doi.org/10.52095/gp.2021.4395.1036

Arafat, S. M. Y., Amin, R., Baminiwatta, A., Hussain, F., Singh, R., Kar, S. K., & Mubashir, A. S. (2022b). Gender distribution of editors in psychiatry journals of South Asia. *Psychiatry Research, 317*, 114819. https://doi.org/10.1016/j.psychres.2022.114819

BCPS. (2021). *Notification for introducing new fellowship program in Medical Oncology, Palliative Medicine, Child and Adolescent Psychiatry, Paediatric Endocrinology & Metabolism, Paediatric Critical Care Medicine.* http://bcps.edu.bd/bcpscms/upload/Notification_for_introducing_new_fellowship_program_in_Medical_Oncology,_Palliative_Medicine,_Child_and_Adolesent_Psychiatry,_Paediatric_Endocrinology_Metabolism,_Paediatric_Critical_Care_Medicine.pdf (accessed on 30 October, 2024).

BCPS. (2022). *Notification for counting two years training in MCPS.* http://bcps.edu.bd/bcpscms/upload/Notification_for_counting_two_years_training_in_MCPS.pdf (accessed on 30 October, 2024).

BMDC. (2002). *BM&DC, MBBS Curriculum – 2002.* https://www.bmdc.org.bd/curriculum-2002 (accessed on 29 October, 2024).

BMDC. (2012). *MBBS Curriculum Update – 2012.* https://www.bmdc.org.bd/curriculum-2012 (accessed on 29 October, 2024).

BMDC. (2021). *MBBS Curriculum Update – 2021.* https://www.bmdc.org.bd/curriculum-2020 (accessed on 29 October, 2024).

Chowdhury, N. F., Fariduzzaman, A. M., & Arafat, S. M. Y. (2024). Prominent figures in psychiatry in Bangladesh. In S. M. Y. Arafat (Ed.), *Mental health in Bangladesh*. Springer. https://doi.org/10.1007/978-981-97-0610-5_1

Enam Nursing College. (2024). *Master of science in nursing.* https://enc.edu.bd/msc-in-nursing/ (accessed on 29 October, 2024).

Government of the People's Republic of Bangladesh. (2022). *National Mental Health Strategic Plan, 2020–2030*. https://dghs.gov.bd/sites/default/files/files/dghs.portal.gov.bd/notices/e27171cb_a80b_42d4_99ad_40095adef31b/2022-08-16-08-42-af8622e2c4936593dd45601b84f4920f.pdf (accessed on October 29, 2024).

Hasan, M. K., Aktar, M. T., Ara, S. A., Kabir, F. R., & Islam, M. R. (2021). Doctors' view about status of Teaching & Learning of Psychiatry at Undergraduate Medical Education in Bangladesh. *Bangladesh Journal of Medical Education, 12*(2), 18–22. https://doi.org/10.3329/bjme.v12i2.54449

Karim, M. R., Shaheed, F., & Paul, S. (2006). Psychiatry in Bangladesh. *International Psychiatry: Bulletin of the Board of International Affairs of the Royal College of Psychiatrists, 3*(3), 16–18.

Majumder, M. A. (2003). Medical education in Bangladesh: Past successes, future challenges. *Bangladesh Medical Journal, 32*(1), 37–39.

Morning News. (1970). *Mental Health*. Published on March 03, 1970.

Mullick, M. S. I. (2007). Teaching and training in psychiatry and the need for a new generation of psychiatrists in Bangladesh: Role of the Royal College of Psychiatrists. *International Psychiatry: Bulletin of the Board of International Affairs of the Royal College of Psychiatrists, 4*(2), 29–31.

Roy, S., & Arafat, S. Y. (2018). Recent changes in MBBS curriculum in psychiatry in Bangladesh: A call for attention. *Bangladesh Journal of Psychiatry, 32*(2), 24–25. https://doi.org/10.3329/bjpsy.v32i2.55125

Universal Nursing College. (2024). *Master of science in nursing*. https://unc-bd.com/msc-in-nursing/ (accessed on 29 October, 2024).

World Health Organization. (2022). *Mental Health Atlas 2020 Country Profile: Bangladesh*. https://www.who.int/publications/m/item/mental-health-atlas-bgd-2020-country-profile (accessed on March 30, 2023).

# Chapter 6
# Psychiatry Teaching and Training in India

**M. Kishor, Arghya Pal, and Varchasvi Mudgal**

**Abstract** Psychiatry education in India has undergone significant evolution in response to the growing burden of mental illness and the urgent need for trained mental health professionals. This chapter provides a comprehensive overview of the current structure, challenges, and opportunities within undergraduate and postgraduate psychiatry training in India. At the undergraduate level, the introduction of competency-based medical education (CBME) has standardized learning objectives and enhanced clinical exposure, though disparities in implementation and faculty shortages persist. Postgraduate training, offered through MD, DNB, and DPM programs, continues to expand in scope but faces issues such as regional imbalance, insufficient psychotherapy training, and enthusiasm of trainee-trainer. Faculty development remains a cornerstone for sustaining quality education, with national-level programs and innovative platforms like Indian Teachers of Psychiatry (IToP) playing key roles. This chapter also explores emerging trends, including digital learning tools, interdepartmental collaborations, and artificial intelligence in medical education. A vision for the future emphasizes the need for equitable distribution of training opportunities, enhanced infrastructure, standardized assessments, and continual faculty upskilling. Strengthening psychiatry education is essential to bridging India's mental health treatment gap and ensuring a competent and compassionate psychiatric workforce for the future.

M. Kishor (✉)
Department of Psychiatry, JSS Medical College & Hospital, JSS Academy of Higher Education & Research, Mysuru, Karnataka, India
e-mail: kishorm@jssuni.edu.in

A. Pal
Department of Psychiatry, All India Institute of Medical Sciences, Kalyani, West Bengal, India

V. Mudgal
Department of Psychiatry, MGM Medical College, Indore, Madhya Pradesh, India



S. K. Kar et al. (eds.), *Teaching and Training in Psychiatry in South Asia*, South Asian Perspectives in Mental Health and Psychology,
https://doi.org/10.1007/978-981-95-1845-6_6

**Keywords** Psychiatry education · Undergraduate medical education · Postgraduate psychiatry training · Competency-based medical education (CBME) · Faculty development · Medical curriculum reform

## 1 Introduction

Psychiatry, a branch of medicine, focuses on understanding, diagnosing, and managing mental, emotional, and behavioral disorders. Mental disorders are a leading cause of global morbidity and mortality, often complicating other medical conditions. In India, with over one-sixth of the world's population, mental health is a growing concern, impacting development indicators and featuring high suicide rates. Insufficient psychiatry training for medical undergraduates contributes to a lack of competence in diagnosing and managing common mental health issues like depression and anxiety. Mental health conditions, such as depression, anxiety, and substance use disorders, are leading contributors to the global disease burden. They significantly impact quality of life, emphasizing the importance of psychiatry in healthcare systems worldwide (Kishor et al., 2016; Prince et al., 2007).

In India, the need for psychiatry education has grown due to the country's vast mental health treatment gap, exacerbated by a shortage of trained professionals. Effective psychiatry education aims to address this gap by equipping medical graduates with essential skills to recognize, treat, and manage mental health conditions.

Psychiatry as a medical specialty has gained significant prominence in India, with growing recognition of mental health's critical role in overall well-being. The training pathway for psychiatry in India encompasses undergraduate and postgraduate levels, each designed to equip medical professionals with the skills to address the country's diverse mental health challenges. At the undergraduate level, exposure to psychiatry is integrated into the MBBS curriculum, aiming to provide foundational knowledge about mental health conditions, their diagnosis, and treatment. Postgraduate psychiatry training, pursued as a Diploma in Psychological Medicine (DPM), MD or DNB (Diplomate in National Board) in Psychiatry, offers in-depth clinical exposure, research opportunities, and advanced therapeutic techniques. Over the years, advancements in curriculum design, teaching methodologies, and the increasing availability of specialized training institutes have strengthened psychiatry education in India. This chapter delves into the structure, objectives, and challenges of psychiatry training at both levels, exploring how it shapes competent professionals to meet India's mental health needs (Raju, 2022).

# 2 Undergraduate Psychiatry Education

## 2.1 Historical Background

The inclusion of psychiatry in undergraduate medical education in India began during the mid-twentieth century, reflecting global trends emphasizing mental health awareness. Psychiatry was initially introduced as part of general medicine, with a limited focus in the MBBS curriculum. The Medical Council of India (now National Medical Commission) mandated dedicated teaching of psychiatry in the 1970s, recognizing the growing burden of mental health disorders. Early efforts were driven by pioneers who advocated for psychiatry's importance in holistic medical training. Over time, teaching evolved from didactic lectures to interactive clinical exposure, ensuring graduates could identify, manage, and refer mental health conditions effectively (Reddy, 2007).

The evolution of undergraduate psychiatry training in India has been marked by key milestones that reflect a growing acknowledgement of mental health's importance. Beginning with the Bhore Committee in 1946, which advocated for dedicated psychiatry departments, subsequent reforms addressed deficiencies in teaching and infrastructure. Seminars like those held at the Central Institute of Psychiatry, Ranchi (1965) and workshops at Jawaharlal Institute of Postgraduate Medical Education and Research (1983) and The National Institute of Mental Health and Neuro Sciences (1989) highlighted the need for curriculum updates, innovative methods, and faculty expansion. The National Mental Health Program (1982) emphasized the role of medical undergraduates in primary mental health care. By 2011, significant curriculum reforms by the MCI doubled teaching hours, increased clinical postings, and integrated psychiatry with community medicine, ensuring more exposure for future clinicians. These developments underscore the progressive recognition of psychiatry as an integral component of medical education (Kumar et al., 2018).

## 2.2 Current Structure and Curriculum

The National Medical Commission (NMC) has established a competency-based medical education (CBME) framework for psychiatry at the undergraduate level in 2019. This curriculum is designed to prepare Indian medical graduates (IMGs) to identify and manage common mental health issues, focusing on their role in primary care. Psychiatry clinical postings are structured as two-week sessions in Phase III, Part I, and four-week sessions in Phase III, Part II. Additionally, psychiatry is incorporated into final theory examinations, with specific marks allocated in the second paper of Medicine. The training approach integrates various teaching techniques, such as lectures, practical clinical experiences, and discussions based on real-life cases. Students gain hands-on exposure through simulated scenarios, patient interactions, and collaborative teaching with related disciplines like Community

Medicine. The curriculum emphasizes skill-building in areas like mental health assessments and basic interventions. However, psychiatry was not mandatory in evaluation at any phase of MBBS. The 2024 CBME psychiatry has made two certifiable skills mandatory for medical students, one on diagnosis of depression and management in primary care, the other on suicide risk assessment (Narasimha et al., 2024; Sethi et al., 2024).

Undergraduate students are expected to develop the ability to recognize, diagnose, and provide initial treatment for prevalent psychiatric conditions such as depression and anxiety. They should demonstrate effective communication, empathy, and the ability to refer patients needing advanced care. In the CBME curriculum, there are opportunities for students to choose electives in psychiatry, which are designed by the department depending upon the interest and resources available. This is optional for students and is full-time exposure for four weeks. There is a need to evaluate such novel aspects in undergraduate psychiatry. Various components of psychiatry training are described in Table 6.1 (Medical Council of India, 2018).

## 2.3 *Challenges in Undergraduate Psychiatry Education*

Undergraduate psychiatry education in India faces several obstacles that hinder its effective implementation. A significant challenge is disproportionate increase in medical students across India (100-250 per year /institute) for existing staff in addition to decrease in enthusiasm of learners-trainers for various reasons. The other issues are related to administrative burden, which includes a shortage of trained educators, resource constraints, and competing responsibilities for faculty members, such as teaching, research, and clinical duties. Strengthening medical education departments within institutions and offering mentorship programs, workshops, and teacher training initiatives—like those introduced by the Indian Teachers of Psychiatry (IToP)—can help address these gaps. Additionally, attitudinal inertia among educators often leads to reliance on outdated teaching methods, which hampers the adoption of CBME. Empowering teachers with proper orientation, support,

**Table 6.1** Components of psychiatry training for undergraduates

| Component of psychiatry training | Quantity/division |
|---|---|
| Competencies in psychiatry | 17 (2 are certifiable skills) |
| Topics | 13 |
| Competencies for horizontal and vertical integration in teaching hours | 40 hrs (13 lectures,17 Small Group, 10 self-directed learning) |
| Total postings | 2 + 4 weeks (divided across semesters) |
| Assessment as a part of medicine (Dermatology + Psychiatry) | 15 marks in internal assessment<br>25 marks for psychiatry in final exams |
| Internship | 2 weeks (mandatory) + 4 weeks (optional-electives in Psychiatry) |

and recognition for implementing CBME can motivate them to modernize their approaches. Another critical issue is the disproportionate student-to-teacher ratio, which makes personalized mentorship and skill-based training challenging. Strategies like engaging psychiatry residents, interdisciplinary teaching collaborations, and digital platforms such as the National Knowledge Network could mitigate this disparity (Gupta & Menon, 2022; P. Kumar et al., 2018).

## *2.4 Opportunities for Improvement*

Innovative approaches present significant opportunities to enhance undergraduate psychiatry education. Increasing the use of blended learning methods, which combine digital tools and traditional teaching techniques, can enrich the curriculum while addressing faculty shortages. Low-supervision tasks, such as learning psychiatric theory through online modules, can be complemented with high-touch, supervised activities like interviewing and psychoeducation.

Limited time allocated to psychiatry in India's undergraduate medical curriculum necessitates innovative teaching approaches. One example is a rural medical college where interactive lectures (using cases, MCQs, and student participation), personalized learning (tailoring content to student interests), interdepartmental collaboration, and a student-faculty newsletter ("MINDS") were implemented. These strategies effectively engaged students and enhanced their learning within the time constraints. The authors advocate for wider adoption of such methods until psychiatry becomes a mandatory, examined subject (Kishor & Vinay, 2015).

Furthermore, digital simulations and interactive tools can offer safe, controlled environments for students to practice critical skills, such as patient communication and mental health assessments. Psychiatry clubs in medical colleges can also serve innovate approach to enhancing teaching-learning. There is also emerging role of learning from various platforms initiated by psychiatry teachers who are passionate in teaching. Addressing stigma against psychiatry through multidisciplinary teaching and early exposure to behavioral sciences during foundation courses can foster greater interest in the field. Enhancing formative and summative assessments using techniques like Objective Structured Clinical Examination (OSCEs), case-based discussions, and innovative evaluation methods will ensure students develop the competencies required for modern psychiatry practice. These strategies, combined with regular curriculum evaluations and updates, can significantly improve psychiatry education in India (Kavoor & Mitra, 2015; Sethi et al., 2024).

# 3 Postgraduate Psychiatry Education in India

## *3.1 Introduction to Postgraduate Psychiatry Training*

Postgraduate (PG) training forms the cornerstone of competency in psychiatric practice. This chapter undertakes a comparative analysis of PG psychiatry training in India and Western nations, exploring similarities, differences, strengths, and areas for improvement within these distinct educational frameworks. Psychiatry and mental health have historically received insufficient emphasis, particularly impacting training opportunities in low- and middle-income countries where PG programs are often scarce. The adoption of competency-based training models and novel assessment methods for PG trainees reflects a growing focus on demonstrable skills. Effective PG psychiatry education necessitates an integrated approach encompassing diverse domains such as psychotherapy, pharmacotherapy, and neuroscience.

In India, postgraduate psychiatry education plays a crucial role in developing the skilled mental health professionals needed to address the nation's substantial treatment gap. The primary pathway is a three-year Doctor of Medicine (MD) specialization in Psychiatry, offering comprehensive training across theoretical, clinical, and research domains. Alongside the MD, alternative routes include the Diplomate of National Board (DNB) in Psychiatry and the DPM. The DNB, overseen by the National Board of Examinations (NBE), provides equivalent recognition to the MD but is often situated in private or smaller institutional settings. The DPM is a two-year program focusing predominantly on clinical exposure. These diverse training options aim to enhance flexibility for aspiring psychiatrists and collectively strive to meet the increasing demand for specialized mental health services throughout India. At present, postgraduate psychiatry training in India is offered through approximately 331 institutions providing an MD degree, with an annual intake of around 1293 seats. Additionally, 13 institutions offer a Diploma in Psychiatry (DPM) with 31 seats per year, while 26 Diplomate of National Board (DNB) seats are available at hospitals accredited by the National Board of Examinations (NBE) (*National Medical Commission*, n.d.).

## *3.2 Admission Process and Challenges*

Admission to postgraduate psychiatry programs is primarily through two national-level entrance examinations: the National Eligibility cum Entrance Test for Postgraduates (NEET-PG), which governs admissions to MD and DNB programs across government, private, and deemed universities, and the Institutes of National Importance Combined Entrance Test (INI-CET), which manages admissions to prestigious institutions such as the All India Institute of Medical Sciences (AIIMS), the National Institute of Mental Health and Allied Neurosciences (NIMHANS), and other institutes of national importance. Despite an increase in available seats, psychiatry remains relatively undersubscribed compared to other medical specialties. This underrepresentation is likely influenced by persistent stigma surrounding mental illness and the perception of psychiatry as a less lucrative career path. Furthermore, a significant geographical imbalance exists in seat distribution, with urban centers and southern states holding a disproportionate share of training institutions. This disparity creates a critical shortage of trained mental health professionals in rural and underserved areas, perpetuating inequities in mental healthcare access and delivery (Mudgal et al., 2024). It should also be noted here; there are other challenges in admission that impact quality training for example NMC has diluted the NEET-PG selection by making admission possible by zero percentile criteria in recent years!! The high fee structure in non-government institutions also makes it possible for postgraduates who can afford to pay fee rather than those postgraduates who are more qualified but cannot afford.

### *3.3 Curriculum and Training: A Competency-Based Approach*

The postgraduate psychiatry curriculum in India adopts a competency-based model designed to cultivate clinical expertise, research proficiency, and teaching skills. Clinical exposure is gained through rotations in outpatient (OPD) and inpatient settings, community psychiatry, and consultation-liaison psychiatry. Trainees encounter a wide range of psychiatric conditions, including psychoses, neurotic disorders, substance use disorders, and organic mental disorders. Rotations often include specialized clinics focusing on child and adolescent mental health, addiction treatment, and sexual medicine, providing diverse clinical experiences. Research training involves the completion of a dissertation, fostering skills in research methodology, critical analysis, and evidence-based practice. Workshops on biostatistics, study design, and scientific writing are typically integrated into the curriculum to enhance research capabilities. The integration of technology, including telepsychiatry and artificial intelligence (AI) applications, is increasingly emphasized, particularly in premier institutions like NIMHANS. However, access to these technologies remains uneven across institutions, leading to disparities in training quality. Finally, teaching and interactive learning are promoted through small group discussions, journal clubs, and clinical case presentations, encouraging critical thinking and peer learning (Mudgal et al., 2024; Narasimha et al., 2024; National Medical Commission, 2019).

## 3.4 Subspecialization Opportunities: Addressing Evolving Needs

Recognizing the increasing specialization within mental health care, postgraduate psychiatry education in India offers a range of subspecialization opportunities. Fellowships in areas such as child and adolescent psychiatry, addiction psychiatry, geriatric psychiatry, and forensic psychiatry are widely available. Notably, premier institutes like the National Institute of Mental Health and Neurosciences (NIMHANS) provide advanced Doctorate of Medicine (DM) super-specialization programs in Child and Adolescent Psychiatry and Addiction Medicine, catering to the need for deeper expertise in these domains.

In line with these developments, the NIMHANS ECHO model represents a significant innovation in subspecialty skill dissemination. Based on the Extension for Community Healthcare Outcomes (ECHO) framework, this initiative leverages telementoring to extend the reach of expert knowledge to mental health professionals across India. Through its virtual platform, the NIMHANS ECHO model offers short-term certificate courses and modular programs in a variety of niche areas such as psychotherapy, perinatal psychiatry, school mental health, neurodevelopmental disorders, and geriatric mental health. These programs emphasize capacity building among general psychiatrists and other mental health professionals especially in remote areas by facilitating access to structured learning, case-based discussions, and real-time mentorship from domain experts (Mehrotra et al., 2018).

These courses plays a crucial role in bridging the treatment gap, especially in underserved and remote regions, by equipping practitioners with the subspecialty competencies required to manage complex and population-specific psychiatric presentations. As highlighted by Narasimha et al. (2024), such targeted training initiatives are integral to meeting the evolving mental health needs of India's diverse population, particularly in specialized populations like children, older adults, and individuals with substance use disorders.

## 3.5 Challenges in Postgraduate Psychiatry Training: A Multifaceted Perspective

Postgraduate psychiatry training in India faces several significant challenges. Regional disparities in training opportunities persist, with premier institutions in metropolitan areas and southern states offering superior resources and clinical exposure compared to smaller colleges, which often lack adequate infrastructure and diverse clinical experiences. This imbalance hinders the equitable distribution of trained psychiatrists across the country. Resource deficiencies are also prevalent, with many institutions lacking access to advanced diagnostic and therapeutic tools, such as neuroimaging and neuromodulation equipment. Access to newer modalities like repetitive transcranial magnetic stimulation (rTMS) is often limited to high-resource settings. Overreliance on pharmacotherapy and minimal focus on psychotherapy remains a challenge in PG psychiatry training currently. Prevalent use of traditional teaching training methods and focus on summative assessment are major hurdles as well. The research work done by postgraduates still fall short of international standard owing to various responsibilities shouldered by them. Finally, burnout among trainees is a serious concern. The demanding workload, coupled with academic and research responsibilities, can lead to significant stress and burnout. The lack of adequate mental health support systems within training programs exacerbates these challenges (Kakunje et al., 2019; Narasimha et al., 2024).

## *3.6 Proposals for Enhancing Postgraduate Psychiatry Training: A Path Forward*

Several proposals can enhance postgraduate psychiatry training in India. Standardizing clinical exposure across all institutions, ensuring uniform access to advanced therapies like rTMS, electroconvulsive therapy (ECT), and neuroimaging, can significantly improve training quality. Expanding multidisciplinary training through collaborations with neurology, psychology, and social work departments can foster a more holistic and comprehensive approach to mental healthcare. Encouraging regional development by establishing well-equipped psychiatry departments in underserved regions is essential for addressing disparities in training opportunities and mental health service provision. Promoting global collaboration and research through exchange programs and international partnerships can expose trainees to global best practices and enhance their research output. Finally, establishing robust trainee support systems, including structured wellness programs and readily accessible mental health resources, is crucial for mitigating burnout and promoting trainee well-being and performance. Implementing these proposals can significantly strengthen postgraduate psychiatry training in India, ultimately leading to improved mental healthcare access and outcomes for the population (Gupta & Menon, 2022; O. P. Singh, 2022).

### 3.6.1 Insights

Innovations in psychiatry education are pivotal for advancing training quality and improving mental healthcare delivery. Integrating technology, such as online modules, telepsychiatry training, and virtual reality simulations, provides accessible learning resources and enhances training, particularly in underserved regions. Simulation-based learning, through standardized patient encounters and virtual scenarios, offers a safe platform for trainees to develop clinical and decision-making skills. Interprofessional education, involving collaboration with psychologists, nurses, and social workers, fosters a holistic approach to patient care.

Community-based training enables learners to address social determinants of mental health while gaining experience in diverse settings. Personalized learning approaches, tailored to individual preferences and interests, enhance engagement and retention. Focusing on specific competencies, such as cultural sensitivity, communication, and ethical practice, ensures readiness for real-world challenges. Innovative assessment methods, including Mini-CEX, OSCEs, and portfolios, provide a more comprehensive evaluation of skills. Faculty development programs equip educators with modern teaching methods, ensuring effective knowledge transfer. Global collaboration facilitates the exchange of best practices and accelerates the adoption of advanced training models. Additionally, incorporating preventive strategies and public health principles into psychiatry education empowers future psychiatrists to address mental health challenges at both individual and population levels, promoting a proactive approach to care.

# 4 Psychiatry Faculty Training in India

## *4.1 Microsystem of Medical Education and Faculty Roles*

To understand the psychiatry teachers' training in the country, it is imperative that we understand the medical education microsystem in India. As of September 2024, there are more than 750 medical colleges that are registered under the National Medical Commission (NMC), an apex body under government of India. Among these, majority institutes, and the medical curriculum must adhere to the CBME as laid down by the NMC (Sharma & Sharma, 2017). However, there are a few other institutions which are autonomous in terms of framing their curriculum and need not mandatorily follow the NMC guidelines. There are about 30 medical colleges in various stages of functioning, which are deemed the status of Institutes of National Importance (INI). Though most of the INIs are autonomous, there are a few like JIPMER, Puducherry; which follow the NMC guidelines. Traditionally, Psychiatry has been approached as a fringe subject in the past editions of the curriculum as was designed by the Medical Council of India (MCI) (the erstwhile governing body, that was autonomous and in 2020 autonomous status was dissolved, NMC was formed). The situation did improve substantially in 2019 when MCI introduced the competency-based medical curriculum, when there was a definite increase in the weightage of Psychiatry as an undergraduate subject. However, despite the changes, experts of the field felt that there was a need for more focus on psychiatry education at the undergraduate levels. Being outside the governance of NMC has enabled the autonomous institutes such as INIs to introduce innovations in the Psychiatry curriculum. Prime examples of this can be AIIMS Rishikesh and AIIMS Deoghar, who have introduced a summative evaluation in Psychiatry, which is rather unique in the country. However, as we will be discussing subsequently, the scope of training of the faculty members in Psychiatry varies across India.

Differences of responsibilities of Faculty members in Psychiatry across institutes:

In 2009, the MCI felt it is important to train all medical teachers in teaching methods and started program across India, something that was not existent before. It is important to look at responsibility of medical teachers in India. The responsibilities of faculty members differ to a certain extent based on the nature of the college that they are working. While all medical colleges of India usually recruit applicants for the position of faculty members as full-time employment, the *National Medical Commission Postgraduate Medical Education Board* in 2021 has allowed employment of visiting faculty members with a part-time limited role. However, all medical colleges and INIs recruit most of the faculty members on full-time employment.

Another notable difference in the recruitment of faculty members in non-INIs is that it is mandatory for any recruitment in an NMC affiliated medical college for all staff, assistant professor onward to have training in basic medical education technologies, whereas such an experience is informally considered desirable in INIs. However, training in medical education has not been mentioned as an explicit criterion in any recruitment notifications of autonomous INI. A recent change adopted by NMC for non-INI is mandatory facial recognition based attendance which is in effect since first May 2025 for ease of use and ascertaining proper faculty presence at their respective workplaces.

## 4.2 Generic Training Opportunities for Psychiatry Faculty

Training courses available in the NMC affiliated colleges:

There are several courses that are available specifically in the NMC affiliated colleges, which are conducted in the NMC-designated regional centers and nodal centers under the supervision of expert co-ordinator. The components of these courses are uniform across the various centers where they are held. It is noteworthy that it is mandatory for all faculty members of the NMC affiliated colleges to complete these courses and is an essential criterion for their promotion.

- Revised basic course workshop in medical education technologies:
  This course is the basic course that introduces faculty members to the concepts of medical education conducted at nodal center or medical education unit of respective medical college under supervision of nodal center. The course is usually conducted over 3 days and provides comprehensive exposure to the concepts with provision of hands-on exposure. With the advent of the competency-based curriculum, the course underwent a revision to incorporate the demands of the new curriculum.
- Training in attitude, ethics, communication (AETCOM) module:
  This training is usually held after the basic course as an additional day-long component. The objective of this course is to enable the medical teachers to impart training on the aspects of attitude, ethics, and communication, which has been

conceptualized as the cornerstone of successful implementation of the new medical curriculum.

- Curriculum implementation support program:
  The objective of this course was to provide handholding to the faculty members to the nuances of the competency-based curriculum. The course provides specific training to the stakeholders of interpreting the curriculum and designing the learning objectives, teaching-learning methods and designing their evaluation strategies from the competencies.

  These courses to be imparted to all faculties in India are extremely time consuming and may take many years. Interestingly NMC also made Basic Course in Biomedical Research (BCBR) and Good Clinical Practice (GCP) certificate also mandatory for faculty seeking promotion.

Training courses in autonomous colleges:

All the autonomous medical colleges have established a medical education unit with trained faculty members heading the units. These medical education units provide training to the faculty members on the basic concepts of medical education. There is an amount of variation in the components of these courses though in principle they tend to borrow the basic elements of the revised basic course and the AETCOM module. These courses are considered desirable in these institutes however, they are not mandatory for the promotion of faculty members. However, various institutes explicitly mention that experience in medical education is given weightage in the annual appraisal of faculty members.

Advanced courses in medical education:

The advanced course in medical education is imparted under the ambit of National Medical Council for faculty members who have completed the basic course. It is a one-year course usually held in a hybrid model with predominantly online sessions with contact programs at pre-decided schedule, which is usually two five-day contact sessions. These sessions are held in the nodal centers of the NMC and also include a project submission (Zodpey et al., 2016). These are usually for enthusiastic faculty and or those keen to be part of medical education units or departments of respective medical college.

Foundation for Advancement of International Medical Education and Research (FAIMER):

The Foundation for Advancement of International Medical Education and Research (FAIMER) is an internationally accredited fellowship course that is held over two years. Overall, worldwide there are seven FAIMER centers out of which three are in India. These centers are situated at Seth G S Medical College, Mumbai; Christian Medical College at Ludhiana, Punjab, and PSG Institute of Medical Sciences and Research in Coimbatore. Each of these centers caters to the whole of South Asian region and every year 16 applicants are selected for this course. The FAIMER course curriculum includes advanced medical education techniques, leadership skills, and focus of developing professional bonds (1). In FAIMER, participants can take up subject-specific teaching-learning methodology, thus benefiting psychiatry faculty who are keen to pursue this fellowship.

## 4.3 National Teacher Training Center

The National Teacher Training Centre (NTTC) was established in JIPMER, Puducherry, by the Ministry of Health and Family Welfare, Government of India, with the assistance of World Health Organization (WHO) in 1975 (Zayapragassarazan & Dharanipragada, 2022). The center was established in lines with the effort of the WHO to promote global training of medical educators in educational science and technology, for which, the University of Illinois was identified as the nodal agency. Subsequent to the establishment of NTTC at JIPMER, further centers were also inaugurated at the Postgraduate Institute of Medical Education and Research (PGIMER), Chandigarh, Institute of Medical Sciences, Banaras Hindu University, Varanasi, and Maulana Azad Medical College, New Delhi. However, currently only the NTTC at JIPMER remains functional.

The NTTC at JIPMER conducts the National Course on Educational Science for Teachers of Health Professionals (NCESTHP) twice a year which is an initiative to train the medical educators in educational science and technology, educational planning and in conducting educational research. The course is executed by the Department of Medical Education at JIPMER which is comprised of full-time faculty members from the Department of Medical Education and adjunct faculty members from preclinical, paraclinical, medical, and surgical disciplines of JIPMER. Prior to 2013, the course was a comprehensive 10-day course. But since 2013, the course has been customized to a 6-day course, which is predominantly offline. During the COVID-19 pandemic, the course was held online as well.

The broad aim of the course is to train the participants to apply the principles of medical education in undergraduate training. The course comprises 26 sessions that cover most of the major domains of medical education ranging from taxonomy of domains of learning, teaching-learning methods, evaluation, feedback, curriculum designing, etc. The program is evaluated on a 4-level framework for the evolution and customization of the program.

## 4.4 Specific Training Opportunities for Psychiatry Faculty

Indian Teachers of Psychiatry (IToP):

The Indian Teachers of Psychiatry forum was created in 2016, which focussed on imparting the requisite skills of teaching and conducting research for faculty members in Psychiatry. The forum is funded by the Mysore based charitable trust named Minds United for Health Sciences and Humanity Trust and the trust has raised funds from individuals and organizations such as the Infosys foundation. IToP currently provides two distinct kinds of support to the faculty members working in the Department of Psychiatry in any medical college of India. These are as follows:

- ITоP-STEPS (Scholarship for Teachers toward Enrichment of Psychiatry Teaching Skills):
  The Scholarship for Teachers toward Enrichment of Psychiatry Teaching Skills was initially launched as an online course spanning over 20 sessions with the scholars being exposed to cutting-edge developments in the field of medical education, specifically for Psychiatry (Kishor et al., 2023). Subsequently, as the program became popular and the effects of the COVID-19 pandemic waned, the program started running on a hybrid mode with a contact session to commence the proceedings and another contact session at the end for award of certificates. The call for the scholarship goes out to any faculty member in Psychiatry. However, the selection panel usually tends to have an equal representation of private and government medical colleges while selecting the scholars. The awardees and peer faculty members of the program are also provided with a financial award of 10,000 INR. After the completion of the course, the scholars are asked to join the team as peer educators and mentors for the next year.

  The development of curriculum for the course was a rigorous affair. Other than an expert committee meeting scheduled on this purpose, the expert drew ideas from the basic course workshop as designed by the erstwhile Medical Council of India and also from the survey of felt needs of Psychiatry teachers. Overall, it was decided that the course will comprise 20 sessions, 16 of which will be structured and pre-decided, whereas 4 sessions will be customized and based on the choices of the scholars.

  The program has a rigorous evaluation strategy where the program is evaluated on the benchmarks of reaction, learning, impact, and outcome and the feedback is used to evolve the curriculum to make it more appealing and useful for the next year.
- ITоP MUST (Minds United Scholarship for Teachers in Psychiatry) Enrich Research Grant:
  The ITоP MUST (Minds United Scholarship for Teachers in Psychiatry) Enrich Research Grant is a competitive grant that is offered to Psychiatry faculty members for conducting research in psychiatry education (Verma et al., 2024). This grant provides the necessary handholding for psychiatry teachers by expert peer faculty and guidance exclusively in the field of psychiatry education and a one-time research grant of 10,000 INR is provided for this purpose. This grant has been influential in driving the research in psychiatry education in the country and has provided training in various methodologies to the recipients (Kishor, 2022).

  Other Initiatives of ITоP Forum

  The ITоP forum also provides multiple platforms for psychiatry teachers to upskill themselves at regional, zonal, and national conferences. Such programs have been held in Bihar, Uttar Pradesh, Uttarakhand, West Bengal, Jammu Kashmir, Karnataka, Kerala, Telangana, and Andhra Pradesh. In every annual conference of IPS (ANCIPS) since 2016, one or other workshops have been carried out on Psychiatry CBME by ITоP forum, this is in addition to exclusive national CMEs and Conference of IToP Forum, latest was in 2024 November at Bengaluru. In this conference, taking a step forward, exclusive workshop for psychiatry teaching skills was held for postgraduates and senior residents, where more than 30 participants were trained in half day program.

IToP forum provides annual awards for psychiatry teachers and or departments of psychiatry for best initiatives or research in undergraduate and postgraduate section since 2018, thereby motivating teachers to enhance their skill in teaching-learning in a unique way (Narasimha et al., 2024).

Interestingly, exclusively for psychiatry teachers a YouTube channel has been floated that has also recorded every session of Sunday Special 60 mins with Psychiatry Teachers program, which was a joint initiative of IToP forum and IPS UG & PG education subcommittee and IPS Faculty Training Task Force.

The IToP forum has also established website, and all resources for psychiatry teachers are made available for free. It is indeed heartening to note that these strategies are new model for subject-specific teaching-learning enhancement, both in India and rest of the world.

To conclude, though in the yesteryears, representation of Psychiatry as a subject has been under-represented, the situation has undergone significant changes in the recent past. A number of initiatives specifically for the psychiatrists have commenced which has garnered commendable attention. This domain has also been a field of innovation which has changed the landscape of medical education in the country. There is no doubt that Psychiatry has been receiving more importance in the medical curriculum, though there is a need for further investment in Psychiatry education. But it can be said that the developments in this field have been complementary to the renewed attention.

## 5 The Future of Psychiatry Training in India

### *5.1 The Future of Undergraduate Medical Education*

The primary focus toward enhancing mental health services in the community shall always remain with the training of upcoming doctors. The plan to increase medical seats from 1,25,000 to 1,75,000 per year in coming years in India, should be seen as challenge from various perspectives and planning should begin now. There is already great concern about exponential increase in number of students who join medical institutions sometime sheerly because of financial affordability rather than knowledge and or keen interest (Kishor et al., 2020). With each medical education institution in India enrolling 100 to 250 students annually, faculty are likely to have uphill task to imbibe required competencies in every student. Psychiatry faculty have to continuously devise innovative strategies so that every upcoming doctor has competencies in psychiatry as notified in Indian Medical Graduate (IMG) CBME guidelines of NMC (Khanna & Kishor, 2025; Kishor et al., 2024; Kishor & Vinay, 2015).

It is in this context that every student becomes important and students in India need both motivation and mandatory regulations for psychiatry learning. It is expected that medical students are more likely to choose technology-based approach to learn psychiatry, hence the authenticity of sources and skill of the information provider shall play a role. Hence, there is need to monitor such platforms.

Artificial intelligence (AI) is the future of education, and this has to be incorporated in psychiatry education and optimized for learning. Human experience is the soul of psychiatry training and services, and every undergraduate should have opportunity to interact and learn from patient experiences. AI should augment the experience of learning not replace human interaction for psychiatry learning. Medical students should be made aware of limitations of AI and importance of socio-cultural aspects of patient experiences.

Psychiatry curriculum for undergraduates should be examined periodically to incorporate the new developments (Tekkalaki & Kishor, 2020). The curriculum should encourage the medical graduate to think, listen, observe, and examine appropriately so as to optimize skills in psychiatry. Ability to critically evaluate and apply thorough principles of science is essential. Hence, information from real-world scenarios is continuously required in curriculum to build more competencies in preventive psychiatry.

## 5.2 *The Future of Postgraduate Psychiatry Education*

As the psychiatry seats increased exponentially in the last decade and likely take a big leap from current 1000 plus seats to more than double the number in India, meticulous work toward enhancing every psychiatry resident's skill is required. The quality of medical education and the of late zero percentile rule from NMC to enroll in postgraduate courses in India shall be a challenge for every passionate psychiatry teacher. This is in addition to mere financial resources of undergraduate as means to gain entry to postgraduate program in most of private institutions. The robust psychiatry postgraduate training strategies are the need of the hour. Every faculty should be trained to make assessment of postgraduates' interest and efforts to learn psychiatry. Academic evaluation of postgraduate should be continued in visible manner and planned periodically. More and more research are needed to examine the postgraduate in 360-degree evaluation process (A. Kumar et al., 2024). The sanctity of the postgraduate training with the patient-based learning should never be sacrificed. Evaluation should be double blind in formative and summative assessment, where examiners provide objective feedback. The future of postgraduate program could be about all information related to training that is available with public for scrutiny so that every upcoming psychiatrist in India has rigorous training to meet the challenges of optimal services in mental health. Furthermore, there have been initiatives from various stakeholders like the Indian Academy of Child and

Adolescent Mental Health Academy (IACAM academy) and the National Institute of Mental Health and Neurosciences (NIMHANS) Digital Academy has been instrumental in capacity building in various sub-specialties of the subject. These options are useful because of it being delivered remotely and has been well-accepted by the psychiatry teachers for capacity building (Govindan et al., 2024; Malhotra & Gupta, 2022).

Artificial Intelligence (AI) based learning in postgraduate psychiatry will grow in amazing speed. The analytical ability of psychiatry residents should come from unique individual experiences of patients. Collaborative approach with patients in understanding the manifestation and management of conditions should become hallmark in the world with AI. The expansion in AI, development of 3D printing, gene modification, and advent of artificial neuronal networks are likely to be complimentary to one another, and postgraduate training should quickly adapt to these changes that are likely to unfold in few years from now. In the same period, poverty and disparity, animal instincts that have shaped human experiences shall continue to play a role in psychiatry. Residents should continue to have open mind in accepting the changes and constants of life, even in the era of AI.

Postgraduates in psychiatry are likely to learn from outside parental educational institutions due to various reasons that can range from a mismatch in felt needs to better opportunities elsewhere. How does personalized approach benefits postgraduate psychiatry learning needs to be discussed and deliberated. More super-specialization demand is expected, and more rigorous strategies are needed to carry out optimal postgraduate training, which shall be foundation for every psychiatrist in India irrespective of higher learning interest (A. Singh et al., 2024).

## 5.3 The Future of Psychiatry Faculty Training

Psychiatry faculty training needs to overcome many challenges that are currently affecting optimal psychiatry education in India. The issue of ghost faculty is still a concern in all branches of medicine including psychiatry. Absence of psychiatry faculty who is not engaging the students but is recorded as present in the institution has serious repercussion on competencies of upcoming doctors and psychiatrist who render service to affected patients with mental illness. Although NMC has made numerous policies and regulation, the problem persists. In addition, there are faculty who are present in the institutions who do not engage students either because of lack of interest or skill in teaching. Hence, a robust groundwork is needed to ensure ghost faculties are eliminated and all faculties who are enrolled in institutions are available for engaging the undergraduates and postgraduates. The training of such faculty can be carried out by regional medical education experts in psychiatry, who can periodically, at least twice in year carry out workshops in psychiatry education. Many advances in technology including AI can be used for training psychiatry teachers. India needs at least one center for psychiatry faculty training for a cluster of 10–15 medical colleges; such clusters can have a state or regional center for further enhancement of psychiatry faculty training. These centers should be affiliated to universities and or professional bodies (Kishor, 2022). One national and international conference in psychiatry education and a midterm meet are required for nation which has nearly 1.5 billion population and is growing.

It is important that psychiatry faculty training opportunities are available for faculty all through the year and such programs should be designed by the professional bodies and universities from India and abroad (Narasimha et al., 2024). A faculty should be able to enroll in any desired area of psychiatry education and upskill (Kishor et al., 2023). The future is about multiple platforms for psychiatry faculty to continuously find avenues in offline and online platforms for enhancing teaching skills. There has to be robust psychiatry education research linked with faculty training (Verma et al., 2024).

Funds and scholarship should be specifically provided for such initiatives. Incentives for psychiatry faculty with awards and scholarships go a long way to secure future of psychiatry teachers' training programs that directly benefit psychiatry education in India.

## 6 Conclusion

Psychiatry education in India stands at a critical juncture, shaped by historical underrepresentation and contemporary efforts toward reform and innovation. Over the past two decades, there has been a marked evolution in both undergraduate and postgraduate psychiatry training, primarily driven by the introduction of the competency-based medical education (CBME) framework and the increasing prioritization of mental health within national health agendas. At the undergraduate level, the integration of psychiatry into the CBME curriculum—with designated competencies, structured clinical exposure, and certifiable skills—has significantly enhanced the scope and quality of training. Nevertheless, disparities in implementation, faculty shortages, and limited student engagement continue to hinder the uniform realization of these educational objectives.

Postgraduate psychiatry education in India, offered through MD, DNB, and DPM programs, has expanded in breadth and complexity. It now incorporates diverse clinical exposure, subspecialty training, and research components. However, systemic challenges such as unequal regional distribution of training institutions, inadequate psychotherapy training, and limited access to advanced technologies persist. Innovative models like the NIMHANS ECHO initiative and telementoring platforms demonstrate the potential to bridge these gaps, particularly in underserved regions. Faculty development remains a linchpin for sustainable improvement. National-level initiatives, including the IToP-STEPS program, FAIMER fellowships, and structured faculty development workshops, have introduced promising frameworks for enhancing pedagogical and research capabilities among psychiatry educators. Despite these efforts, there is a pressing need for scale, standardization, and sustained institutional support to ensure widespread impact.

Looking to the future, the anticipated expansion in medical student and post-graduate seat intake necessitates a proactive and well-resourced response. Psychiatry training must leverage technological innovations, including artificial intelligence and virtual simulation, while maintaining the essential humanistic and socio-cultural dimensions of psychiatric practice. Faculty training should be continuous, adaptive, and incentivized, with robust governance mechanisms to ensure accountability and effectiveness. In conclusion, the transformation of psychiatry education in India is both a reflection of and a response to the country's growing mental health needs. A coordinated, multi-stakeholder approach—encompassing curricular reform, faculty empowerment, digital integration, and equity in training access—is imperative to build a competent, compassionate, and future-ready psychiatric workforce. Such an approach will be instrumental in addressing India's mental health treatment gap and establishing a globally relevant model of psychiatry education.

## References


Govindan, R., Gandhi, S., Nattala, P., Ramu, R., & Marimuthu, P. (2024). Effectiveness of digital learning in community mental health care among nurses in India. *Indian Journal of Community Medicine, 49*(2), 334–341. https://doi.org/10.4103/ijcm.ijcm_619_22

Gupta, S., & Menon, V. (2022). Psychiatry training for medical students: A global perspective and implications for India's competency-based medical education curriculum. *Indian Journal of Psychiatry, 64*(3), 240–251. https://doi.org/10.4103/indianjpsychiatry.indianjpsychiatry_187_22

Kakunje, A., Punnoose, V. P., Ponnusamy, K. P., Mysore, A. V., & Daniel, S. J. (2019). Revisiting Postgraduate (PG) psychiatry training in India. *Indian Journal of Psychological Medicine, 41*(4), 380–387. https://doi.org/10.4103/IJPSYM.IJPSYM_15_19

Kavoor, A. R., & Mitra, S. (2015). Psychiatry at undergraduate level in India: What is needed? *Journal of Neurosciences in Rural Practice, 6*(03), 449–450. https://doi.org/10.4103/0976-3147.158804

Khanna, A., & Kishor, M. (2025). Establishing psychiatry clubs: Novel approach to enhance psychiatry teaching learning in India. *Digital Journal of Clinical Medicine, 7*(1). https://doi.org/10.55691/2582-3868.1236

Kishor, M. (2022). A center for psychiatry education, faculty training, and research. *Indian Journal of Psychiatry, 64*(5), 518–519. https://doi.org/10.4103/indianjpsychiatry.indianjpsychiatry_170_22

Kishor, M., Chandran, S., & Kumar, A. (2020). Coronavirus disease-19: Is it time to reflect on the entrance process for medical profession in India? *Journal of Medical Sciences and Health, 6*(2), 66–67. https://doi.org/10.46347/JMSH.2020.v06i02.014

Kishor, M., Isaac, M., Ashok, M., Pandit, L., Rao, T., & S. (2016). Undergraduate psychiatry training in India; past, present, and future looking for solutions within constraints!! *Indian Journal of Psychiatry, 58*(2), 119. https://doi.org/10.4103/0019-5545.183794

Kishor, M., Manohar, S., & MR, M. (2024). Clinical teaching methods in psychiatry for undergraduates. In *Psychiatry in medical education* (Vol. 10, 1st ed., pp. 49–54). Indian Psychiatric Society South Zonal Branch. https://ipsszb.org/publications/

Kishor, M., Menon, V., Vinay, H., Shah, H., Isaac, M., & Arun, M. (2023). The IToP-STEPS: A unique scholarship program to upskill teachers of psychiatry. *Indian Journal of Psychiatry, 65*(3), 381–384. https://doi.org/10.4103/indianjpsychiatry.indianjpsychiatry_428_22

Kishor, M., & Vinay, H. (2015). Innovative ways and customizing psychiatry training for undergraduates. *Indian Journal of Psychiatry, 57*(4), 431. https://doi.org/10.4103/0019-5545.171850

Kumar, P., Jangid, P., & Sethi, S. (2018). Undergraduate psychiatry in India: A SWOT analysis. *Asian Journal of Psychiatry, 33*, 46–51. https://doi.org/10.1016/j.ajp.2018.02.018

Kumar, A., Singh, L. K., Somani, A., & Laxmi, N. P. (2024). What we know, we see and do: Formative assessments practices of psychiatry: Postgraduate residency from a general hospital psychiatry unit in India. *Indian Journal of Psychological Medicine, 46*(5), 466–470. https://doi.org/10.1177/02537176241273711

Malhotra, S., & Gupta, N. (2022). IACAM academy: An Initiative of Indian Association for Child and Adolescent Mental Health (IACAM). *Journal of Indian Association for Child and Adolescent Mental Health, 18*(4), 270–271. https://doi.org/10.1177/09731342231166432

Medical Council of India. (2018). *Competency based undergraduate curriculum for the indian medical graduate*. MCI. https://www.nmc.org.in/wp-content/uploads/2020/01/UG-Curriculum-Vol-II.pdf

Mehrotra, K., Chand, P., Bandawar, M., Rao Sagi, M., Kaur, S., Aurobind, G., Raj, A., Jain, S., Komaromy, M., Murthy, P., & Arora, S. (2018). Effectiveness of NIMHANS ECHO blended tele-mentoring model on Integrated Mental Health and Addiction for counsellors in rural and underserved districts of Chhattisgarh, India. *Asian Journal of Psychiatry, 36*, 123–127. https://doi.org/10.1016/j.ajp.2018.07.010

Mudgal, V., Gupta, S., & Issac, M. (2024). PG psychiatry training in India and the West. In *Psychiatry in medical education* (Vol. 10, pp. 85–100). Indian Psychiatric Society South Zonal Branch. https://ipsszb.org/wp-content/uploads/2024/11/dr-Anil-book.pdf

Narasimha, V. L., Suhas, S., Kishor, M., Dixit, A., & Murthy, P. (2024). Advances in psychiatry training and faculty development in India. *Indian Journal of Psychological Medicine, 46*(5), 391–399. https://doi.org/10.1177/02537176241284348

National Medical Commision. (n.d.). *College course and search*. Retrieved April 17, 2025, from https://www.nmc.org.in/information-desk/college-and-course-search/

National Medical Commission. (2019, September). *Guidelines for competency based postgraduate training programme for MD in psychiatry*. NMC. https://www.nmc.org.in/wp-content/uploads/2019/09/MD-Psychiatry.pdf

Prince, M., Patel, V., Saxena, S., Maj, M., Maselko, J., Phillips, M. R., & Rahman, A. (2007). No health without mental health. *The Lancet, 370*(9590), 859–877. https://doi.org/10.1016/S0140-6736(07)61238-0

Raju, N. N. (2022). Psychiatry training in India. *Indian Journal of Psychiatry, 64*(5), 433–439. https://doi.org/10.4103/indianjpsychiatry.indianjpsychiatry_649_22

Reddy, I. R. (2007). Undergraduate psychiatry education: Present scenario in India. *Indian Journal of Psychiatry, 49*(3), 157–158. https://doi.org/10.4103/0019-5545.37311

Sethi, S., Tekkalaki, B., Shah, N., Smitha, C., & Kumar, R. (2024). Undergraduate psychiatry CBME curriculum revision: The process and the way ahead. *Indian Journal of Psychiatry, 66*(11), 1066–1069. https://doi.org/10.4103/indianjpsychiatry.indianjpsychiatry_821_24

Sharma, S., & Sharma, G. (2017). Medical education in India. *Annals of the National Academy of Medical Sciences (India), 53*(04), 179–193. https://doi.org/10.1055/s-0040-1712806

Singh, O. P. (2022). Postgraduate psychiatry training in India – National Medical Commission competency-based PG curriculum. *Indian Journal of Psychiatry, 64*(4), 329–330. https://doi.org/10.4103/indianjpsychiatry.indianjpsychiatry_426_22

Singh, A., Kishor, M., & Kar, S. K. (2024). A survey among psychiatrists to assess the need for psychiatry sub/super-specialization courses in India. *Indian Journal of Psychological Medicine, 46*(5), 425–428. https://doi.org/10.1177/02537176241273934

Tekkalaki, B., & Kishor, M. (2020). Medical Council of India module on pandemic management: Neglecting mental health training a major lacuna. *Indian Journal of Psychiatry, 62*(6), 750. https://doi.org/10.4103/psychiatry.IndianJPsychiatry_1019_20

Verma, N., Gupta, S., & Shatadal, P. (2024). Research in psychiatry medical education through "MUST Enrich Grant": A scoping review. *Indian Journal of Psychological Medicine, 46*(5), 382–390. https://doi.org/10.1177/02537176241265742

Zayapragassarazan, Z., & Dharanipragada, K. (2022). Forty-five years of faculty development: The Experience of the National Teacher Training Centre, Jawaharlal Institute of Postgraduate Medical Education and Research, India. *International Journal of Advanced Medical and Health Research, 9*(1), 4–12. https://doi.org/10.4103/ijamr.ijamr_94_22

Zodpey, S., Sharma, A., Zahiruddin, Q. S., Gaidhane, A., & Shrikhande, S. (2016). Faculty development programs for medical teachers in India. *Journal of Advances in Medical Education & Professionalism, 4*(2), 97–101.

# Chapter 7
# Psychiatry Teaching and Training in Nepal

**Pawan Sharma, Sagun Ballav Pant, and Devavrat Joshi**

**Abstract** Nepal, a landlocked Himalayan Nation, has a large unmet burden of mental health problems. The National Mental Health Survey has shown a prevalence of mental disorders of around 10%. Though there has been steady improvement in the service delivery and trained manpower over the last decade, Nepal faces a severe shortage of mental health professionals, with only a small number of psychiatrists, clinical psychologists, and psychiatric nurses available, predominantly in urban areas. The training in mental health, mainly postgraduation in psychiatry and M.Phil. in psychology, has started only recently, two decades back. Though undergraduate psychiatry teaching is now a mandatory component in all medical colleges, there is heterogeneity in the duration of teaching hours and percentage of curriculum among universities. In this chapter, we aim to discuss the historical background, current context, challenges, and ways out in the context of undergraduate, postgraduate psychology teaching and training along with other nonspecialized mental health training in the context of Nepal.

**Keywords** Psychiatry · Psychology · Mental health · Psychiatry teaching · Mental health training · Nepal

P. Sharma (✉)
Department of Psychiatry, Patan Academy of Health Sciences, Lalitpur, Nepal
e-mail: Pawansharma@pahs.edu.np

S. B. Pant
Department of Psychiatry and Mental Health, Institute of Medicine, Tribhuvan University, Kathmandu, Nepal

D. Joshi
Mental Hospital Lagankhel, National Academy of Medical Sciences, Lalitpur, Nepal



S. K. Kar et al. (eds.), *Teaching and Training in Psychiatry in South Asia*, South Asian Perspectives in Mental Health and Psychology,
https://doi.org/10.1007/978-981-95-1845-6_7

## 1 Introduction

Nepal, a landlocked federal republic nation in South Asia, is home to a diverse population representing multiple ethnicities, languages, and religions. With a population of approximately 30 million, bordered by China to the north and India to the south, the Nepalese population is influenced by both neighbors over centuries of migration, trade, and cultural exchange (Devkota & Khanal, 2024). Mental health issues have been a major public health concern in Nepal. According to the National Mental Health Survey conducted from 2019 to 2020, the prevalence of mental disorders among adults was found to be 10% over their lifetime, with 4.3% currently experiencing a mental disorder. Among adolescents, the prevalence of mental disorders was 5.2%, with neurotic and stress-related disorders being the most common. Suicidality is also a critical issue, with 7.2% of adults experiencing some form of suicidality in their lifetime (Dhimal et al., 2022).

Depression and anxiety were the most frequently diagnosed mental health conditions in the country in 2019 (Dhungana et al., 2023). A meta-analysis of prevalence studies of Depression found out that the pooled prevalence of 13.75% among the adult population (Sharma et al., 2025). Anxiety disorders are similarly widespread, affecting around 17.7% of the population, ranging from mild to severe cases (Pandey et al., 2024). Alcohol use disorder also poses a major challenge, with prevalence estimates varying between 1.5% and 25% among adults (Rathod et al., 2018). These statistics highlight the urgent need for mental health interventions and support systems in Nepal.

Despite the widespread prevalence of mental health issues, Nepal faces a substantial gap in mental health treatment, with a vast majority of individuals unable to access necessary care. Around 85% of people with severe mental health conditions receive no treatment, a disparity that is even more severe in rural areas where mental health services are scarce, as per a review of 2015 (Luitel et al., 2015). There are around 250 psychiatrists and around 40 clinical psychologists registered in Nepal as of 2025, which suggests a wide treatment gap (Sharma et al., 2024). The stigma and low mental health awareness further widen the gap, as many individuals avoid seeking help due to fear of discrimination or a lack of understanding about mental health issues. Financial barriers also play a crucial role, as high out-of-pocket costs and minimal insurance coverage make treatment unaffordable for many (Sharma et al., 2024). Nepal has had a National Mental Health Policy in place since 1996 and a Mental Health Strategy and Action Plan, 2020, and a national plan (15th Five-Year plan, 2019–2024) which aim to ensure universal access to mental health services to all Nepalese citizens. The important components of all these national documents are decentralization of services, integration of mental health services into general health settings, advocacy and awareness on mental health, capacity building of the mental health workforce, enhancing community participation and mental health research (Singh & Khadka, 2021). The implementation of mental health policies and action plans in Nepal has been progressing at a slow pace due to multiple challenges. Furthermore, mental health services remain largely concentrated in urban centers, leaving rural and remote populations with minimal access to even basic mental health care. Addressing these barriers requires a multi-pronged approach, including increased investment, awareness campaigns, and decentralization of services to ensure equitable mental health care across the country (WHO, 2022).

The need for trained mental health professionals in Nepal is critical, given the high prevalence of mental health issues and the limited availability of mental health services. Currently, Nepal faces a severe shortage of mental health professionals, with only a small number of psychiatrists, clinical psychologists, and psychiatric nurses available, predominantly in urban areas (Luitel et al., 2015). This shortage leaves rural and remote populations with minimal access to mental health care. Additionally, existing training programs are limited in scope and resources, making it difficult to produce enough qualified professionals to meet the growing demand for services. While there has been yearly increase in the number of psychiatrists, psychiatric nurses, and clinical psychologists, this is not enough to address the widespread need for care (Rai et al., 2021a, b; Sharma et al., 2024). To address these gaps, several approaches are being considered in Nepal, including the implementation of task-sharing strategies for integration of mental health care into primary health care settings, where primary health care workers are trained to identify and manage common mental health conditions based on the adaptation of the Mental Health Gap Action Programme—mhGAP (Angdembe et al., 2017; Jordans et al., 2013; Upadhaya et al., 2020).

## 2 History of Medical Education and Psychiatry Training in Nepal

The history of medical education in Nepal began with the introduction of Western medicine during the Rana regime, with the establishment of the Civil Medical School in 1934 to train compounders and dressers. The Institute of Medicine (IOM) was established in 1972 under Tribhuvan University (TU), initially focusing on middle-level health workers before starting the MBBS program in 1978. Postgraduate medical education began with the MD General Practice in 1982, expanding to various specialties over the years (Dixit, 2017). Currently, there are 24 medical colleges in Nepal, whose qualifications are recognized by the Nepal Medical Council and regulated by the Medical Education Commission (Government of Nepal, 2025; Nepal Medical Council, 2025). These include both public and private institutions. The government has continued to expand medical education through various universities, specialized academies, and private hospitals to meet the growing healthcare needs of the country.

The Department of Psychiatry at IOM, TU, played a crucial role in advancing psychiatric training and services in Nepal. Psychiatric outpatient services at Tribhuvan University Teaching Hospital (TUTH) began in 1986, followed by inpatient services in 1987. In 1997, the IOM started the postgraduate specialization

(MD) in Psychiatry program, followed by the M.Phil. in Clinical Psychology in 1998 and the Bachelor in Psychiatric Nursing in 2000 (Sharma, 2013). These programs helped produce specialized mental health professionals and catalyzed similar initiatives in other institutions, with BP Koirala Institute of Health Sciences (BPKIHS) starting MD psychiatry in 1999 and Masters in Nursing program in psychiatry in 2008. Since the last decade, government hospitals, academy, and private medical colleges have been key in scaling up postgraduate programs in psychiatry (Singh et al., 2021).

Likewise, training of mid-level and lay health workers in mental health, supported by organizations like the United Mission to Nepal (UMN), played a significant role in mental health training for lay health workers, faith healers, and nurses, which expanded mental health services to rural areas of Nepal (Sharma, 2013). Overall, the development of psychiatry training in Nepal has been marked by gradual expansion, increased training opportunities, and efforts to integrate mental health into primary care and community settings.

## 3 Undergraduate Teaching of Psychiatry

Traditionally, in the Indian subcontinent, including Nepal, psychiatry has often been regarded as a minor subject within the MBBS curriculum. Several factors contribute to this perception, including limited curriculum time, stigma, availability of research, and clinical experience during placements, which affects their choice and interest in psychiatry (Bhugra, 2016). In Nepal, for instance, the teaching duration for mental health in medical schools ranges from 25 to 92 hours, significantly less than other major subjects like internal medicine and surgery. The weight of psychiatry in summative assessments is also minimal, ranging from just 0.21% to 2.4% across different universities. Traditional didactic lectures are the primary teaching method, which may not engage students as effectively as more interactive approaches (Marahatta et al., 2021). There are also significant disparities in mental health education across Nepalese medical universities, in regard to coverage of priority mental health conditions, substance use disorders, and child and adolescent mental health conditions. Despite the Nepal Medical Council's (NMC) requirement for a psychiatry department in medical schools, it does not mandate specific teaching durations or assessment methods. Additionally, the weightage of 1.1% (2 marks out of 180 marks) in the MBBS licensing examination affects both student exposure and career interest in the field (NMC, 2017). This has led to the situation where graduated MBBS doctors have low confidence in independent execution of important pre-service skills like screening of common mental health conditions, assessment and brief intervention for harmful use of alcohol and tobacco which are important skills for MBBS doctors for working in primary health care center (Pradhan et al., 2022). Efforts are being made to address these issues, including increasing the time allocated to psychiatry, adopting modern teaching methods, and integrating mental health into primary care, with the goal of reducing stigma and improving mental health education and training.

## 4 Postgraduate Teaching of Psychiatry

The postgraduate (PG) medical training in Nepal, including post-graduation in Psychiatry, is usually of 3 years' duration with either a Doctor of Medicine (MD) or Master of Surgery (MS) degree provided at the end. The eligibility criteria for postgraduate include: Nepal Medical Council (NMC) license, a year of service after the undergraduate MBBS degree, and a merit score in the common PG entrance exams conducted annually by the Medical Education Commission (MEC) (Nepal Medical Council, 2017; Government of Nepal, 2025).

### *4.1 Department of Psychiatry at the Institute of Medicine, Kathmandu*

The Institute of Medicine (IOM) under the Tribhuvan University established a 400-bed Tribhuvan University Teaching Hospital (TU-Teaching Hospital), in the year 1983. At the TU-Teaching Hospital, the Psychiatric Outpatient Service was started in February 1986, followed by the addition of a 12-bed psychiatric inpatient unit in December 1987. Later, a ten-bed deaddiction unit was added to the Psychiatric Inpatient setup, thus totaling a current strength of 22 beds in the department. MD Psychiatry courses were started in 1997 (Sharma, 2013; Aich, 2010). Subsequently, a two-year M.Phil. course in Clinical Psychology was started in 1998, and a Bachelor of Psychiatric Nursing was started in 1999, at the same center. Indian faculty from AIIMS, New Delhi, and other postgraduate institutes in India actively collaborated with their counterpart in the Department of Psychiatry, IOM, during the initial years of MD Psychiatry training, teaching, and examination programs (Aich & Giri, 1997; Aich, 2010). Currently, 4 to 5 Psychiatry residents are enrolled annually in this program (Government of Nepal, 2025).

### *4.2 BP Koirala Institute of Health Sciences, Dharan*

BP Koirala Institute of Health Sciences (BPKIHS) at Dharan was established in 1993, as a part of the joint Indo–Nepal collaboration on developing an international standard of teaching and training, and a research-oriented medical institute, similar to All India Institute of Medical Sciences (AIIMS), New Delhi. Outpatient psychiatric service at BPKIHS was started in 1995, after Dr. HP Jhingan and Dr. SK

Khandelwal joined the institute on a short-term deputation from AIIMS, New Delhi. A 20-bed psychiatric ward was started in February 2000. The department started an MD course in Psychiatry in the same year. Since the beginning of the PG course, visiting faculties from India and other countries have formed an integral part in imparting teaching and training to PG residents in psychiatry. At present, every year, five to six students enroll in the MD psychiatry course (Shakya, 2014; Government of Nepal, 2025).

### 4.3 National Academy of Medical Sciences, Kathmandu

The government of Nepal reached a significant milestone with the establishment of the Postgraduate Medical Education Coordination Committee (PGMECC) under the Ministry of Health in 1994 AD. Thus, post graduate programs in various medical specialties began in the same year by utilizing the hospitals of Kathmandu valley. Building upon these experiences and based on the national need, the National Academy of Medical Sciences (NAMS) Act was passed by the parliament in 2002 with the aim to establish a government academy mainly working to produce trained human resources with the priority of training and deploying doctors of the government healthcare system (National Academy of Medical Sciences, 2025). Bir Hospital was assigned as main hospital of the National Academy of Medical Sciences (NAMS) along with other affiliated hospitals including Mental Hospital. Postgraduate MD Psychiatry program of NAMS was started at the Mental Hospital from the year 2012 (Karki & Dixit, 2004; Dixit et al., 2018). A minimum of two postgraduate residents were enrolled annually in this program and recently the number of seats has been increased to five (Government of Nepal, 2025).

### 4.4 Patan Academy of Health Sciences, Lalitpur

The erstwhile Patan Hospital which had been involved in postgraduate medical training for three decades, starting with the PGMECC in 1994 and later as a major training site of NAMS (Bir Hospital was developed into Patan Academy of Health Sciences (PAHS), a public not for profit health science university, starting medical school with a competency-based undergraduate (MBBS) program in a hybrid model utilizing problem-based learning (PBL) in basic science years and clinical presentation (CP) in clinical years (Baral et al., 2016). The postgraduate MD/MS programs started in PAHS in 2017 (Shah et al., 2021). It differs from the traditional medical education in all other institutes in Nepal as it offers Competency-Based Medical Education (CBME) giving a significant weightage to formative assessment and continuous effective feedback (Shrestha et al., 2021). Postgraduate Psychiatry program started in 2018 with two to four residents being trained annually (Government of Nepal, 2025).

## 4.5 *Kathmandu University Medical School, Dhulikhel*

The first postgraduate programs of Kathmandu University (KU) were in Pathology and Psychiatry, being conducted at Bangalore, Mangalore, and Manipal, India, in collaboration with the Manipal Education and Medical Group (MEMG) in 2004. Other MD programs in Medicine were started later at KU-affiliated private colleges at Pokhara, Bharatpur, and Nepalgunj from 2007. MD Psychiatry program commenced at Kathmandu University Medical School, Dhulikhel, from 2018, with two residents being trained annually (Dixit et al., 2018; Government of Nepal, 2025).

## 4.6 *Private Medical Colleges in Nepal*

During the last three decades, a number of privately run medical colleges have come up in Nepal, affiliated to either the Tribhuvan University or the Kathmandu University. With functioning teaching hospitals attached to each of these medical institutes, the In- and Outpatient Departments of Psychiatry were also established in most of them. Of late, a postgraduate course (MD) in psychiatry has been started in all of these private medical institutes. These institutes are the Manipal College of Medical Sciences, Pokhara, the Universal College of Medical Sciences, Bhairahawa, National Medical College, Birganj. Nobel Medical College, Biratnagar, Birat Medical College, Biratnagar, Gandaki Medical College, Pokhara, Nepalgunj Medical College, Nepalgunj, Nepal Medical College, Kathmandu, Kathmandu Medical College, Kathmandu, Kist Medical College, Lalitpur, and Lumbini Medical College, Palpa (Aich, 2010; Aich & Giri, 1997; Dixit et al., 2018).

Over the last two decades, there has been a substantial increase in the number of institutes providing postgraduate psychiatry training. There are approximately 50 Psychiatry residency training positions in various institutions throughout the country. These institutions have already trained non-national residents as well, including residents from India and Maldives. However, the postgraduate training program is not nationally standardized as there is no uniform curriculum and process of evaluation (Koirala, 2013). There are currently five different MD Psychiatry curricula in practice across the country, namely, MD Psychiatry curriculum of Tribhuvan University (TU), Kathmandu University (KU), B.P. Koirala Institute of Medical sciences (BPKIHS), National Academy of Medical Sciences (NAMS), and Patan Academy of Health Sciences (PAHS). The initial four curricula follow the traditional format, which is prevalent in the South Asian region, whereas the last one, followed by PAHS is the only curriculum which is competency-based (Shrestha et al., 2021; Dangal, 2020). In the PAHS curriculum, the trainees are required to be certified for pre-sets Entrustable Professional Activities (EPAs), and to cover the 8-Core Competencies in various domains in: Professionalism, patient-centered care, procedural skills, clinical reasoning, communication, scholarship, leadership, and community orientation (Shah et al., 2021). Though the training methods may differ, all psychiatry residency programs in Nepal focus mainly on training in general adult psychiatry, and exposure to training in psychiatric subspecialties is lacking due to the absence of training sites (Aich, 2010).

## 5 Specialized Training of Psychiatry

There is a shortage of psychiatrists with sub-specialty trainings in Nepal with only four formally trained child and adolescent psychiatrists within the whole country (U. Karki et al., 2020). Specialized child and adolescent psychiatry inpatient/outpatient services are available in the Kanti Children's Hospital, Kathmandu, since 2015, and in the Mental Hospital, Lalitpur, since 2023. However, no sub-specialty trainings in Child and Adolescent Psychiatry are available within the country till now (Republica, 2024).

A clinical fellowship in Addiction Psychiatry program has recently started at the Department of Psychiatry under the Institute of Medicine, Tribhuvan University from 2024. The PhD program in mental health is on pipeline to be started in 2025 in the same institute and clinical fellowship in geriatric psychiatry is on pipeline at the Patan Academy of Health Sciences, Lalitpur. Besides these, there are no other formal specialty training programs as yet in Nepal.

## 6 Psychology Training/Academic Programs

Modern psychology entered in Nepalese academia in the mid-1900s. The history of psychology training in Nepal can be traced back to 1947 when it was introduced at Tri-Chandra College, Kathmandu, in the intermediate level as part of humanities stream with affiliation from Patna University (Regmi, 1987). The Tribhuvan University (TU) started its teaching, research, and other academic activities on July 14, 1959 under the Tribhuvan University Act promulgated in the same year. The T.U granted recognition to governmental and non-governmental colleges conducting Intermediate and Bachelor level courses of study and Tri-Chandra College, the first college of the country, launched its Bachelor of Psychology programs. After the establishment of TU, courses including psychology intermediate and bachelor level were already introduced at four colleges by the mid-1960s, which provided momentum for the initiation of Master's level courses in psychology in 1980 (Sujen, 2012).

By the 1980s, the graduates of psychology were largely involved in university teaching or in government jobs. However, this era failed to produce professional clinical psychologists dedicated to mental health. Despite this, the academia in psychology and the graduates of the Master's program in psychology from Tribhuvan University provided strong groundwork for establishment of M.Phil. Clinical Psychology course at the TU Institute of Medicine in the late 1990s. Availability of substantial number of psychology graduates, but lack of clinical training/exposure among them, and the gradually increasing need to provide mental health services made it crucial for initiation of clinical psychology training in Nepal. After one year of initiation of the MD Psychiatry program at the Institute of Medicine, TU, the M.Phil. Clinical Psychology was also started in 1998. The minimum requirements, i.e., dissertation, supervision, assessments, number of hours of various therapies, etc., were similar to Indian curriculum. Regular Clinical Psychology OPD services along with a Child Guidance Clinic also came into functioning from the same year. The annual intake capacity of this program was two students per year which has further increased to four students since 2022 (Rana & Shakya, 2022).

At present there are more than 40 professionally registered Clinical psychologists in Nepal, majority of them being graduates from M.Phil. Clinical Psychology program at IOM, TU. This number is insufficient and limited because only one institution runs this professional course in clinical psychology till date. There is a lack of specialization and further training in the form of fellowships, doctoral and post-doctoral programs, and skill-based trainings focusing on superspecializations in different forms of psychological assessment, psychotherapy, neuropsychological approaches, indigenous therapies, transcultural approaches, and so on (Rana & Shakya, 2022).

## 7 Nonspecialized Training

The community mental health services started in 1983 with training of health workers in Bhaktapur after which in 1984, five-year mental health project was started in Lalitpur (Singh et al., 2022). Christine S. Wright, then director of mental health at United Mission to Nepal (UMN), and Prof. Dr. Mahendra K. Nepal, then head of Department of Psychiatry and Mental Health at the Institute of Medicine in 1987, set up the Mental Health Project (MHP) with technical assistance of UMN and financial assistance of Redd-Barna Nepal, an international NGO working in Nepal (Aich, 2010; Acland, 2002). This project aimed to expand Mental Health services outside Kathmandu Valley in 1991 through the approach of task sharing. The World Health Organization (WHO) launched the Mental Health Gap Action Programme (mhGAP) and the mhGAP Intervention Guide (mhGAP-IG) with the aim of providing evidence-based clinical guidance to primary healthcare workers. WHO mhGAP was first tested by the PRIME project which included a consortium of six countries one of which was Nepal (Jordans et al., 2019). Later, the mhGAP-IG (V2.0) was translated and adapted under the leadership of National Health Training Centre (NHTC). It has also developed different modules and has been providing training for medical practitioners and paramedic professionals. The training modules currently implemented in Nepal has been tabulated in Table 7.1.

**Table 7.1** Different training modules at National Health Training Centre

| Module | Target manpower | Days | Areas covered |
|---|---|---|---|
| 1 | Nurses | 6 days (Optional 2 days) | • Psycho-education of mental disorders that are included in adapted Nepali version of WHO mhGAP, basic psychosocial support and behavioral activation for depression.<br>• (Optional two days for psychological support for alcohol use disorder) |
| 2<br>2a<br>2b | Medical Doctors<br>Paramedic professionals | 5 days | • Based on the Nepali adapted version of WHO mhGAP V2 for mental, neurological, and substance use disorders in nonspecialized settings.<br>• Also contains the curriculum for training of trainers (ToT).<br>• Capacity building of healthcare providers on assessment, management, treatment, follow-up, and referral of patients with MNS disorders. |
| 3 | Medical doctors<br>Nurses<br>Paramedic professionals | 5 days | • Training on assessment, management, follow-up, and referral of children and adolescents with developmental, behavioral, and emotional disorders. |
| 4 | Female community health volunteers (FCHVs) | 2 days | • Capacity building of on screening and referral of individuals with MNS disorders in the communities.<br>• Teaches on how to use standard validated community informant detection tool (CIDT) for screening of mhGAP disorders. |
| 5 | Public health professionals including managers and administrators | 2 and half days | • Capacity building on conceptualization, designing, implementation, and evaluation of community-based mental health programs. |
| 6 | Health Assistants<br>Nurses within government health care delivery system | Three phases<br>• Basic.<br>• Advanced 1.<br>• Advanced 2.<br>(Each phase of 10 days) | • Derived from the para-professional counselor training developed and used by several non-government organizations working on MHPSS in Nepal.<br>• The participants of the training must appear in online tests and evaluation and must complete the field assignments before accreditation. |

# 8 Challenges and Way Out

## *8.1 Inadequate Competency in Sub-Specialties During Postgraduate Training*

In the postgraduate training, the subspecialty trainings are provided and there is adequate exposure of cases of child and adolescents, geriatric, substance abuse, and consultation liaison psychiatry. However, the trainees perceive their trainings to be inadequate and the competency has not been defined by most of the universities (Karki et al., 2020; Rai et al., 2020). The case is similar in terms of psychotherapy. An online survey among early career psychiatrist revealed that only one-third of them had received psychotherapy training and it was inadequate (Rai et al., 2021a, b). Hence, there is a need to have a competency-based training program with a defined competency in the subspecialties of psychiatry.

## *8.2 Inadequate Competency and Poor Training Coverage Among Primary Health Worker*

A qualitative study of focus group discussion at three isolated district hospitals in rural Nepal where there was no access to mental health professionals showed that Primary care providers reported limited training, lack of knowledge and skills, and discomfort in delivering mental health care (Acharya et al., 2016). Though the trainings are provided, there is a lack of proper supervision. Also, the trainings have not covered the whole health system of the country. Hence, there is need to assure the quality with proper supervision and 100% coverage so that the transfer of staffs won't hamper the services. One of the modality that could be useful considering large coverage rural population could be video lectures and on-site skills training for clinicians (Acharya et al., 2017).

## *8.3 Curriculum Differences and Modality of Teaching Among Different Universities for Undergraduate Medical Training*

There is a need to compare the different aspects of the curriculum such as the topics covered, skills imparted, methods of teaching, must-know areas, and assessment methods in this region. Another important area to explore is the outcome of psychiatry training exposure in each country that will give us an in-depth idea. There is heterogeneity among the medical schools regarding the curriculum of psychiatry; hence, we emphasize competency-based homogenous curriculum all over the nation.

## *8.4 Research on Psychiatry Training Curriculum*

One of the major challenges is the lack of research and funding in the research of the impact of curriculum. There has not been any major research regarding the leaning impact and competency of the ongoing curriculum. Hence, there is a need to invest in this education research area. The need assessment survey needs to be conducted to find out what contextual requirements are there in sector of Nepalese mental health.

### 8.5 *Lack of Competency-Based Structured Curriculum*

One of the challenges has been the heterogenous curriculum across the universities in Nepal in both undergraduate psychiatry teaching and postgraduate psychiatry training. The role of curriculum development and implementation was previously taken by Nepal Medical Council; however, after the establishment of Medical Education Commission (MEC) as per provision of the National Medical Education Act 2019, this role has been taken up by MEC. There has been gradual improvement in this area, for example, the formulation of a dynamic guide, National framework of Medical National Curriculum Framework for Undergraduate Health Professionals Education in Nepal (Medical Education Commission, 2025). The similar structure is being planned for the postgraduate medical education in Nepal. Once the framework is implemented this challenge can be addressed.

### 8.6 *Lack of Collaboration*

There is a gross lack of collaboration among the stakeholders working in the field of mental health regarding the scope and limitations of the trained manpower. Hence, there should be consensus among the universities and the non-government organizations and associations for a well-devised mental health training at different levels.

## 9 Conclusion

The teaching and training of psychiatry in Nepal have undergone substantial development over the past three decades. The landmark has been the establishment of the first postgraduate psychiatry and M.Phil. in psychology program at the Institute of Medicine (IOM), Tribhuvan University. Over the years, several universities—including BP Koirala Institute of Health Sciences (BPKIHS), Kathmandu University, and Patan Academy of Health Sciences (PAHS)—have initiated their own MBBS and MD Psychiatry programs, significantly expanding the capacity for mental health education and workforce development. Undergraduate psychiatry teaching is now a mandatory component in all medical colleges, although the depth and quality of exposure still vary. There is a need to develop and implement a competency-based homogenous curriculum throughout the universities that is in par with other countries. There is a need of continued and coordinated efforts to ensure that psychiatry teaching and training in Nepal can meet the growing mental health needs of the population and contribute meaningfully to the global mental health landscape.

## References


Acharya, B., Hirachan, S., Mandel, J. S., & van Dyke, C. (2016). The Mental Health Education Gap among Primary Care Providers in Rural Nepal. *Academic Psychiatry: The Journal of the American Association of Directors of Psychiatric Residency Training and the Association for Academic Psychiatry, 40*(4), 667–671. https://doi.org/10.1007/s40596-016-0572-5

Acharya, B., Tenpa, J., Basnet, M., Hirachan, S., Rimal, P., Choudhury, N., Thapa, P., Citrin, D., Halliday, S., Swar, S. B., van Dyke, C., Gauchan, B., Sharma, B., Hung, E., & Ekstrand, M. (2017). Developing a scalable training model in global mental health: Pilot study of a video-assisted training Program for Generalist Clinicians in Rural Nepal. *Global Mental Health, 4*, e8. https://doi.org/10.1017/gmh.2017.4

Acland, S. (2002). Mental health services in primary care. In A. Cohen, A. Kleinman, & B. Saraceno (Eds.), *World mental health casebook: Social and mental health programs in low-income countries* (pp. 121–152). Springer US. https://doi.org/10.1007/0-306-47686-X_5

Aich, T. K. (2010). Contribution of Indian psychiatry in the development of psychiatry in Nepal. *Indian Journal of Psychiatry, 52*(Suppl1), S76–S79. https://doi.org/10.4103/0019-5545.69216

Aich, T. K., & Giri, D. (1997). *Psychiatry in Nepal: Training and Training Centre and its Relevance to India.*

Angdembe, M., Kohrt, B. A., Jordans, M., Rimal, D., & Luitel, N. P. (2017). Situational analysis to inform development of primary care and community-based mental health services for severe mental disorders in Nepal. *International Journal of Mental Health Systems, 11*(1), 69. https://doi.org/10.1186/s13033-017-0176-9

Baral, K. P., Upadhyay, S. K., Bhandhary, S., Gongal, R. N., & Karki, A. (2016). Development of community-based learning and education system within undergraduate medical curriculum of Patan Academy of Health Sciences.

Bhugra, D. (2016). Medical students choice of psychiatry – An international survey. *European Psychiatry, 33*, S29. https://doi.org/10.1016/j.eurpsy.2016.01.850

Dangal, G. (2020). *An overview and changing scenario of post-graduate medical education in Nepal: What Is the Way Forward?*

Devkota, K. L., & Khanal, G. K. (2024). Nepal. In N. Steytler (Ed.), *The Forum of federations handbook on local government in federal systems* (pp. 347–376). Springer. https://doi.org/10.1007/978-3-031-41283-7_12

Dhimal, M., Dahal, S., Adhikari, K., Koirala, P., Bista, B., Luitel, N., Pant, S., Marahatta, K., Shakya, S., Sharma, P., Ghimire, S., Gyanwali, P., Ojha, S. P., & Jha, A. K. (2022). A Nationwide Prevalence of Common Mental Disorders and Suicidality in Nepal: Evidence from National Mental Health Survey, 2019–2020. *Journal of Nepal Health Research Council, 19*(4), 740–747. https://doi.org/10.33314/jnhrc.v19i04.4017

Dhungana, R. R., Pandey, A. R., Joshi, S., Luitel, N. P., Marahatta, K., Aryal, K. K., & Dhimal, M. (2023). The burden of mental disorders in Nepal between 1990 and 2019: Findings from the Global Burden of Disease Study 2019. *Global Mental Health (Cambridge, England), 10*, e61. https://doi.org/10.1017/gmh.2023.55

Dixit, H. (2017). History of Health Professional Education in Nepal. *Journal of Kathmandu Medical College, 6*(4), Article 4.

Dixit, S. M., Ranjit, E., & Dixit, H. (2018). Post-graduation in medicine and allied health sciences in Nepal. *Journal of Kathmandu Medical College, 7*(3), Article 3.

Government of Nepal. (2025). *Medical Education Commission*. https://www.mec.gov.np/en.

Jordans, M. J., Luitel, N. P., Tomlinson, M., & Komproe, I. H. (2013). Setting priorities for mental health care in Nepal: A formative study. *BMC Psychiatry, 13*(1), 332. https://doi.org/10.1186/1471-244X-13-332

Jordans, M. J. D., Luitel, N. P., Kohrt, B. A., Rathod, S. D., Garman, E. C., De Silva, M., Komproe, I. H., Patel, V., & Lund, C. (2019). Community-, facility-, and individual-level outcomes of a district mental healthcare plan in a low-resource setting in Nepal: A population-based evaluation. *PLoS Medicine, 16*(2), e1002748. https://doi.org/10.1371/journal.pmed.1002748

Karki, D. B., & Dixit, H. (2004). An overview of undergraduate and postgraduate medical education in Nepal and elsewhere. *Kathmandu University Medical Journal (KUMJ), 2*(1), 69–74.

Karki, U., Rai, Y., Dhonju, G., Sharma, E., Jacob, P., Kommu, J. V. S., & Seshadri, S. P. (2020). Child and adolescent psychiatry training in Nepal: Early career psychiatrists' perspective. *Child and Adolescent Psychiatry and Mental Health, 14*(1), 13. https://doi.org/10.1186/s13034-020-00319-5

Koirala, N. R. (2013). Psychiatrists' Association of Nepal-Future of psychiatric services in Nepal-A mission and vision document. *Journal of Psychiatrists' Association of Nepal, 2*(2), 3–5.

Luitel, N. P., Jordans, M. J., Adhikari, A., Upadhaya, N., Hanlon, C., Lund, C., & Komproe, I. H. (2015). Mental health care in Nepal: Current situation and challenges for development of a district mental health care plan. *Conflict and Health, 9*(1), 3. https://doi.org/10.1186/s13031-014-0030-5

Marahatta, K., Pant, S. B., Basnet, M., Sharma, P., Risal, A., & Ojha, S. P. (2021). Mental health education in undergraduate medical curricula across Nepalese universities. *BMC Medical Education, 21*(1), 304. https://doi.org/10.1186/s12909-021-02743-3

Medical Education Commission. (2025). *National Curriculum Framework For Undergraduate Health Professionals Education in Nepal*. Retrieved May 6, 2025, from https://mec.gov.np/en/detail/national-curriculum-framework-for-undergraduate-health-professionals-education-in-nepal

*National Academy of Medical Sciences*. (2025). Retrieved April 28, 2025, from https://nams.edu.np/en

Nepal Medical Council. (2017). Retrieved April 28, 2025, from https://nmc.org.np/regulations-for-postgraduate-medical-education-md-ms-program-2017

Pandey, A. R., Adhikari, B., Bista, B., Lamichhane, B., Joshi, D., Saugat Pratap, K. C., Sharma, S., & Baral, S. (2024). Prevalence, determinants and care-seeking behaviour for anxiety and depression in Nepalese population: A secondary analysis of data from Nepal Demographic and Health Survey 2022. *BMJ Open, 14*(8), e078582. https://doi.org/10.1136/bmjopen-2023-078582

Pradhan, P. M., Adhikari, B., Pant, S. B., Ranjit, N., Rawal, S., & Basnet, S. (2022). Self-assessment of non-communicable diseases related competencies among Interns of a Medical Institute of Nepal. *Journal of Institute of Medicine Nepal, 44*(2), Article 2. https://doi.org/10.59779/jiomnepal.1216

Rai, Y., Karki, U., Thapaliya, S., & Molina, R. (2020). Neuropsychiatry training in Nepal: Experiences of trainees and psychiatrists. *Journal of Psychiatrists' Association of Nepal, 9*(1), Article 1. https://doi.org/10.3126/jpan.v9i1.31312

Rai, Y., Gurung, D., & Gautam, K. (2021a). Insight and challenges: Mental health services in Nepal. *BJPsych International, 18*(2), E5. https://doi.org/10.1192/bji.2020.58

Rai, Y., Karki, U., & da Costa, M. P. (2021b). Psychotherapy training in Nepal: Views of early career psychiatrists. *BJPsych International, 18*(2), E6. https://doi.org/10.1192/bji.2020.50

Rana, M., & Shakya, S. (2022). Towards professional training in clinical psychology in Nepal. *Nepalese Psychology, 1*, 47–67.

Rathod, S. D., Luitel, N. P., & Jordans, M. J. D. (2018). Prevalence and correlates of alcohol use in a central Nepal district: Secondary analysis of a population-based cross-sectional study. *Global Mental Health, 5*, e37. https://doi.org/10.1017/gmh.2018.28

Regmi, M. P. (1987). Historical Development of Psychology in Nepal. In *Psychology Moving East*. Routledge.

Republica. (2024). *First adolescent mental health unit established in Nepal*. https://myrepublica.nagariknetwork.com/news/first-adolescent-mental-health-unit-established-in-nepal

Shah, J. N., Shah, J., Shah, J., Shrestha, A., & Pradhan, N. M. S. (2021). Postgraduate medical education: The history and development of competency-based training program in Nepal. *Journal of Patan Academy of Health Sciences, 8*(1), Article 1. https://doi.org/10.3126/jpahs.v8i1.36243

Shakya, D. R. (2014). Department of psychiatry, BPKIHS and its contribution to mental health literature of Nepal. *Journal of Psychiatrists' Association of Nepal, 3*(1), Article 1. https://doi.org/10.3126/jpan.v3i1.11354

Sharma, V. D. (2013). Department of psychiatry, IOM up to 2013: Contributions and achievements. *Journal of Psychiatrists' Association of Nepal, 2*(2), Article 2. https://doi.org/10.3126/jpan.v2i2.9731

Sharma, P., Gautam, K., & Marahatta, K. (2024). Access to Mental Health Care in Nepal: Current status, potential challenges, and ways out. In S. M. Y. Arafat & S. K. Kar (Eds.), *Access to Mental Health Care in South Asia: Current status, potential challenges, and ways out* (pp. 91–111). Springer Nature. https://doi.org/10.1007/978-981-99-9153-2_6

Sharma, P., Singh, S., Parajuli, A., Dhungel, O., & Pathak, P. (2025). View of prevalence and associated factors of depression in Nepal: A systematic review and meta-analysis. *JNMA: Journal of the Nepal Medical Association, 63*(284), 286–297. https://doi.org/10.31729/jnma.8960

Shrestha, S., Shrestha, A., Shah, J. N., & Gongal, R. N. (2021). Competency based post graduate residency program at patan academy of health sciences, Nepal. *Journal of Nepal Health Research Council, 19*(1), 189–195. https://doi.org/10.33314/jnhrc.v19i1.3263

Singh, R., & Khadka, S. (2021). Mental health law in Nepal. *BJPsych International, 19*(1), 24–26. https://doi.org/10.1192/bji.2021.52

Singh, R., Gupta, A. K., Singh, B., Basnet, P., & Arafat, S. M. Y. (2021). History of psychiatry in Nepal. *BJPsych International, 19*(1), 7–9. https://doi.org/10.1192/bji.2021.51

Singh, R., Gupta, A. K., Singh, B., Basnet, P., & Arafat, S. M. Y. (2022). History of psychiatry in Nepal. *BJPsych International, 19*(1), 7–9. https://doi.org/10.1192/bji.2021.51

Sujen. (2012). *State of psychology in Nepal*. Sujen Man Maharjan. Retrieved April 20, 2025, from https://sujenman.wordpress.com/2012/02/28/state-of-psychology-in-nepal-2012/

Upadhaya, N., Regmi, U., Gurung, D., Luitel, N. P., Petersen, I., Jordans, M. J. D., & Komproe, I. H. (2020). Mental health and psychosocial support services in primary health care in Nepal: Perceived facilitating factors, barriers and strategies for improvement. *BMC Psychiatry, 20*, 64. https://doi.org/10.1186/s12888-020-2476-x

*WHO*. (2022) *Nepal—WHO Special Initiative for Mental Health*. Retrieved February 17, 2025, from https://www.who.int/publications/m/item/Nepal_country_assessment_SIMH_2022

# Chapter 8
# Psychiatry Teaching and Training in Pakistan

**Nazish Imran, Ali Madeeh Hashmi, Irum Aamer, and Jawed Akbar Dars**

**Abstract** Pakistan is a Low- and Middle-Income Country (LMIC), located in South Asia. Like many LMICs, mental health has long been a neglected area in Pakistan's healthcare system, despite the high burden of common psychiatric disorders. However, over the years, psychiatric education and clinical services have gradually evolved. Psychiatry is now recognized as a mandatory component of undergraduate medical education, with teaching of both behavioral sciences and psychiatry. At the postgraduate level, psychiatry training is offered through a two-year membership program and a more comprehensive four-year fellowship program. Pakistani institutions have increasingly placed a greater emphasis on aligning psychiatric training with international standards, aiming to enhance the quality and relevance of psychiatric education. Child and adolescent psychiatry is currently the only formally established subspecialty. Several challenges persist, such as stigma associated with mental illness, lack of resources, insufficient exposure of medical students to Psychiatry, and a shortage of faculty trained in modern teaching methods. The key recommendations for the future include enhancing the exposure of psychiatry among medical students, incorporating bio-psycho-social perspectives into curricula, tackling social stigma, and fostering international collaboration and research partnerships. Strengthening advocacy efforts is also essential for building a workforce that can deliver evidence-based mental health care.

N. Imran (✉)
Department of Child and Family Psychiatry, King Edward Medical University/Mayo Hospital, Lahore, Pakistan

A. M. Hashmi
Department of Psychiatry and Behavioral Sciences, King Edward Medical University/Mayo Hospital, Lahore, Pakistan

I. Aamer
Fatima Jinnah Medical University/Sir Ganga Ram Hospital, Lahore, Pakistan

J. A. Dars
Jinnah Sindh Medical University/ National Institute of Child Health, Karachi, Pakistan



S. K. Kar et al. (eds.), *Teaching and Training in Psychiatry in South Asia*, South Asian Perspectives in Mental Health and Psychology,
https://doi.org/10.1007/978-981-95-1845-6_8

**Keywords** Mental health · Psychiatry · Psychiatry education · Stigma · Pakistan · Training · Curriculum

## 1 Introduction

Pakistan, situated in South Asia and classified as "Low- and Middle-Income Country" category by the World Bank, is the world's fifth most populous country with a population of around 240 million according to the 2023 census (Bureau of Statistics, Government of Pakistan). Approximately 22% of the population lives below the poverty line (World Bank, 2023). A majority (64%) of the population lives in rural areas, and Islam is the most practiced religion. The main languages spoken in Pakistan are Urdu, English, Punjabi, Pushto, Sindhi, Balochi, and Saraiki. The literacy rate for males is 70% and for females is 48%. Approximately 25% of Pakistan's population is under the age of 15, a huge young population. Despite political and economic challenges, Pakistan continues to prioritize development in all key sectors, including Healthcare, while facing a huge burden of communicable and non-communicable diseases. The country's health budget remains relatively low, with less than 1% of gross domestic product (GDP) being spent on health. Health indices like maternal and infant mortality rates, although improving, remain a cause of concern. Poor access to health services, safe drinking water, sanitation and hygienic conditions and limited access to primary education are amongst some of Pakistan's most acute health related challenges (Shaikh, 2024).

## 2 Mental Health in Pakistan

Like most low- and middle-income countries, mental health has remained a neglected area in Pakistan. With no dedicated allocation for mental health in the national healthcare budget, it has not been a priority for successive governments. However, the COVID-19 pandemic highlighted the importance of mental health in the overall healthcare landscape, leading to increased focus on it in various policy initiatives in the country. Rapid urbanization, prolonged economic and political instability, terrorism, and geopolitical tensions alongside environmental changes and climate related stressors (rising temperatures, floods, air pollution, etc.) have likely contributed to the rising prevalence, disability, and mortality associated with mental health disorders in the country (Javed et al., 2020; Noorullah et al., 2024). The country has a suicide mortality rate of 9.7 per 100,000 individuals (Dayani et al., 2024). In the first nationally representative study of psychiatric morbidities in Pakistan, the lifetime prevalence of psychiatric disorders was noted to be 37.91%, while the current prevalence was 32.28%. Common mental health conditions included anxiety and stress-related disorders (24.81%), mood disorders (19.62%), psychotic disorders (4.52%), and substance use disorders (0.85%). Mental illnesses were more common among women, older individuals, urban residents, those with lower incomes, and divorced individuals. Additionally, 6.17% of participants reported experiencing suicidal thoughts in the past month, and 1.05% had attempted suicide at some point in their lives (Rahman et al., 2024). Despite the high prevalence of psychiatric illnesses in the country, a huge proportion of patients do not seek help due to prevailing stigma, poor health and mental health literacy, scarcity of specialized mental health services and professionals especially in rural areas, where most of the population lives, and limited financial resources (Siddiqui & Khan, 2021). At present, the number of qualified psychiatrists in the country is less than 1000. WHO Mental Health Atlas 2020 reported only 11 large-scale psychiatric hospitals in the country, with 578 residential care facilities and 800 psychiatric units in general hospitals, and just over 600 community-based psychiatric inpatient units. The number of Psychiatric inpatient beds in the population was 2.1/100,000. Almost all tertiary care hospitals usually have mental health outpatient clinics integrated within them. There are approximately 3729 outpatient mental health facilities, with only 1% for children and adolescents (World Health Organization, 2020). There has been more emphasis on smaller psychiatric units in general hospitals as well as community-based services in recent years.

Psychiatric services, education and training in Pakistan have evolved over the years with more emphasis on smaller psychiatric units in general hospitals, integration of psychiatric services in primary care and the community as well as structured programs for teaching and training of undergraduate and postgraduate medical students. This chapter will provide an in-depth exploration of psychiatry teaching and training in Pakistan, offering a comprehensive understanding of the current scenario, the context in which psychiatric services are operating, the challenges faced, and the way forward.

## 3 Psychiatry Teaching and Training in Pakistan

### *3.1 Undergraduate Psychiatry Education*

"The curriculum should be responsive to the needs of the society it serves, ensuring that medical graduates are equipped with the knowledge, skills, and attitudes relevant to the healthcare challenges of their own communities." *Ronald M. Harden.*

The Pakistan Medical and Dental Council (PMDC) regulates medical education in Pakistan by setting standards, licensing practitioners, and accrediting institutions to ensure quality training. (https://online.pmdc.pk/). Operating under the Pakistan Medical and Dental Council Ordinance, 1962, the PMDC recently gained accreditation from the World Federation for Medical Education (WFME), reinforcing its commitment to high educational standards. In Pakistan, students are admitted to medical colleges after completing 12 years of education, and embark on a five-year undergraduate medical education journey, following a curriculum designed by the

Pakistan Medical and Dental Council (PMDC) in collaboration with the Higher Education Commission (HEC) and implemented by each medical college's Department of Medical Education (DME).

Psychiatry is currently regarded as a required field for undergraduate medical education. Behavioral sciences were introduced in 2007 and are being taught as a subject from the first year onward in Bachelor of Medicine and Bachelor of Surgery (MBBS), a move welcomed by the psychiatric community (Table 8.1). Typically taught by faculty from the Psychiatry department, the course covers essential topics such as behavior, emotions, memory, personality, stress management, doctor–patient relationships, and medical ethics. In many Institutions, third-year medical students appear in the subject of behavioral sciences annually in their professional examination, which includes a written paper and an objectively structured performance exam (OSPE). Teaching behavioral sciences to undergraduate medical students in Pakistan faces several challenges due to curriculum limitations,

**Table 8.1** PMDC-recommended curriculum: Psychiatry & Behavioral Sciences for MBBS

| Component | Topics/contents | Teaching hours | Clinical rotation hours | Teaching-learning methodologies | Assessment methods |
|---|---|---|---|---|---|
| Psychiatry | Mood disorders, anxiety disorders, obsessive compulsive disorder, schizophrenia, bipolar, psychosis, substance use, deliberate self-harm (DSH), dementia, child and adolescent psychiatry. | 40 | 4 weeks during fourth year MBBS +2 weeks community psychiatry rotation (recommended)* | Lectures, clinical rotations, role-plays, and case-based learning | Multiple choice questions (MCQs), short answer questions (SAQs), objective structured clinical examination (OSPE), logbook, and case presentations(final year professional exam) |
| Behavioral Sciences | Perception, memory, cognition, personality, communication, counseling, grief, psychosocial aspects of health/illness | 50 | Three weeks in Psychiatry department during third year MBBS, Integrated in all rotations | Lectures, small group discussions, problem-based learning, and role-plays | MCQs, SAQs, OSPE (Third year professional exam) |

Communication skills, medical ethics, and professionalism are reinforced across all clerkships
Community psychiatry is recommended as an additional 2-week component where feasible
Nutrition, communication, evidence-based practice, and behavioral sciences are also taught in fourth year MBBS as a component of Community Medicine

programmatic's structure, duration and composition issues, lack of motivation and time constraints faced by clinical teachers, and, finally, gaps in faculty training in interactive teaching methodologies (Javed et al., 2020).

The subject of Psychiatry is taught in clinical years through theoretical lectures and clinical placements (Table 8.1). Undergraduate psychiatric education in Pakistan differs significantly from that in the West, where assessments of psychiatric knowledge are highly valued. As per the curriculum for medical education 2024 by PMDC, the discipline of psychiatry and behavioral sciences has been given 150 hours out of 6200 hours of complete teaching of 5-year medical education. There is a 4–6-week mandatory rotation of students in Psychiatry departments of attached teaching hospitals, where biopsychosocial history, physical examination, and mental state examination are taught to them through bedside teaching, supervised case conferences, and role-play exercises. However, since Psychiatry is not an essential subject in final examination, undergraduate medical students have little motivation to study this crucial discipline in depth (Javed et al., 2020). Given the growing mental health burden, there is a critical need to strengthen undergraduate psychiatry education to equip future doctors with the essential skills to recognize and manage common psychiatric conditions in the community.

### *3.2 Postgraduate Psychiatry Training Pathways*

The College of Physicians and Surgeons of Pakistan (CPSP), established in 1962, is the country's leading postgraduate medical institute. CPSP oversees all postgraduate medical education in Pakistan in all specialties (CPSP, 2025). It offers two postgraduate programs for the field of psychiatry: a 2-year membership program and a 4-year intensive fellowship program. Both the programs have competency-based curricula, and the college offers various mandatory workshops (prerequisites to appear in the exit examination) in communication skills, research and biostatistics, and computer skills along with basic life support courses, to enhance trainees' professional skills. CPSP also accredits all training sites where postgraduate trainees work (hospitals and clinics), although it has no hospital of its own.

To enter specialist psychiatry training, candidates must have registered with the Pakistan Medical and Dental Council (PMDC) after completing his/her 5 years of medical education and 1 year of mandatory internship (Javed et al., 2020). CPSP offers part 1 (entry) examination four times a year which is required to enroll in the fellowship program (the 2-year Membership of College of Physicians and Surgeons Pakistan (MCPS) does not have an entry exam).

Following registration with the college, the postgraduate trainee must pass each hospital's entry test (if applicable) for an available training slot or a centralized test (varies in different provinces of the country) to be appointed in different hospitals. During these 4 years of rigorous training, postgraduate trainees need to complete mandatory rotations, 3 months each, in medicine, neurology, and psychology (Rana et al., 2008) (Fig. 8.1).

The workshops, rotations, and a research proposal approval are mandatory to qualify for Intermediate module examination, for which the student is eligible after 2 years of training. During these 4 years, trainees go through extensive hands-on training for in-patient and out-patient work, emergency cases, liaison visits, and special cases of addiction, forensic, and child & adolescent patients along with internal and external assessments. Following completion of 4 years of training and after fulfilling all other training requirements including publishing a high-quality research paper, candidates are eligible to appear for a final exit exam (FCPS-II) to become Fellows of CPSP. The Exit Exam has two parts: theory and clinical. There are two theory papers consisting of MCQs. The clinical examination consists of a long case, short cases, and TOACS (Task Oriented Assessment of Clinical Skills) stations. They can then also register as specialists with PMDC.

Parallel to the program run by CPSP, several universities across the country offer 2-year Diploma in Psychological Medicine (DPM) programs and also offer Doctor of Medicine (MD) a 4-year structured program in the field of psychiatry (Javed et al., 2020) (Table 8.2).

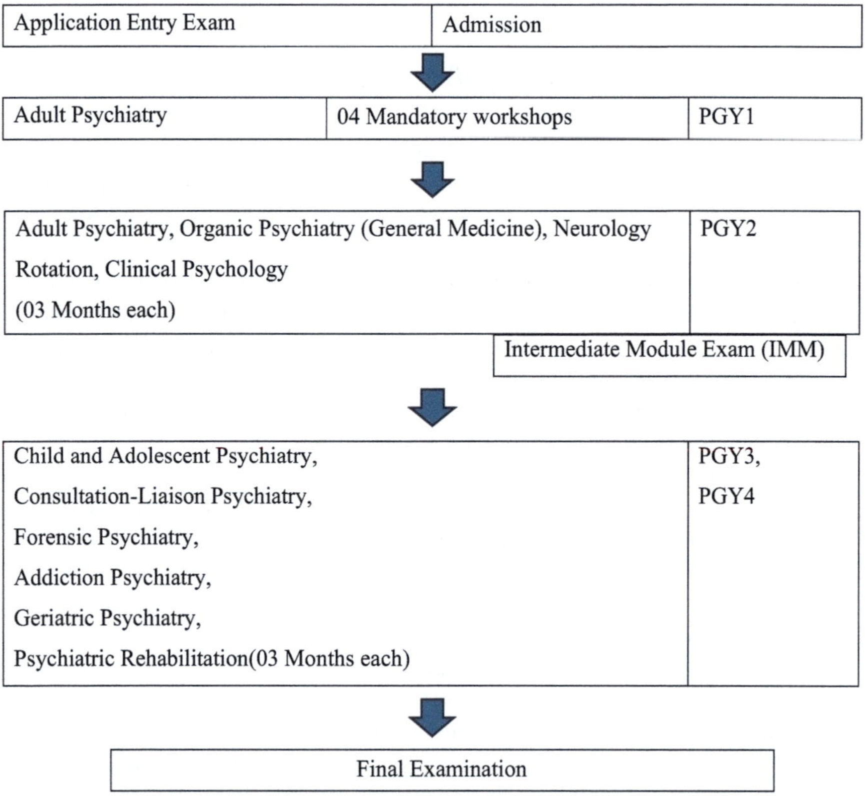


**Fig. 8.1** Duration and scheme of course of FCPS Psychiatry Training

Postgraduate trainees enrolled in CPSP programs and University programs work and train side by side and efforts are underway to align their curricula to provide uniformity and standardization of training as well as to remove discrepancies in training and certification after completion of training. Due to the College of Physicians and Surgeons' extensive national network as well as strong linkages regionally and internationally, FCPS is still the preferred training route for most postgraduate trainees in Pakistan. However, University MD programs are gaining in popularity due to continuous improvement in their curricula and training standards, as well as a huge need for more trained specialists across Pakistan.

## 3.3 *Teaching Methodologies and Training Approaches Including Clinical Training Exposure*

Medical education has taken a huge leap forward in the last few years in Pakistan with changes in teaching methodologies and examination patterns. In a situation where the country is lagging in achieving the UN's millennium development goals in education (education for all) CPSP and Pakistani universities are making strong efforts to bring higher education in psychiatry at par with international standards.

**Table 8.2** Curriculum content for postgraduate MD training in Psychiatry

| Training year | Semester/ module | Title | Duration | Didactic hours |
|---|---|---|---|---|
| PGY1 | Semester 1 | Introduction to Adult Psychiatry | 0–9 months | 10 (5.5 + 4.5) |
| | Semester 2 | Rotation in General Medicine | 9–12 months | 3 (1 + 2) |
| | Workshop 1 | Research Methodology & Biostatistics | 05 days | – |
| | Workshop 2 | Synopsis Writing | 03 days | – |
| | Workshop 3 | Communication Skills | 03 days | – |
| | Workshop 4 | Introduction to Computer Information Technology and Software Program | 03 days | – |
| | Synopsis | Submission of Synopsis | – | – |
| PGY2 | Semester 3 | Adult Psychiatry | 13–24 months | 7 (4.5 + 2.5) |
| | Semester 4 | | | 7 (4.5 + 2.5) |
| PGY3 | Semester 5.1 | Clinical Psychology | 25–27 months | 3 (2 + 1) |
| | Semester 5.2 | Substance Abuse Psychiatry | 28–30 months | 3 (2 + 1) |
| | Semester 6 | Rotation in Neurology | 31–36 months | 6 (4 + 2) |
| PGY4 | Semester 7.1 | Child & Adolescent Psychiatry | 37–39 months | 3 (2 + 1) |
| | Semester 7.2 | Consultation-Liaison Psychiatry | 40–42 months | 3 (2 + 1) |
| | Semester 8.1 | Forensic Psychiatry | 43–45 months | 3 (2 + 1) |
| | Semester 8.2 | Geriatric Psychiatry | 46–48 months | 3 (2 + 1) |

**Table 8.3** Assessment methods in postgraduate training in Psychiatry

| Continuous internal assessment(CIS) | Generic competency training and assessment | Speciality specific competency | Intermediate module exam (IMM) | Procedure-based assessment, multisource feedback evaluation | Annual review report |
|---|---|---|---|---|---|
| Workplace-based assessments | • Patient care<br>• Medical knowledge and research<br>• Practice and system-based learning<br>• Communication skills<br>• Professionalism as per Hippocratic Oath | • Observer status<br>• Assistant status<br>• Performed under supervision<br>• Performed independently | Is it possible to format this in a way that last 3 columns both sections are merged in green colur as looks empty in current format as if text is missing , other option is to add content. In that case add written and clinical examonation for this column | Workplace-based assessments | Log Books, Formal evlauation of trainees, feedback etc |

Modern methods of medical education, including moving away from rote learning and transforming the role of teachers into facilitators, are being incorporated into medical curricula. CPSP, through its competency-based model, tries to ensure that the students are capable and competent professionals well-versed in the principles of pedagogy, advocacy, and professionalism. Using modern teaching methods such as case-based learning (CBL), problem-based learning (PBL), workplace-based assessments (WPBA), and other techniques, medical education in Pakistan is slowly being aligned with international standards (Table 8.3, Box 8.1).

However, significant challenges remain with the total number of psychiatrists in the country still standing at less than 1000, with only a fraction of these formally trained in medical education. Continued migration to more economically advanced countries ("brain drain"), low pay in academic settings, combined with multiple clinical and administrative responsibilities, mean job burnout is quite common. This will be difficult to correct unless the current health budget of the country is revised drastically upward (Hassan, 2023).

As the trend of medical education changes from obtaining highest marks to clinical competence and professional behavior in clinical environment, WPBA remain an essential component in creating a self-directed learning environment (Liu, 2012).

**Box 8.1 Teaching learning methodology in postgraduate training in Psychiatry**
**Teaching learning methodologies**

- Seminars.
- Case conferences.
- Journal clubs.
- Psycho-somatic rounds.
- Case presentations.
- Research forum.
- Psychotherapy tutorials.
- Electroconvulsive therapy (ECT) training.
- Training in ECT administration.
- Extra-mural activities.

WPBA is now mandatory for all trainees in training programs across the country and initial feedback from postgraduate trainees is positive as it fosters reflective practices in the educational setting besides improvement in clinical training (Fatima et al., 2023).

The 4 years psychiatry fellowship training by CPSP, despite having structured rotations in general medicine, neurology, and psychology still lacks an appropriate curriculum for community psychiatry, which is an essential component of holistic care (Rehman et al., 2022). When it comes to subspecialty training in Psychiatry, only child and adolescent psychiatry is currently established as a discipline in Pakistan. Digital learning after Covid has become a norm and every medical university is supposed to have a complete IT sector with necessary facilities to carry out online teaching as well as assessments. The logbook for case entries, feedback by supervisors has been digitalized by the college. The trainees must publish two scientific papers in a reputable journal during their training period of 4 years.

## 3.4 *Psychiatric Subspecialties Training in Pakistan*

Psychiatric Subspecialty Training is at a very early stage in Pakistan. Due to the limited number of trained specialists and services, General Adult Psychiatrists provide most services for children and adolescents, learning disability, old age, addiction, forensic patients and those needing rehabilitation services within limited resources. Training in General Adult Psychiatry requires trainees to gain experience in various subfields. In addition to general adult psychiatry, which includes both outpatient and inpatient care, trainees must also develop some expertise in psychotherapy, child psychiatry, learning disabilities, substance abuse, geriatric psychiatry, organic psychiatry, forensic psychiatry, liaison psychiatry, neurology, and psychometry (Naeem & Ayub, 2004). This diverse exposure ensures comprehensive training and prepares them for a wide range of psychiatric conditions and patient needs.

However, there have been significant recent advancements in the establishment of psychiatric subspecialties, particularly in the nation's largest public and private hospitals and academic departments (Javed et al., 2020). Literature suggests that countries with the largest percentage of children and adolescents in their population are those that lack both a policy for children and adolescents' mental health and services for that population. Due to unmet needs and a huge gap in services for the large young children and adolescent population, the first subspecialty training started in Pakistan is that of second fellowship in Child & Adolescent psychiatry. In its official notification on December 15, 2014, the College of Physicians and Surgeons Pakistan (CPSP) announced the approval of the Child and Adolescent Psychiatry fellowship in the country. This was a multi-center collaborative effort with many people playing a major role in this development nationally and internationally, by helping with the 2 years child and adolescent psychiatry curriculum development and multiple-choice question bank requirements needed for the start of training (Azeem et al., 2015). The second fellowship was due to start in three centers in the country including King Edward Medical University (Lahore), Rawalpindi Medical University (Rawalpindi), and Agha Khan University (Karachi) simultaneously in 2015. However, due to various logistical challenges and the COVID-19 pandemic, its implementation was delayed for several years. Efforts to restart the fellowship resumed during Pandemic, with revision of the curriculum, and training site visits and supervisors' approval. In 2020, King Edward Medical University (Child and Family Psychiatry Department) became the first institution in the country to be officially recognized and accredited for CPSP-accredited training in Child and Adolescent Psychiatry. Later four more centers (Agha Khan Medical University & Liaquat University of Medical and Health Sciences in Sindh, Rawalpindi Medical University (Punjab) and Baluchistan Institute of Psychiatry & Behavioural Sciences (Baluchistan) have been recognized, and training is currently underway in three of these centers with first exit exam planned in summer 2025. Alongside FCPS second fellowship, Universities have also begun offering MD postgraduate training in child and adolescent psychiatry with a curriculum similar to CPSP. In actual practice, both FCPS and MD trainees work and learn side by side in the same hospitals.

The Child and Adolescent (C&A) second fellowship is a 2-year training program in child and adolescent psychiatry after 4 years of FCPS training in General Psychiatry. Candidates have to undertake two years training in a recognized institute under an approved supervisor before becoming eligible for the C&A exam. The supervisor is responsible for ensuring training in accordance with college standards. Trainees need to maintain a logbook of training, attend mandatory workshops, and get an article published in a recognized journal during the training period. Like Psychiatry primary fellowship, the Exam of second fellowship in Child & Adolescent Psychiatry has two parts: theory and clinical. There are two theory papers consisting of 100 problem-based MCQs each. The clinical examination consists of one long case and four short cases and up to 16 TOACS stations.

Plans are underway to start subspecialty training in Forensic and Addiction psychiatry in the near future in Pakistan. To support learning in subspecialties, several other ongoing initiatives have been introduced, such as the Child & Adolescent Mental Health Certificate (CAMH-C) course by CorTeach in collaboration with Baqai Medical University Karachi, which offers an interactive online program for practitioners interested in child mental health. Other opportunities include courses by APPNA Merit Academy on addiction and old-age psychiatry, and few other short-term courses.

## 4 Challenges in Psychiatry Teaching and Training in Pakistan

Training as a Psychiatrist and teaching Psychiatry as a subject in Pakistan are challenging due to multifaceted systemic and social challenges.

- One major hurdle is the need for clinical acumen to recognize the local customs, traditions, and belief systems, which influence the presentation of mental illnesses. Psychiatrists must be able to align contextual pathology with modern scientific understanding and effectively communicate with patients and their families, requiring skills such as empathy, cultural sensitivity, and the ability to navigate diverse experiences. Furthermore, Psychiatrists also need to be competent in assessing and managing a variety of subspecialties. Despite the need for strong leaders to advocate for mental health, residency programs often lack leadership training. Residents also need to be taught reflective practice and spiritual altruism, qualities that transcend traditional curricula but are necessary for effective Psychiatric practice (Williams, 2024).
- *Psychiatry as a Career Choice During Medical Years*
  Psychiatry remains an unpopular career choice among medical students in Pakistan due to prevailing stigma and misconceptions. Many students perceive it as less prestigious, financially unrewarding, and emotionally exhausting compared to other medical specialities. Negative stereotypes, lack of exposure to Psychiatry during early medical education, discouragement from parents to opt for Psychiatry, and limited mentorship further discourage students from pursuing this field (Dars et al., 2024).
- *Challenges Faced by Residents Opting for Psychiatry*
  Psychiatry residents in Pakistan face significant training challenges, including reliance on a single supervisor who may be unavailable or disinterested, limiting mentorship and learning opportunities. To compensate, these adult learners seek external resources and peer support, but many still struggle with confidence in prescribing due to inadequate hands-on experience. Most training programs lack

structured psychotherapy supervision, leaving residents to rely on theoretical knowledge rather than hands-on experience (Kahn & Ahmed, 2024).

- *Shortage of Trained Faculty and Psychiatrists*
  Over the last 10 years, the number of consultant Psychiatrists in Pakistan has increased, primarily due to the hiring of Psychiatrists who have completed two-year MCPS and diploma programs, particularly in primary and secondary care settings. However, Pakistan still falls short of the WHO standard of one Psychiatrist per 10,000 people. The availability of supervisors for Psychiatry training and teaching programs across the country remains limited. Supervisors are selected through a rigorous process established by the College of Physicians and Surgeons Pakistan (CPSP) and local universities offering MD programs. Since this role does not offer monetary compensation, many trained Psychiatrists, including those with MD or FCPS qualifications, are reluctant to become trainers. While some Psychiatrists are eager to teach, the lengthy selection process often results in only one or two supervisors per department. As a result, these supervisors are burdened with overseeing 10 to 12 trainees, placing significant strain on their time and resources and ultimately impacting the quality of mentorship and training. Despite various challenges, supervisors in Psychiatry training programs across Pakistan remain committed to imparting knowledge, skills, and professional attitudes to their residents.
  Gaps in Research Training and Evidence-Based Practice
- *Undergraduate Factors:*
  Research is essential for medical progress, but medical students in Pakistan often lack practical exposure to it. They view original research as time-consuming and complex, deterring them from engaging in such activities. Funding for meaningful research, such as randomized controlled trials (RCTs), is scarce, and access to international psychiatric journals is limited. High publication fees further hinder the dissemination of local research, restricting students' exposure to global advancements in the field.
- *Postgraduate Factors:*
  At the postgraduate level, psychiatry residency programs struggle with insufficient research training and funding. Residents often have limited opportunities to conduct or publish research, and the lack of mentorship discourages them further.

CPSP and local universities offer workshops for basic research methodologies, biostatistics, and medical writing and have now made it compulsory for residents to publish at least one original research paper in recognized journals during the residency program.

- *Infrastructural and Funding Limitations in Psychiatric Education*
  While all medical schools and universities have Psychiatry inpatient and outpatient units, many are not purpose built and lack essential facilities like child and adolescent units, dedicated spaces for psychotherapy clinics, isolation rooms, and adequate space for treatment. In rural areas, Psychiatric services are even scarcer, with little to no resources for training and service delivery. Exposure to enrichment activities, such as special study modules, electives, and university

Psychiatry clubs, plays a crucial role in increasing students' interest in psychiatry and encourages them to pursue it as a career (Farooq et al., 2014). These activities enhance overall engagement with Psychiatry education and training, fostering a deeper understanding and appreciation for the field. However, most Psychiatry departments in Pakistan are unable to offer these enrichment opportunities due to limited funding, hindering the ability to attract and retain students in the specialty. Staff positions often remain vacant due to insufficient funding. As a result Psychiatric hospitals and teaching facilities are often understaffed, underfunded, and ill-equipped to offer comprehensive training for residents and students.

## 5 Opportunities

Despite various challenges, postgraduate Psychiatry training in Pakistan continues to flourish, driven by the dedication of passionate supervisors and motivated trainees. The commitment to excellence is evident in the increasing number of trainees seeking international exposure and higher qualifications. The College of Physicians and Surgeons Pakistan (CPSP) has entered into an agreement with the Health Service Executive (HSE) and the Forum of Postgraduate Training Bodies in Ireland to offer a postgraduate scholarship program. This initiative allows Pakistani Psychiatry trainees to complete part of their training in Ireland, enhancing their clinical skills, expanding their knowledge base, and gaining insight into alternative healthcare delivery models. Many trainees also pursue the Membership Examination of the Royal College of Psychiatrists (MRCPsych) in the UK to strengthen their clinical expertise and improve their professional portfolios. These opportunities reflect the resilience and ambition of Pakistani Psychiatry trainees, ensuring that the field continues to progress despite existing challenges.

## 6 Role of Professional Organizations and International Collaborations

As a low- and middle-income country (LMIC), Pakistan lags behind the developed world in training techniques and cutting-edge research. LMICs are home to a majority of the world's population. At the same time, they produce a miniscule proportion of global high-quality research and consequently lag behind the rest of the developed world in multiple indices including the latest teaching and training methods (Sahdra et al., 2024). The role of professional organizations, both national and international as well as collaborations with leading global institutions, therefore, becomes all the more important for LMICs like Pakistan.

Pakistan Psychiatric Society (PPS) is the national representative organization of psychiatrists in Pakistan. Founded in 1969 (Ahmed, 2023), PPS is now a vibrant nationwide organization boasting active representation from all four provinces of Pakistan as well as its administrative territories of Gilgit Baltistan and Azad Jammu/ Kashmir. All academic training centers in Pakistan are strongly linked to PPS with faculty members serving as office bearers of the organization after being elected to office every two years. In addition, most of Pakistan's 800+ psychiatrists are active dues-paying members of PPS. While being an academic psychiatrist is not a prerequisite for being elected to PPS office, college and university faculty members usually share other networks as well including serving as postgraduate supervisors and examiners for the College of Physicians and Surgeons of Pakistan as well as individual colleges and universities. PPS also holds several national and international conferences each year where in addition to having a chance to rub shoulders with leading Pakistani academicians, psychiatry trainees also have a chance to meet and interact with distinguished international researchers and academicians as well as present their own original research to a national audience. In recent years, PPS has also begun awarding travel and research grants to psychiatry trainees to encourage more active research involvement by under-training psychiatrists. Plans are also in the works to create a sub-category of "Trainee members" of PPS to encourage psychiatry trainees to participate more actively in the awareness, advocacy, and policy-making activities of PPS both locally and nationally.

PPS is a component society of the World Psychiatric Association (WPA) representing 147 psychiatric societies in 123 countries (WPA, www.wpanet.org). In recent years, the link between PPS and WPA has been considerably strengthened after the election of Dr. Afzal Javed, a Pakistan origin psychiatrist in the UK as President of the WPA from 2020 to 2023. Pakistani psychiatrists have participated actively in research collaborations with the WPA both individually and via the PPS and these collaborations are ongoing. One of our authors (NI) was a member of the WPA Working Group on medical students from 2020 to 2023.

Multiple institutions in Pakistan also work closely with international organizations like the World Health Organization and UNICEF to promote mental health awareness, advocacy, and research training. A recent example is the "Being" project of Shifa Tameer-e Millat University, King Edward Medical University and several international partners, including UNICEF and Johns Hopkins University (GIHD, gihd.stmu.edu.pk/being). "Being" is a multi-country youth mental health initiative to promote mental health awareness and education in young people at risk in partner countries. Many institutions in Pakistan including King Edward Medical University in Lahore also maintain strong links with US based physician organizations. The Association of Physicians of Pakistani Descent of North America (APPNA), King Edward Medical College Alumni Organization of North America (KEMCAANA), and Pakistani American Psychiatric Association of North America (PAPANA) are some of the organizations which regularly design and deliver continuing education courses, exchange programs, workshops, trainings, symposia, and conferences for Pakistan-based psychiatry trainees.

## 7 Future Directions and Recommendations

Improving Psychiatric education and training in low- and middle-income countries like Pakistan is a crucial component of reforming and enhancing medical training to improve population health. While countries like Pakistan grapple with numerous economic, political, and social challenges, it is essential that health for a young and growing population remains a priority to ensure future development in all spheres of national life. The following ideas regarding psychiatric education in the medical context can provide a road map toward this goal.

- Psychiatric curricula in medical colleges and universities are nominally organized around the "Biopsychosocial" model as recommended by international best practices. In actual practice, the curricula remain heavily "biomedical" with scant attention paid to psychological competence and very little to social factors. For a country like Pakistan, real-time immersion of psychiatry students and trainees in the social milieu prevalent in the country is essential to learn about actual problems facing patients and their families. One way to accomplish this is to mandate community psychiatry rotations during training and to incorporate knowledge and competence about the role of social factors in mental illness into both ongoing formative assessments, such as WPBA as well as summative assessments of all trainees.
- Psychiatric subspecialty training to develop and enhance the competence of psychiatric specialists in forensics, child and adolescent psychiatry, geriatric psychiatry, substance abuse, and addiction psychiatry, to name a few, is essential to allow the growth of psychiatry as a specialty and to improve the standard of care for these vulnerable populations. Child and Adolescent Psychiatry is already a well-established discipline thanks to the efforts of a handful of pioneering psychiatrists in Pakistan. Other psychiatric specialties need to be developed all over the country with international collaboration.
- The ever-present stigma around mental illness is gradually beginning to recede especially in the young, urban, educated population, thanks to continuous awareness and advocacy efforts and the increasing use of social media. While this is encouraging, the use of misinformation is also rampant on social media. Efforts must continue both at the government and non-government levels to continue educating the public about mental health and its evidence-based treatment and support. Basic mental health education should be embedded in school curricula starting in kindergarten. Medical school curricula must be further reformed to integrate mental health into medical studies starting in the first year of medical college and combining it with career guidance and planning to maintain student interest.
- Psychiatry as a career choice for medical students and aspiring future specialists is undergoing a sea change. From a heavily stigmatized career field in a country steeped in ignorance about mental health and mental illness, an increasing number of medical students are now beginning to be interested in pursuing a career as a psychiatrist. With the development of increasing scientific knowledge about

mental illness and new and exciting treatment options in the field, combined with increasing income opportunities and career options within psychiatry, many bright young medical students now envision themselves as future psychiatrists. This is a welcome development given the critical shortage of psychiatrists in Pakistan and other low- and middle-income countries. Incorporating career counseling and guidance strategies into medical curricula beginning in the clinical years is a good strategy to encourage young people who want to pursue a career in Psychiatry and help relieve some of the human resource constraints in the field.

- Strengthening research capacity and encouraging global collaboration are essential for advancing psychiatry training in Pakistan. International organizations like the World Psychiatric Association (WPA) can play a key role by facilitating knowledge sharing, mentorship, and capacity-building initiatives. Collaborative research initiatives and international training opportunities can enhance local expertise and align psychiatric education with global best practices.

## 8 Conclusion

To conclude, improving psychiatric education and training to deliver robust evidence-based mental health interventions to improve population health is an essential part of meeting Pakistan‘s commitment to the United Nations Sustainable Development Goals and "Health for all."

**Acknowledgments** The authors acknowledge the assistance of Dr. Rabiya Rasheed, postgraduate trainee in our department, for her help with the tables and figures in the manuscript.

## References

Ahmed, S. H. (2023). Pakistan psychiatric society: A reflection of early years. *Journal of Pakistan Psychiatric Society, 20*(04), 38–41. https://jpps.pk/index.php/journal/article/view/314

Azeem, M. W., Rana, M. H., & Stubbe, D. (2015). New Era for child psychiatry in Pakistan. *Journal of Pakistan Psychiatric Society, 12*(01), 6–7. https://jpps.pk/index.php/journal/article/view/499

College of Physicians and Surgeons Pakistan. (2025, April 13). https://www.cpsp.edu.pk/

Dars, J. A., Syed, I. A., Abbas, K., Ali, N., & Asad, A. (2024). The socioeconomic and training influences on medical students' psychiatry career choices. *Annals of Jinnah Sindh Medical University, 10*(2), 54–58.

Dayani, K., Zia, M., Qureshi, O., Baig, M., & Sabri, T. (2024). Evaluating Pakistan's mental healthcare system using World Health Organization's assessment instrument for mental health system (WHO-AIMS). *International Journal of Mental Health Systems, 18*(1), 32. https://doi.org/10.1186/s13033-024-00646-6

Farooq, K., Lydall, G. J., Malik, A., Ndetei, D. M., & Isosccip Group, & Bhugra, D. (2014). Why medical students choose psychiatry-a 20-country cross-sectional survey. *BMC Medical Education, 14*, 1–13. https://doi.org/10.1186/1472-6920-14-12

Fatima, S., Ul Abideen, M. Z., Siddiqui, A. A., Khan, F. F. S., Gillani, S. W., Hussain, M. W., et al. (2023). Perception, attitude, and preference of trainees towards workplace-based assessment in dental education at a tertiary care institute in Multan, Pakistan. *Work, 75*(2), 703–710. https://doi.org/10.3233/WOR-220132

Hassan, W. (2023). Mandatory mental health education in Pakistan: A proposal. *The Lancet Psychiatry, 10*(5), 318–319. https://doi.org/10.1016/S2215-0366(23)00108-6

Javed, A., Khan, M. N. S., Nasar, A., & Rasheed, A. (2020). Mental healthcare in Pakistan. *Taiwanese Journal of Psychiatry, 34*(1), 6–14. https://doi.org/10.4103/TPSY.TPSY_8_20

Khan, A., & Ahmed, R. A. (2024). Psychiatry residents' views on quality of psychotherapy training in Pakistan: A cross-sectional survey. *BJPsych Open, 10*(S1), S94–S95. https://doi.org/10.1192/bjo.2024.276

Liu, C. (2012). An introduction to workplace-based assessments. *Gastroenterology and Hepatology from Bed to Bench, 5*(1), 24.

Noorullah, A., Asad, N., Pirani, S., Iqbal, S., & Khan, M. M. (2024). Mental health care in Pakistan. In S. M. Y. Arafat & S. K. Kar (Eds.), *Access to mental health care in South Asia*. Springer. https://doi.org/10.1007/978-981-99-9153-2_7

Naeem, F., & Ayub, M. (2004). Psychiatric training in Pakistan. *Medical Education Online, 9*(1), 4369. https://doi.org/10.3402/meo.v9i.4369

Rahman, R., Sheehan, D., Javed, A., Ahmad, S. H., Shafiq, K., Kanwal, U., Afridi, M.I., Nizami, A.T., Rasool, G., Taj, R., Ansari, M., & Ayub, M. (2024). The National Psychiatric Morbidity Survey of Pakistan (2022): Prevalence, socio-demographic and disability correlates. *medRxiv*, 2024-07.

Rana, M. H., Farooq, S., Ali, S., & Afridi, M. I. (2008). An outline of structured training programme for FCPS in psychiatry. *Journal of Pakistan Psychiatric Society, 5*(2), 58–64. https://www.jpps.pk/index.php/journal/article/view/639

Rehman, R., Quraishy, S., & Siddiqi, N. (2022). Postgraduate community psychiatry training in Pakistan. *Journal of Pakistan Psychiatric Society, 19*(02), 44–47. https://www.jpps.pk/index.php/journal/article/view/158

Sahdra, B. K., King, G., Payne, J. S., Ruiz, F. J., Kolahdouzan, S. A., Ciarrochi, J., & Hayes, S. C. (2024). Why research from lower-and middle-income countries matters to evidence-based intervention: A state of science review of ACT research as an example. *Behavior Therapy*. https://doi.org/10.1016/j.beth.2024.06.003

Shaikh, B. T. (2024). Universal health coverage in Pakistan: Exploring the landscape of the health system, health seeking behaviours, and utilization of health services. *The Lancet Regional Health-Southeast Asia, 27*, 100440. https://doi.org/10.1016/j.lansea.2024.100440

Siddiqui, F., & Khan, Q. (2021). Barriers and challenges to mental health care in Pakistan. *Pakistan Journal of Neurological Sciences (PJNS), 16*(3), 1–2.

Williams, S. S. (2024). Fine-tuning postgraduate psychiatry training in South Asia. *Indian Journal of Psychological Medicine, 46*(5), 380–381. https://doi.org/10.1177/02537176241280284

World Bank Group. Poverty & Equity Brief, South Asia, Pakistan. Updated 2023. https://databankfiles.worldbank.org/public/ddpext_download/poverty/987B9C90-CB9F-4D93-AE8C-750588BF00QA/current/Global_POVEQ_PAK.pdf. Accessed 9/2/2025.

World Health Organization. Mental Health Atlas 2020 Country Profile: Pakistan; https://www.who.int/publications/m/item/mental-health-atlas-pak-2020-country-profile

World Psychiatric Association. WPA. Available at: https://www.wpanet.org/ (Accessed: 02 April 2025).

# Chapter 9
# Teaching and Training in Psychiatry in Sri Lanka

**Anuradha Baminiwatta and Janith Galhenage**

**Abstract** Psychiatric education and training in Sri Lanka have evolved significantly, particularly since the 1990s, with notable changes in the undergraduate and postgraduate medical curricula. The introduction of the national core curriculum in 2017 has created greater consistency across the country's medical faculties, improving exposure to mental health issues for medical students. However, despite these advances, the country still faces challenges, such as the scarcity of qualified psychiatric professionals and the migration of trained specialists. These issues, coupled with the underrepresentation of key areas like child psychiatry and psychotherapy training, highlight the need for further reforms. The training of allied health professionals, including nurses, psychologists, social workers, and occupational therapists, has also advanced, but shortages persist. Upskilling health staff in primary care and the use of digital tools for continuing professional development are promising strategies for addressing treatment gaps. This chapter explores the progress, challenges, and future directions in psychiatric education in Sri Lanka, emphasizing the need for increased investment in faculty, infrastructure, and training for subspecialties.

**Keywords** Medical education · Mental health literacy · Health care · Undergraduate · Postgraduate · Allied health · Professional development

A. Baminiwatta (✉)
Department of Psychiatry, Faculty of Medicine, University of Kelaniya, Ragama, Sri Lanka
e-mail: baminiwatta@kln.ac.lk

J. Galhenage
Teaching Hospital, Polonnaruwa, Sri Lanka



S. K. Kar et al. (eds.), *Teaching and Training in Psychiatry in South Asia*, South Asian Perspectives in Mental Health and Psychology,
https://doi.org/10.1007/978-981-95-1845-6_9

## 1 Introduction

Psychiatric education and training form the cornerstone of a nation's response to its mental health needs. In Sri Lanka, where the burden of mental illness is substantial, the importance of strengthening the mental health workforce cannot be overstated. A meta-analysis of community-based studies estimated that 19% of the general population in Sri Lanka experience depressive symptoms, while a national survey in 2007 found that 15% of Sri Lankans suffered from a mental disorder within a single month, most commonly depressive disorders (Alwis et al., 2024; Institute for Research and Development, 2007). Although large-scale, up-to-date national data are lacking, recent trends in suicide rates offer a window into the growing mental health burden. Following a marked decline in suicide rates from 47 per 100,000 in 1995 to 19 in 2011, a concerning rise has been observed again, with the rate increasing from 14.0 in 2020 to 15.3 in 2023 (Rajapakse, 2017; Sustainable Development Council, 2025). These figures underscore the urgent need to build mental health capacity across the island.

The provision of mental health services in Sri Lanka is primarily led by psychiatrists, supported by a network of doctors, nurses, and allied health professionals (Amarasinghe & Rajapakse, 2024). Most care is delivered through the public health system, which provides services free-of-charge. However, with only 0.47 psychiatrists per 100,000 people and significant regional disparities—particularly in areas like the Northern Province—access to specialized mental health care remains limited (Pathirathne & Kulathilake, 2024). Migration of psychiatrists continues to hinder the expansion of services (Chandradasa & Kuruppuarachchi, 2024). Despite these challenges, 23 out of 24 districts now have acute inpatient units (Amarasinghe & Rajapakse, 2024). Given the shortage of specialists, the role of primary care physicians in identifying, treating, and managing mental disorders has become increasingly critical.

There is a growing recognition of the need to equip not only doctors but also nurses, midwives, and allied health professionals with the skills to provide mental health care. This aligns with the recommendations of the World Health Organization (WHO) for task-shifting and task-sharing to address the mental health gap in low- and middle-income countries (WHO, 2016). Comprehensive, well-structured training programs at undergraduate and postgraduate levels, as well as ongoing professional development, are essential to meet these demands. This chapter explores the evolution, current status, and future directions of psychiatric education and training in Sri Lanka—spanning medical students, postgraduate trainees, allied health professionals, and the broader community.

## 2 Undergraduate Psychiatry Education

### 2.1 *Historical Developments*

Undergraduate psychiatric education in Sri Lanka has undergone a transformative journey over the past few decades (Hapangama et al., 2023). Although undergraduate medical education in Sri Lanka dates back to 1870 when the Colombo Medical School was established during the British colonial period, psychiatric teaching was not introduced until the 1960s, and its role in the curriculum remained marginal for much of the twentieth century (Amarasinghe, 2024). Until the 1990s, psychiatry was generally confined to a few lectures and a short clinical attachment during the third or fourth year of study. The subject was not independently examined; instead, it was assessed through a single structured essay and a few multiple-choice questions (MCQs) as part of the final medicine paper. As a result, many graduates completed their training with minimal understanding of psychiatry, often perpetuating stigma and diagnostic inaccuracy in clinical practice (Gambheera & Williams, 2011).

A landmark shift occurred in 1995 when the Faculty of Medicine at the University of Colombo introduced a separate Mental Health Module and expanded the clinical attachment in psychiatry to two months in the final year. This reform also introduced an independent final-year examination in psychiatry. These changes aligned with the WHO's call for the reorientation of medical education at the time (Amarasinghe, 2024). These progressive steps elevated the status of psychiatry in medical education and influenced other state universities in Sri Lanka to revise their curricula accordingly.

Another major milestone was the introduction of the national core curriculum in psychiatry in 2017 (Hanwella & De Silva, 2024; Hapangama et al., 2023). Approved by the University Grants Commission of Sri Lanka, this curriculum created a unified framework for undergraduate psychiatry teaching and assessment across all state medical faculties (University Grants Commission, 2017). While individual universities have retained unique approaches, this core curriculum has ensured consistency in learning outcomes and assessment standards throughout the country. Since 2018, psychiatry has been recognized as one of the five final-year clinical specialties contributing to the merit ranking for internship placement, alongside medicine, surgery, obstetrics and gynecology, and pediatrics. This has significantly increased students' motivation to engage meaningfully with the discipline.

### 2.2 *Current Training and Assessment*

Today, all state medical faculties in Sri Lanka provide 8–10 weeks of dedicated clinical training in psychiatry. Students rotate through inpatient and outpatient settings under supervision, gaining hands-on experience in diagnosing and managing a range of mental health conditions. Exposure to community-based mental health services adds further depth to their training. For instance, at the University of Kelaniya, medical students spend one week in the field, visiting community-based organizations and rehabilitation centers supporting people with mental illness, dementia, and substance use disorders. Teaching methods in Sri Lankan medical schools have gradually shifted away from traditional didactic lectures toward more student-centered and interactive approaches (Rodrigo et al., 2012). These include small group discussions, problem-based learning (PBL), student-led seminars, and case-based teaching. Some faculties incorporate elements of medical humanities, such as reflective essays, film discussions, or drama, to enhance students' empathetic engagement with mental illness. For instance, a film related to dementia has been used successfully to provide an empathetic understanding of this condition to medical students (Baminiwatta et al., 2023).

Assessment is both comprehensive and rigorous, and follows the core curriculum recommendations (University Grants Commission, 2017; Hapangama et al., 2023). All students sit for a theory examination consisting of structured essay questions (SEQs) and a standardized MCQ paper common to all universities. Students answer six SEQs, including one on child and adolescent psychiatry, and 50 MCQs. The clinical component includes a long case examination, two mini-observed clinical examinations (MOCEs), and continuous assessment. In the long case, a student spends 30 minutes with a patient taking the history and performing a mental state examination, before discussing the case with a panel for over 15 minutes. The theory and clinical components each contributes to 50% of the total marks. Importantly, students are required to pass both theory and clinical components independently to qualify. This ensures that graduates possess a baseline competence in psychiatric diagnosis, communication, and management.

## 2.3 *Outcomes of Undergraduate Psychiatry Education*

Evidence suggests that these curricular changes have had a positive impact. Rodrigo et al. (2012) found a significant increase in positive attitudes toward psychiatry after an eight-week psychiatry clerkship. de Alwis et al. (2013) similarly found enhanced empathy and understanding toward schizophrenia, depression, and heroin use following a clerkship. A nationwide survey further confirmed that final-year students who had completed their psychiatry rotation demonstrated more favorable attitudes toward psychiatry than those who had not (Baminiwatta et al., 2020). A survey among recent medical graduates of a single university reported that, out of the five final-year professorial attachments, the highest satisfaction was for psychiatry, and that, in the final examination, clinical decision-making was best discussed in the psychiatry cases (Karunathilake et al., 2022).

Compared to the structure and extent of psychiatric exposure within medical curricula in other South Asian countries, Sri Lanka appears to stand out (Arafat et al., 2021). There is greater uniformity in the training and assessment methods across universities. The greater duration of clinical exposure to psychiatry, lasting 8–10 weeks, has been a major achievement, and positive effects on students' attitudes have been observed. However, whether the students' interest in psychiatry is retained after they graduate and start working as doctors is questionable. Although some academics have suggested introducing an internship rotation in psychiatry to help graduates sharpen their practical skills in psychiatry and carry the interest forward, this has not yet materialized (Hapangama et al., 2023).

### *2.4 Challenges in Undergraduate Psychiatry Education*

Despite this progress, important challenges remain. One of the most pressing issues is the shortage of academic psychiatrists to facilitate education. The migration of psychiatrists abroad continues to impact both service delivery and education, limiting the pool of experienced faculty available for undergraduate teaching (Chandradasa & Kuruppuarachchi, 2024). In many institutions, existing faculty are overburdened with clinical duties, leaving limited time for curriculum development or educational innovation. Infrastructure limitations also hinder the adoption of more advanced teaching technologies.

Moreover, some important areas of psychiatry remain underrepresented in undergraduate training. These include child and adolescent psychiatry, addiction psychiatry, geriatric psychiatry, and community mental health. Strengthening these components is essential to prepare graduates for the complex and diverse mental health needs of the Sri Lankan population. There is also a need for greater incorporation of interprofessional education and collaboration with allied health disciplines.

The COVID-19 pandemic had a significant impact on medical education. A survey among medical students from eight universities in Sri Lanka reported that there was a substantial impact from the pandemic on the acquisition of skills in mental state examinations, developing rapport with, and diagnosing patients (Baminiwatta et al., 2022). Understandably, peer learning and self-study were less affected. Exams were also affected, more so in the clinical component. Despite these challenges, the pandemic led to the widespread adoption of online education, and may have propelled innovative educational approaches into action—"a blessing in disguise" (Karunathilake & De Abrew, 2021).

## 3 Postgraduate Psychiatry Education

The first Sri Lankan psychiatrist started treating patients in 1940 (Gambheera, 2011). Until the 1980s, medical graduates who wanted to specialize in psychiatry had to go to the UK to receive training as specialists (Chandradasa & Champika, 2019). The Postgraduate Institute of Medicine (PGIM) was established in 1980 and started to offer a five-year program leading to an MD in psychiatry (Gambheera & Williams, 2011). Currently, there are two pathways for postgraduate studies in Psychiatry as MD Psychiatry and Diploma in Psychiatry.

### 3.1 Training of Specialists in Psychiatry

The structure and requirements of the MD Psychiatry program are outlined in a prospectus published by the PGIM, last revised in 2013, and are summarized below (Postgraduate Institute of Medicine, 2013). Any medical officer who successfully completes the PGIM selection test can enroll in the MD Psychiatry training program. The selection examination consists of an MCQ paper and SEQ paper. Candidates are required to obtain a minimum of 50% in each component to be successful in the selection examination. Once enrolled, three years are spent in Stage I (Pre-MD training) as a Registrar before the MD Psychiatry examination. The focus of this period is training in general adult psychiatry, with brief exposures to forensic psychiatry, and child and adolescent psychiatry (three months each). Additionally, registrars receive some exposure to addiction and old age psychiatry at the National Institute of Mental Health, and some tertiary care centers (Gambheera & Williams, 2011). The PGIM conducts formal lectures for trainees, typically once a month, covering key areas in psychiatry.

The training outcomes expected of the trainee are competence for the roles of a medical expert, communicator, collaborator, health advocate, manager, scholar, and a professional (Postgraduate Institute of Medicine, 2013). The supervising consultant must complete a progress report for the trainee at the end of each placement. Trainees are required to have 80% attendance in each major component of training.

Stage I trainees must take an objective structured clinical examination (OSCE) following their first 12 months of training. This assesses their skills in mental state examination, cognitive assessments, psychoeducation, and communication. Trainees must pass the OSCE to be eligible for the MD Psychiatry exam. Additionally, the trainee should submit a casebook of ten case discussions on patients seen during the first 24 months of training, which is assessed by an examiner. Acceptance of the case book by the Board of Study is also a prerequisite for the MD Psychiatry examination.

The MD (Psychiatry) examination comprises two main components: theory and clinical. The examination carries a total of 1000 marks, with 400 allocated to the theory component and 600 to the clinical component. The theory component includes an MCQ paper, SEQ paper, and an essay paper. The clinical component comprises one long case, two observed short cases, and a viva voce examination on patient management problems.

The MD (Psychiatry) degree will be awarded to trainees who successfully complete the examination in both the theory and clinical components. Upon passing, trainees will be eligible to proceed to Stage II of training, which leads to board certification as a psychiatry specialist. Alternatively, depending on the availability of training positions, they may choose to pursue subspecialty training in child and adolescent psychiatry, old age psychiatry, or forensic psychiatry.

To receive board certification, Stage II trainees must complete further organized, supervised training as well as submit a dissertation and portfolio. Training for senior registrars in Stage II is structured as one year in General Adult Psychiatry in Sri

Lanka and one year in General Adult Psychiatry overseas. Historically, most Sri Lankan trainees have traveled to either Australia or the UK for their post-MD overseas training. Hospital-sponsored placements in Australia are perhaps the most sought-after, but some trainees are accepted through the Medical Training Initiative program in the UK. This period of overseas training in an accredited station provides the trainees with the opportunity to learn from a more advanced, high-resource health system, and facilitates the transfer of that knowledge and experience back to Sri Lanka. Once having returned to Sri Lanka from overseas training, the trainee needs to undergo a pre-board certification assessment (PBCA). A portfolio forms the basis of the PBCA. All Stage II trainees are required to complete a research project and submit a dissertation or a publication in a recognized peer-reviewed journal based on the project before applying for board certification.

### 3.2 *Sub-specialization in Psychiatry*

Sub-specialization within psychiatry was introduced more recently. Forensic psychiatry was introduced in 2013 with the mission of producing a forensic psychiatrist skilled in working with mentally disordered offenders and their families, as well as collaborating effectively with health, legal, correctional, and social services, along with other relevant stakeholders, to ensure the delivery of high-quality, ethical, and responsible care (Postgraduate Institute of Medicine, 2013a). For a long time, general adult psychiatrists have been providing opinions to the courts in relation to legal matters such as fitness to plead and criminal responsibility. Despite forensic psychiatry being introduced in 2013, as of now, there are very few forensic psychiatrists working in Sri Lanka, as many have migrated. Therefore, the burden of conducting forensic psychiatric assessments still falls mostly on general adult psychiatrists distributed across the country. Given the large unmet mental health needs of prison populations, and the outdated legal processes involved, forensic psychiatrists in Sri Lanka have a crucial role to play in addressing these broader issues (De Alwis et al., 2024).

Subspecialty in child and adolescent psychiatry was also introduced in 2013, with the objective of fulfilling the unique mental health needs of the 0–18 years age group (Postgraduate Institute of Medicine, 2013b). The objective was to produce a child and adolescent psychiatrist who is competent in working with children, adolescents and their families and with health, educational, legal and social agencies and other stakeholders involved in the care of children and adolescents, and to provide optimum care in a responsible and ethical manner. As with forensic psychiatry, the number of child and adolescent psychiatrists remaining in Sri Lanka has been dwindling, making it challenging to develop specialized services to address the rising mental health needs of this population (Shoib et al., 2022). Lack of human resources, particularly in the peripheral parts of the country, and the lack of inpatient facilities for young people have also been major barriers (Chandradasa & Champika, 2019). There may be some reluctance from trainees to take up this subspecialty, as it involves an additional year of training and has fewer opportunities for overseas training.

Old age psychiatry was introduced as a subspecialty in 2017 (Postgraduate Institute of Medicine, 2017). Sri Lanka has one of the world's fastest-aging populations, and it has been projected that the proportion of Sri Lankans above the age of 60 years will increase from 16.4% in 2022 to 23.5% by 2042 (De Silva & de Silva, 2023). Suicide rate in Sri Lanka is highest in those above 65 years, especially among males (Baminiwatta, 2024). The burden of dementia management is expected to expand. To address these growing needs, advanced professional training in old age psychiatry is necessary. However, as with the other two subspecialties, owing to similar reasons, the interest among trainees remains low, and retention of those who complete training in this subspecialty has been difficult.

### *3.3 Non-Specialist Qualifications in Psychiatry*

In 2007, to mitigate the gap due to the lack of qualified specialists in psychiatry and to improve community-based mental health care, the PGIM introduced a new training program known as the Diploma in Psychiatry (Hapangama et al., 2023). This is a postgraduate training program spanning one year, but it does not enable the holder to claim specialist or consultant status (Postgraduate Institute of Medicine, 2023). Training includes clinical training, lectures, and field visits. The trainee should submit a case book and maintain a log book. The Diploma in Psychiatry exam is composed of a written component with MCQ and SEQ papers, followed by a clinical component composed of one long case and two short cases. Positions known as Medical Officer of Mental Health (MOMH) have been introduced to provide mental health services to areas not covered by specialists, and they are usually occupied by diploma holders or medical officers with a three-month special training in psychiatry.

### *3.4 Challenges in Postgraduate Psychiatry Training*

There are many challenges facing postgraduate psychiatry training in Sri Lanka. "Brain drain" in the field of psychiatry has been a long-standing issue. This can potentially affect the quality of postgraduate training programs, as experienced psychiatrists are an important asset for the training and assessment of trainees. Although things had started to settle somewhat after the war ended in 2009, there was a major exodus of professionals again during the economic crisis in 2022–2023 (Chandradasa & Kuruppuarachchi, 2024). Perhaps due to the comprehensive nature of the psychiatry training and the exposure to an overseas health system as part of it, Sri Lankan psychiatrists have often been able to find employment overseas without much difficulty. When trainees return to Sri Lanka after their overseas training, they are usually stationed at remote locations in the country with very limited resources, often having to live away from family. Due to limited financial incentives and relatively low salaries, many psychiatrists choose to pursue career opportunities abroad. Better quality of life, social security, and career development opportunities have also been cited as reasons for migrating (De Silva et al., 2013). To discourage this, for every year spent overseas in training, there is a bond between the trainee and the government that requires a specialist to work for a minimum of four years in Sri Lanka, and those who leave within this bonded period need to pay a fairly large sum of money to the government.

Stigma due to working in the mental health field—courtesy stigma—is significantly high among mental health professionals in Sri Lanka (Liyanage et al., 2018). Medical graduates are often discouraged by their families and friends from pursuing careers in psychiatry. However, the expansion of training in psychiatry during the undergraduate years is expected to mitigate stigmatizing attitudes of future doctors. Greater community awareness on mental health may reduce social stigma related to this field in the future.

The use of psychotherapy to treat mental disorders has decreased as biological medicines have become more widely available. Consequently, opportunities for psychotherapy training have decreased (Hanwella, 2012). Yet, psychotherapy remains an important, and for some patients, the only therapy. Improving psychotherapeutic competencies among postgraduate students is vital to improve standards of postgraduate psychiatry training. The shortage of psychiatrists with formal training and/or significant experience in psychotherapy remaining in Sri Lanka makes it difficult to facilitate formal psychotherapy training for the trainees.

## 4 Training of Nurses and Allied Health Professionals

Sri Lanka has made significant strides in developing a multidisciplinary mental health workforce. The following section outlines the training pathways for key professionals involved in mental health service delivery, including nurses, occupational therapists, social workers, and psychologists.

### *4.1 Nurses*

Nursing students receive one month of clinical training in psychiatry and lectures on mental health during the 3-year nursing degree program (Kathriarachchi, 2019). The National Institute of Mental Health (NIMH) houses a nurses' training school that conducts a core program for student nurses over five weeks. In addition, the Ministry of Health offers a six-month training program in community psychiatry nursing (Rajasuriya et al., 2021), where selected nurses receive 18 weeks of English-medium instruction at the NIMH, followed by a clinical placement in a psychiatric unit within an assigned region. Community psychiatry nurses (CPNs) are usually stationed in tertiary care hospitals or the NIMH and assist in conducting community mental health programs.

## 4.2 Occupational Therapists

The School of Physiotherapy and Occupational Therapy, located at the National Hospital of Sri Lanka, has been training occupational therapists since 1976, including training in psychosocial rehabilitation, and offers a diploma in occupational therapy. Additionally, the Faculty of Medicine, University of Kelaniya, offers a Bachelor of Science in Occupational Therapy. Its curriculum, spanning four years, includes more extensive teaching on rehabilitation of mental illnesses, psychosocial disabilities, and community mental health needs. Occupational therapists contribute to the multidisciplinary management in psychiatry units by providing inputs for functional assessment and rehabilitation. However, a shortage of occupational therapists allocated to psychiatric units persists (Jenkins et al., 2012).

## 4.3 Social Workers

Training for psychiatric social workers is currently provided through a three-month program conducted by the Psychiatric Social Work Unit of the NIMH. Since 1978, the Department of Sociology at the University of Peradeniya has offered a Bachelor of Social Work degree. The Postgraduate Institute of Humanities and Social Sciences at the same university offers a Master's degree in Social Work. The National Institute of Social Development (formerly, the School of Social Work) has also trained social workers and was given degree-granting status in 2005. These training programs include some formal teaching on social work related to mental health, and on basic counseling skills.

## 4.4 Psychologists

In Sri Lanka, only a few government universities offer specialized undergraduate degrees in psychology, most of which began in the 1990s. Several private institutions, often affiliated with foreign universities, also provide psychology programs, though the quality of these courses is often questioned. The lack of regulation in psychology education has hindered the discipline's development (Hettigoda & Kularatne, 2024). The first postgraduate program in clinical psychology—a Master of Philosophy (MPhil)—was introduced in 2008 (de Zoysa, 2013). However, currently, there is no designated cadre for clinical psychologists in the state health system, though reforms are underway (Rajasuriya et al., 2021). As a result, most clinical psychologists practice in the private sector. A register of clinical psychologists is maintained by the Sri Lanka Medical Council (SLMC), but it is not yet available online.

### *4.5 Primary Care Workers*

The integration of mental health into primary and community care is a key focus of the 2020–2030 National Mental Health Policy (Ministry of Health, 2021). It promotes the establishment of Primary Community Mental Health Centres (PCMHCs) in each Medical Officer of Health (MOH) area in every district. Primary health services are delivered by teams including the MOH, Public Health Nursing Sister, Public Health Inspector, and Public Health Midwives (PHMs) (Hapangama & Kuruppuarachchi, 2021). PHMs are central to promoting maternal mental health, and their knowledge, skills, and confidence in delivering mental health interventions can be strengthened through pre-service and in-service midwifery education programs. The Maternal Care Package, introduced by the Family Health Bureau, serves as a guideline for field-level healthcare workers, including PHMs, and provides instructions on screening for postpartum depression using the Edinburgh Postnatal Depression Scale.

These capacity-building efforts align with the priorities outlined in the National Mental Health Policy and global initiatives such as the WHO Mental Health Gap Action Programme (mhGAP). However, significant challenges remain, including a shortage of allied health professionals, limited access to postgraduate training, and insufficient continuing professional development opportunities for frontline mental health personnel. Addressing these gaps requires investment in training infrastructure, academic collaboration, and workforce planning.

## 5 Continuing Professional Development (CPD)

CPD is essential for developing a competent and effective health workforce. The future of CPD in Sri Lanka appears promising, especially with the upcoming implementation of a national CPD program for medical officers (Karunathilake et al., 2023). Preliminary investigations have demonstrated stakeholder satisfaction with web-based CPD efforts in terms of cost-effectiveness, productivity, simplicity, flexibility, and information accessibility (Karunathilake et al., 2023). CPD targeting medical officers and postgraduate trainees is conducted regularly by the Sri Lanka College of Psychiatrists (SLCPsych), sometimes in collaboration with other bodies such as the Sri Lanka Medical Association.

A CPD program for Sri Lankan psychiatrists, composed of core outcomes such as knowledge development, skills development, change in attitude and behavior, and personal development, was launched back in 2015 (Kathriarachchi, 2016).

However, the sustainability and practical application of these programs have been difficult given that the country's CPD framework is still being built (Karunathilake et al., 2023). The SLCPsych continues to conduct education and training for medical officers preparing for the selection examination in MD Psychiatry, monthly medical education sessions, and the Annual Academic Sessions with the participation of national and international experts. Shortcomings in our nation's digital infrastructure have been a major barrier to the expansion of CPD initiatives, especially into the rural regions (Karunathilake et al., 2020).

## 6 Raising Public Awareness on Mental Health

Stigma, prejudice, and discrimination against people with mental illness are widespread in Sri Lanka. People often use religious and supernatural explanatory models to understand mental illness. However, with increasing awareness of mental health services, people may be moving away from these cultural models to more medical/biological models. Surveys among the general public, including adolescents, undergraduates, and caregivers, have revealed deficits in mental health literacy (Abesinghe et al., 2023; Attygalle et al., 2017; Ediriweera et al., 2012; Amarasuriya et al., 2015). Mental health is gravely neglected in the school curriculum. Programs designed to improve mental health literacy among school students and teachers have been proposed, but have not yet become mainstream (Ginige et al., 2021; Vithana et al., 2023).

Psychiatrists working in teaching and district general hospitals play an important role in raising public awareness of mental health across the country. The SLCPsych has developed leaflets and YouTube videos for the public and conducts media campaigns to increase awareness and combat stigma (Kathriarachchi, 2019). Some non-governmental organizations also work toward enhancing awareness in the community. As digital literacy is increasing among the public, digital platforms are becoming increasingly important modes of knowledge dissemination.

## 7 Training Infrastructure

Currently, there are 12 medical colleges in Sri Lanka recognized by the Sri Lanka Medical Council. Most of them have a separate department for psychiatry, although in a few schools, academic psychiatrists are attached to general medical departments. These departments are affiliated with a psychiatry unit in a university-affiliated hospital where inpatient and outpatient psychiatric services are provided, and where both undergraduate and postgraduate psychiatric training takes place. Postgraduate training also occurs at the NIMH and a few other centers not affiliated with universities. The university psychiatry units are often teeming with medical students, with up to about 50 students doing a rotation in psychiatry at the same time in some centers. Classroom spaces and teaching/learning equipment are insufficient to meet the demands. Most universities have started to develop e-learning resources, but the limited availability of devices and Internet facilities remains barriers. Typically, about 20 new postgraduate trainee slots are opened every year, distributed across 8–10 centers. There is limited availability of libraries, e-learning resources, or dedicated study spaces for trainees in these centers.

## 8 Way Forward

Although much has already been achieved in undergraduate psychiatry education in Sri Lanka, further effort is required to mitigate stigma and instill positive attitudes toward psychiatry among future doctors. Curricula need to be reviewed and updated regularly to reflect advances in research and technology occurring globally, while retaining cultural relevance. Online learning modules need to be developed to better facilitate remote learning. Novel educational approaches such as AI-based simulation could be explored. However, to support these strategies, the pertinent infrastructure (digital devices, internet facilities, etc.) needs to be put in place. Training university lecturers to design and implement digital educational tools, perhaps through exchange programs with international institutions, would be another crucial step. The needs of both students and faculty should be formally studied.

Postgraduate training should also be further strengthened. As Williams (2024) suggests, psychiatrists working in South Asian countries like Sri Lanka amidst limited resources may need a wider range of knowledge, skills, and attitudes compared to a psychiatrist in a high-income country working within a narrow niche. To this end, he identifies four domains that the postgraduate training in psychiatry in South Asia should address: (a) clinical acumen, particularly a firm grounding in the local culture, and ability to treat a wide range of disorders; (b) training as a teacher and educationist to facilitate task-shifting and task-sharing, and raise public awareness (c) leadership for service development, and (d) skills in conducting locally relevant research.

Furthermore, the digital educational tools mentioned above would be relevant for postgraduate training as well. To meet the mental health needs of the population, the number of trainee positions available for postgraduate training, especially for subspecialties, should be increased. To achieve this, the frequency of entry exams for postgraduate training could be increased from yearly to twice a year (Hanwella & De Silva, 2024). However, infrastructure for postgraduate training should be developed to facilitate this. Leveraging the expertise of Sri Lankan psychiatrists who have migrated abroad can enhance postgraduate psychiatry education. A move toward "brain exchange" to compensate for "brain drain" has been suggested (Altbach, 2015; Chandradasa & Kuruppuarachchi, 2024). This could be a useful strategy to facilitate psychotherapy education, enhance research skills, to foster awareness on international perspectives on patient rights and mental health legislation, and on newer drugs and treatments such as neuromodulation (e.g., transcranial magnetic stimulation) currently not available in Sri Lanka.

Although the psychiatry training units in Sri Lanka have tried to adopt a multidisciplinary approach, the shortage of allied health professionals has been a barrier. Amending this is important to enable both psychiatry trainees and allied health professionals to develop skills in working together effectively within a multidisciplinary space. Training for allied health professionals needs further expansion and refinement. Steps should be taken to standardize clinical psychology education and create a cadre of clinical psychologists within the state health system. Interdisciplinary collaboration in teaching and training of mental health professionals of different categories is required. A comprehensive framework for CPD related to mental health care should be formalized and implemented by the College of psychiatrists. Public awareness programs should be planned and distributed widely across the country, covering both urban and rural areas.

## 9 Conclusion

Sri Lanka has made substantial progress in psychiatric education and training, particularly at the undergraduate and postgraduate levels. With the introduction of the national core curriculum in 2017, there has been greater standardization of undergraduate psychiatric education across universities, leading to improved knowledge and attitudes toward mental health among doctors. However, the country faces significant challenges, including a shortage of qualified academic psychiatrists, and limited training infrastructure. Further investment is needed to enhance faculty development and incorporate innovative teaching methodologies. Strengthening collaborations with allied health professionals, enhancing psychotherapy education, and increasing training opportunities for subspecialties are essential to meet the growing mental health needs of the population. A comprehensive approach to improving mental health literacy, reducing stigma, and enhancing continuing professional development will be crucial for the future of psychiatric education and care in Sri Lanka.

## References

Abesinghe, A. M. I. D., Katuwawela, K. P. D. K. I., Lakmali, K. P. W., Jayanetti, N. L., Munidasa, K. G. P. K., De Silva, B. S. S., & Marikar, F. M. M. T. (2023). Mental health literacy: A survey of the public's ability to recognize mental disorders and their knowledge about the effectiveness of helpful interventions to help the victims. *Journal of Evidence-Based Psychotherapies, 23*(2), 173–202. https://doi.org/10.24193/jebp.2023.2.16

Altbach, P. (2015). Brain drain or brain exchange: Developing country implications. *International Higher Education, 2*. https://doi.org/10.6017/ihe.2013.72.6095

Alwis, I., Baminiwatta, A., & Chandradasa, M. (2024). Prevalence and associated factors of depression in Sri Lanka: A systematic review and meta-analysis. *Social Psychiatry and Psychiatric Epidemiology, 59*(2), 353–373. https://doi.org/10.1007/s00127-023-02495-z

de Alwis, A., Perera, R., Vasantha, H. L., Henegama, T., & Fernando, S. (2013). The attitude of medical students towards the mental mentally ill: The impact of a clinical attachment in Psychiatry. *Sri Lanka Journal of Psychiatry, 3*, 12–15. https://doi.org/10.4038/sljpsyc.v3i2.5132

Amarasinghe, S. (2024). Eminent personalities in the field of psychiatry in Sri Lanka; Emeritus Professor Nalaka Mendis interviewed by College President Dr. Sajeewana Amarasinghe. *Sri Lanka Journal of Psychiatry, 15*(2), 6–12. https://doi.org/10.4038/sljpsyc.v15i2.8603

Amarasinghe, S. C., & Rajapakse, T. N. (2024). Psychiatric morbidity and mental health services in Sri Lanka. In *Access to mental health care in South Asia* (pp. 137–153). Springer Nature Singapore. https://doi.org/10.1007/978-981-99-9153-2_8

Amarasuriya, S. D., Jorm, A. F., & Reavley, N. J. (2015). Depression literacy of undergraduates in a non-western developing context: The case of Sri Lanka. *BMC Research Notes, 8*, 593. https://doi.org/10.1186/s13104-015-1589-7

Arafat, S., Kar, S., Sharma, P., Marahatta, K., & Baminiwatta, A. (2021). A comparative analysis of psychiatry curriculum at undergraduate level of Bangladesh, India, Nepal, and Sri Lanka. *Indian Journal of Psychiatry, 63*(2), 184–188. https://doi.org/10.4103/psychiatry.IndianJPsychiatry_615_20

Attygalle, U. R., Perera, H., & Jayamanne, B. D. W. (2017). Mental health literacy in adolescents: Ability to recognise problems, helpful interventions and outcomes. *Child and Adolescent Psychiatry and Mental Health, 11*(1), 38–38. https://doi.org/10.1186/s13034-017-0176-1

Baminiwatta, A. (2024). *Changing patterns of suicide among the elderly in Sri Lanka from 2015 to 2022: An analysis based on national suicide statistics*. Annual Academic Sessions of the Sri Lanka College of Psychiatrists.

Baminiwatta, A. K. A. B., Bandara, W. A. V. S., Athurugiriya, A. A. I. D., Yangdon, T., Cader, G. R., Bokalamulla, L. A. B., Bandara, W. R. R. D., Bandara, W. M. K. M., Chandradasa, K. A. S. I. P., Athukorala, H. P., & Dias, G. S. S. R. (2020). A nationwide survey of attitudes towards psychiatry among final-year medical students in Sri Lanka. *Asian Journal of Psychiatry, 52*, 102101. https://doi.org/10.1016/j.ajp.2020.102101

Baminiwatta, A., Dayabandara, M., De Silva, J., Gadambanathan, T., Ginige, P., Premarathne, I., Rajapaksha, H., Wickramasinghe, A., Sivayokan, S., & Wijesinghe, C. (2022). Perceived impact of the COVID-19 pandemic on psychiatric training among final-year medical undergraduates in Sri Lanka: An online survey of students from eight universities. *Academic Psychiatry, 46*, 729–734. https://doi.org/10.1007/s40596-022-01667-4

Baminiwatta, A., Fernando, R., & Williams, S. (2023). Improving medical students' understanding of dementia using a movie (*The Father*). *Education for Primary Care, 34*(2), 109–109. https://doi.org/10.1080/14739879.2023.2178333

Chandradasa, M., & Champika, L. (2019). Subspecialisation in postgraduate psychiatry and implications for a resource-limited specialised child and adolescent mental health service. *Academic Psychiatry: The Journal of the American Association of Directors of Psychiatric Residency Training and the Association for Academic Psychiatry, 43*(1), 135–139. https://doi.org/10.1007/s40596-018-0920-8

Chandradasa, M., & Kuruppuarachchi, K. A. L. A. (2024). Brain drain among Sri Lankan psychiatrists. *Sri Lanka Journal of Psychiatry, 14*(2), 1–3. https://doi.org/10.4038/sljpsyc.v14i2.8529

De Alwis, L. A. P., Seneviratne, V. L., Mendis, T. S. S., & Abhayanayaka, C. (2024). The development of laws related to the disposal of forensic patients in Sri Lanka: A historical review. *Sri Lanka Journal of Psychiatry, 15*(2), 13–22. https://doi.org/10.4038/sljpsyc.v15i2.8569

De Silva, W. I., & de Silva, R. (2023). Growth and structural changes of Sri Lankan population during coming decades with special reference to youth and elderly. *Sri Lanka Statistical Review, 2*(1).

De Silva, A. P., Liyanage, I. K., De Silva, S. T. G., Jayawardana, M. B., Liyanage, C. K., & Karunathilake, I. M. (2013). Migration of Sri Lankan medical specialists. *Human Resources for Health, 11*(1), 21. https://doi.org/10.1186/1478-4491-11-21

Ediriweera, H. W., Fernando, S. M., & Pai, N. B. (2012). Mental health literacy survey among Sri Lankan Carers of patients with Schizophrenia and Depression. *Asian Journal of Psychiatry, 5*(3), 246–250. https://doi.org/10.1016/j.ajp.2012.02.016

Gambheera, H. (2011). The evolution of psychiatric services in Sri Lanka. *South Asian Journal of Psychiatry, 2*(1).
Gambheera, H., & Williams, S. (2011). Psychiatric training in Sri Lanka and its relevance to South Asia. *South Asian Journal of Psychiatry, 2*(2).
Ginige, P., Perera, I. B. R. U., Arambepola, S. C. A., Kuruwita, K. A. P. R., & Gunawardena, E. R. N. D. (2021). The impact of a specialized training programme on teacher mental health literacy in Central Sri Lanka. *Sri Lanka Journal of Medicine, 30*(1), 34–34. https://doi.org/10.4038/sljm.v30i1.243
Hanwella, R. (2012). Postgraduate training in psychotherapy in Sri Lanka: The need for a systematic approach. *Sri Lanka Journal of Psychiatry, 2*(2), 49. https://doi.org/10.4038/sljpsyc.v2i2.4039
Hanwella, R., & De Silva, V. (2024). Undergraduate psychiatry education in Sri Lanka: The current situation and the way forward. *Sri Lanka Journal of Psychiatry, 15*(1), 1–4. https://doi.org/10.4038/sljpsyc.v15i1.8565
Hapangama, A., & Kuruppuarachchi, K. A. L. A. (2021). Maternal mental health services in Sri Lanka: Challenges and solutions. *BJPsych International, 18*(4), 100–102. https://doi.org/10.1192/bji.2020.52
Hapangama, A., Kuruppuarachchi, K. A. L. A., & Hanwella, R. (2023). Achievements and challenges in psychiatric education and training in Sri Lanka. *BJPsych International, 20*(1), 2–4. https://doi.org/10.1192/bji.2021.35
Hettigoda, K., & Kularatne, N. (2024). Psychology in Sri Lanka. In *The handbook of international psychology* (2nd ed.). Routledge.
Institute for Research and Development. (2007). *National survey on mental health in Sri Lanka.*
Jenkins, R., Mendis, J., Cooray, S., & Cooray, M. (2012). Integration of mental health into primary care in Sri Lanka. *Mental Health in Family Medicine, 9*(1), 15–24.
Karunathilake, I. M., Bandara, J., Attygalle, D., Gunawardena, C. N., Egodage, T., & Chandrasena, U. (2020). Primary healthcare strengthening through distance education for health professionals. *South-East Asian Journal of Medical Education, 14*(2). https://doi.org/10.4038/seajme.v14i2.281
Karunathilake, I. M., & De Abrew, A. (2021). The Global Pandemic—A blessing in disguise for medical education innovations. *South-East Asian Journal of Medical Education, 15*(2). https://doi.org/10.4038/seajme.v15i2.377
Karunathilake, I. M., Fernando, H. C., & Marambe, K. N. (2023). Continuous professional development in the Sri Lankan health system: Past, present and future. *South-East Asian Journal of Medical Education, 17*(2), 57–63. https://doi.org/10.4038/seajme.v17i2.578
Karunathilake, I. M., Gunawardhane, H. P. M. C., Somaratne, G. T. S. V., & Dias, N. W. G. L. T. L. (2022). Graduate perception on the Undergraduate Medical Curriculum. *South-East Asian Journal of Medical Education, 16*(1), 59–68. https://doi.org/10.4038/seajme.v16i1.430
Kathriarachchi, S. T. (2016). *Continuing professional development for psychiatrists in Sri Lanka.*
Kathriarachchi, S. T. (2019). Development of mental health care in Sri Lanka lessons learned. *Taiwanese Journal of Psychiatry (Taipei), 2019*(33), 55–65.
Liyanage, U. L. N. S., Rowel, W. W. J. S. M., Hewawitharana, U. H., de Silva, V., & Dissanayake, D. M. T. (2018). Stigma due to their work in mental health, among mental health professionals in Sri Lanka. *Sri Lanka Journal of Psychiatry, 9*(1). https://doi.org/10.4038/sljpsyc.v9i1.8174
Ministry of Health. (2021). *National Mental Health Policy 2020–2030.* https://mentalhealth.health.gov.lk/images/2022/NationalMentalHealthPolicy_Final_12.10.2021PRINT-1.pdf
Pathirathne, W. P. K. G., & Kulathilake, S. (2024, July 26). *Survey on available numbers of consultant psychiatrists in the government sector of Sri Lanka [Conference Presentation].* Annual Academic Sessions of the Sri Lanka College of Psychiatrists 2024, Colombo, Sri Lanka.
Postgraduate Institute of Medicine – University of Colombo. (2013a). *Board certification in forensic psychiatry: Postgraduate course conducted by the Board of Study in Psychiatry.*

https://pgim.cmb.ac.lk/wp-content/uploads/2016/07/09.05.2013sub-speciality-in-Forensic-Psychiatry2-1.pdf

Postgraduate Institute of Medicine – University of Colombo. (2013b). *Postgraduate Course Conducted by the Board of Study in Psychiatry for Board Certification in Child and Adolescent Psychiatry*. https://drive.google.com/file/d/1gKrWaY9Qp2W8Y-No7SoSxAwbFQ5UIbkt/view

Postgraduate Institute of Medicine – University of Colombo. (2017). *Board Certification as a Specialist in Old Age Psychiatry*. https://drive.google.com/file/d/18rG-8uTlb5BrwkPfZ60RLe9Suj7EPspX/view

Postgraduate Institute of Medicine – University of Colombo. (2023). *Postgraduate Diploma in Psychiatry*. https://drive.google.com/file/d/1FOOt-kAT1OeFKYI0sYTgjgSJ_g7xfhIn/view

Postgraduate Institute of Medicine University of Colombo. (2013). *MD Psychiatry and Board Certification in Psychiatry: Prospectus*.

Rajapakse, T. N. (2017). A review of the changing patterns of suicide and deliberate self-harm in Sri Lanka. *Sri Lanka Journal of Psychiatry, 8*(1), 3. https://doi.org/10.4038/sljpsyc.v8i1.8132

Rajasuriya, M., Hewagama, M., Ruwanpriya, S., & Wijesundara, H. (2021). Community-based psychiatric services in Sri Lanka: A model by WHO in the making. *Consortium Psychiatricum, 2*(4), 40–52. https://doi.org/10.17816/CP106

Rodrigo, A., Wijesinghe, C., & Kuruppuarachchi, K. (2012). Changes in attitudes toward psychiatry with introduction of a new curriculum: Experiences of a Sri Lankan medical school. *Sri Lanka Journal of Psychiatry, 3*(1), 14–16.

Shoib, S., Chandradasa, M., Rathnayake, L., Usmani, S., & Saeed, F. (2022). Children, adolescent, and youth mental health in Sri Lanka in the context of recent violence, COVID-19, and economic crisis: A call for action. *The Lancet Regional Health – Southeast Asia, 2*, 100021. https://doi.org/10.1016/j.lansea.2022.100021

Sustainable Development Council. (2025). *Status Report on SDG Indicators: Sri Lanka*.

University Grants Commission. (2017). *Core curriculum of psychiatry: Objectives and guidelines for the psychiatry programme of all medical faculties in Sri Lanka*.

Vithana, C., Lokubalasooriya, A., Pragasan, G., Mahagamage, K. L., Nanayakkara, K., Herath, H. P., Karunarathna, P., Perera, N., de Silva, C., Jayawardene, D., & Wickramasinghe, N. D. (2023). Effectiveness of an educational intervention to promote psychosocial well-being of school-going adolescents in Sri Lanka. *BMC Public Health, 23*(1), 2185–2185. https://doi.org/10.1186/s12889-023-17023-6

Williams, S. S. (2024). Fine-tuning postgraduate psychiatry training in South Asia. *Indian Journal of Psychological Medicine, 46*(5), 380–381. https://doi.org/10.1177/02537176241280284

World Health Organization. (2016). *mhGAP intervention guide for mental, neurological and substance use disorders in non-specialized health settings: Mental Health Gap Action Programme (mhGAP): Version 2.0*.

de Zoysa, P. (2013). Clinical psychology in a medical setting in Sri Lanka. *International Psychiatry, 10*(1), 18–19. Cambridge Core. https://doi.org/10.1192/S174936760000357X

# Chapter 10
# Psychiatry Teaching and Training in Bhutan and Maldives

**Ankita Saroj and Sujita Kumar Kar**

**Abstract** South Asia, well-known for its vibrant cultures and rich history, is also one of the most densely populated regions in the world. Unfortunately, this high population density is paired with a significant shortage of trained mental health professionals, many of whom lack adequate training to meet the complex mental health needs of their communities. In this context, education and training in psychiatry emerge as critical pillars within a nation's mental health care framework. Within this region, Bhutan and the Maldives stand out as two small yet unique countries. Both nations face an urgent need for more comprehensive information on the teaching and training of psychiatry, which is often limited. This chapter aims to explore and illuminate the current trends and practices in psychiatric education and training in Bhutan and the Maldives, highlighting the challenges and opportunities that exist for improving mental health care in these countries.

**Keywords** Psychiatry education · Psychiatry teaching · Psychiatry training · Bhutan · Maldives

## 1 Introduction

Teaching and training in psychiatry play a crucial role in the overall mental healthcare framework of a nation. These educational programs are designed to provide healthcare professionals with an in-depth understanding of psychiatric principles, practices, and the latest research developments. Through continuous education, practitioners can refine their clinical skills, stay updated on emerging treatments,

A. Saroj · S. K. Kar (✉)
Department of Psychiatry, King George's Medical University, Lucknow, Uttar Pradesh, India
e-mail: sujitakumarkar@kgmcindia.edu



S. K. Kar et al. (eds.), *Teaching and Training in Psychiatry in South Asia*, South Asian Perspectives in Mental Health and Psychology,
https://doi.org/10.1007/978-981-95-1845-6_10

and learn about new therapeutic approaches tailored to various mental health conditions. Moreover, effective psychiatry training fosters a collaborative environment where knowledge can be disseminated among peers. This exchange of information not only enhances individual competencies but also contributes to improved mental health outcomes for the community. By prioritizing psychiatry education, we can ensure a workforce that is well-equipped to meet the evolving challenges of mental health care, ultimately leading to better support for individuals in need. South Asia is a highly populated region of the world with a paucity of mental health human resources and most of them are undertrained (Gupta & Menon, 2022; Kallivayalil, 2012; Kallivayalil & Enara, 2021; Singh & Ng, 2008; Trivedi & Dhyani, 2007).

Psychiatric education involves teaching and training of:

- Medical undergraduates.
- Medical postgraduates.
- Super-specialization courses in Psychiatry.
- Paramedical, nurses, and social workers.
- General care physicians.
- Volunteers and non-government organizations involved in mental healthcare.

There is a well-laid curriculum for at least the undergraduate and postgraduate medical students in the majority of the South Asian countries (Arafat et al., 2021; Kallivayalil & Enara, 2021; Kar, 2022; Williams, 2024). There is gross heterogeneity in the duration and pattern of training courses across the countries in South Asian region (Arafat et al., 2021; Kallivayalil & Enara, 2021). Bhutan and Maldives are two small countries in the South Asian region. There is a paucity of information related to the teaching and training of psychiatry in Bhutan and the Maldives. This chapter aims at elucidating the trends of teaching and training of psychiatry in Bhutan and the Maldives.

## 2 Psychiatry Teaching and Training in Bhutan

Bhutan is a small Himalayan kingdom renowned for its distinctive approach to development, known as Gross National Happiness (GNH). Over the last few decades, healthcare and education in Bhutan have seen significant improvement. Mental health, which was earlier stigmatized and neglected, is now becoming a more prominent topic of discussion. The teaching and training of psychiatry have evolved over time, similar to the advancements in Bhutan's health system and medical education (Nirola, 2010; Tobgay et al., 2011).

In Bhutan, psychiatry is based on a cultural background that has always seen mental illness through spiritual and karmic lenses. The traditional Bhutanese medical system attributed spirit possession, karma, or imbalances in wind energy to emotional and mental problems for hundreds of years. As a result, the first people to help with mental illness were often religious figures, like lamas, astrologers, and shamans (DORJI, 2004). Even though biomedical research is getting better at understanding mental illness around the world, these beliefs still exist alongside modern psychiatric practice in Bhutan. This coexistence has affected how psychiatry is taught and received in both clinical and community settings (Nirola et al., 2015).

In Bhutan, formal psychiatric services did not start getting established until the late twentieth century. In the early 1990s, the psychiatric unit at the Jigme Dorji Wangchuck National Referral Hospital (JDWNRH) in Thimphu opened (DORJI, 2004). This was a big step forward. At first, the service was basic, mostly for outpatients, and depended on generic psychotropic drugs. It was supported by psychiatrists from other countries, including professionals from Burma and Cuba (Nirola, 2010). Bhutan's first locally trained psychiatrist, Dr. Chencho Dorji, played a significant role in transforming this initial effort into a national psychiatric training framework. Dr. Dorji went back to Bhutan after finishing his postgraduate training in psychiatry in Sri Lanka in 1999. He led several structural and academic changes, including the construction of a proper inpatient ward, detoxification facilities, and the development of teaching modules (Gyeltshen et al., 2024).

The Khesar Gyalpo University of Medical Sciences of Bhutan (KGUMSB) opened in 2013, which was a very important time for psychiatry education in Bhutan. The goal of this university was to improve the education and research of medical and health professionals so that the country does not rely on outside training institutions as extensively. It brought together schools of medicine, nursing, and public health into one place, which made it possible for students to get training that crossed disciplines. In this context, psychiatry was added to both the clinical and academic fields. It was first taught in undergraduate medical school and then in postgraduate medical school (Gyeltshen & Dorji, 2020).

The MBBS curriculum at KGUMSB includes psychiatry as a subject. It is designed to give students both theoretical and clinical experience. The ways of teaching include lectures, bedside clinical teaching, case-based discussions, and role-playing. At JDWNRH and other regional referral hospitals, medical students rotate through psychiatric units. There, they learn about a wide range of mental health conditions and treatment options. Some of these are medication, crisis intervention, basic psychotherapy, and community psychiatry. The education is important because it stresses a biopsychosocial approach, which helps students see psychiatric disease in the bigger picture of social factors and Bhutanese cultural ideas (Tenzin et al., 2023).

Psychiatry postgraduate training has been established in response to the nation's pressing need for mental health professionals. The three-year KGUMSB MD-Psychiatry program offers a comprehensive curriculum that meets international standards. The primary training facility is JDWNRH, the country's central referral hospital, which has gradually expanded its facilities to accommodate advanced mental health services. Graduate students engage in consultation-liaison psychiatry, addiction treatment programs, inpatient care, and outpatient services. The academic program encompasses psychotherapy, child and adolescent psychiatry, forensic psychiatry, neuropsychiatry, and research methodology. Additionally, postgraduate students are advised to complete a dissertation, to provide insights regarding trends of mental health. Local education strategies are complemented by visiting faculty from Australia, Sri Lanka, and India, guaranteeing academic diversity and wide exposure (J. Dorji, 2016; Tenzin et al., 2018).

Bhutan's approach to teaching psychiatry extends beyond medical professionals. To increase mental health capacity across different cadres, the nation has devised a multifaceted approach. The Bachelor of Nursing program includes instruction in psychiatric nursing, with an emphasis on psychosocial interventions, therapeutic communication, and mental status assessment. Additionally, Bhutan has invested in providing short-term certificate programs to train general practitioners and health assistants in mental health care (Gyeltshen & Dorji, 2020). The curriculum is based on the WHO's Mental Health Gap Action Programme (mhGAP). These programs are especially crucial for expanding access to psychiatric care in Bhutan's mountainous and isolated areas, where there are currently few specialized services available (Sharma & Joshi, 2024).

For psychiatric training, Bhutan's cultural setting offers both opportunities and challenges. On the one hand, formal mental health treatment is frequently postponed due to deeply held beliefs in karma, spirit possession, and spiritual healing. A lot of patients turn to astrologers or religious leaders for assistance at first, only turning to doctors when their illness gets beyond control. In addition to making the prognosis worse, this delay puts more strain on tertiary care services. Conversely, Bhutan's spiritual traditions provide ways for promoting mental health in a way that is sensitive to cultural differences. Particularly in wellness programs at work and in schools, practices like mindfulness, meditation, and traditional healing are being incorporated into mental health education. Interest in educating professionals and students in culturally appropriate interventions that integrate the principles of cognitive-behavioral therapy and Buddhist philosophy is expanding (Nirola et al., 2015).

There has been increased awareness of mental health education in the policy environment. The first official framework for growing services and training was offered by the National Mental Health Programme, which was launched in 1997. It placed a strong emphasis on developing human resources, lowering stigma, and integrating mental health into general health services (C. Dorji, 2004). The need for community-based interventions and qualified mental health professionals has been reaffirmed more recently by Bhutan's National Mental Health Strategic Plan (2021–2030) and National Suicide Prevention Strategy. Actionable initiatives have resulted from these policies, including the creation of e-learning platforms for health professionals, the training of school counselors, and the incorporation of mental health education into public health education programs (G. Dorji et al., 2017; Pradhan & Lhamo, 2023).

Even with these developments, there are still a number of challenges. The scarcity of qualified psychiatrists is the most immediate obstacle. Less than ten psychiatrists worked in Bhutan as of the middle of the 2020s, with the majority of them based in Thimphu. The availability of services and the capacity to mentor students in regional areas are both restricted by this maldistribution. The demanding nature of psychiatric work, social stigma, and a lack of role models during early training are some of the causes of the shortage. In addition, there is still a lack of development in psychiatric subspecialties like forensic psychiatry, geriatric psychiatry, and child and adolescent psychiatry. Because there are not enough organized psychotherapy modules or trained supervisors, psychotherapy training is also still in its infancy, and the majority of practitioners rely on pharmaceutical approaches (Gyeltshen et al., 2024; Sharma & Joshi, 2024).

Expanding access, enhancing quality, and promoting contextual relevance are key to the future of psychiatry education in Bhutan. This includes formalizing psychotherapy training, creating sub-specialty training tracks, and expanding the MD program. Additionally, interdisciplinary education that incorporates elements of public health, social work, and psychology needs to be improved.

## 3 Psychiatry Teaching and Training in the Maldives

The Maldives is a small island in the Indian Ocean, with a population of more than half a million by 2021 (WHO, 2022). An earlier conducted mental health survey in the Maldives reported the prevalence of Psychiatric disorders in the Maldives to be close to 30% (WHO, 2022). The government of the Maldives is taking initiatives to strengthen the mental healthcare in the country by developing an integrated mental health law, mental health strategic plan, and mental health program to promote mental health (WHO, 2022). Over the past two decades, there has been an improvement in the mental health scene of the Maldives (WHO, 2006, 2016, 2022). The current major challenges related to mental health in the Maldives are (Mohamed & Mansoor, 2025):

- Governance-related challenges.
- Paucity of trained mental health human resources.
- Limited research in mental health in the Maldives.
- Challenges in the availability and accessibility of mental health services.

In 2019, the Centre for Mental Health was established in the Maldives, which aims to facilitate mental healthcare (WHO, 2022). The trained mental health human resources in the Maldives are scarce in the current scenario. Training programs in psychology, counseling, and nursing are available in the Maldives at present (WHO, 2022). As of 2022, 17 psychiatrists, 7 psychologists, and 2 social workers work in the Maldives in the mental health sector (WHO, 2022). The Mental Health Gap Action Program (mhGAP) supported by the World Health Organization (WHO) is trying to train the doctors, nurses, and social workers of Maldives on mental healthcare (WHO, 2022).

The Mental Health Awareness Foundation (MHAF) is a Non-Government Organization (NGO) in Maldives (MHAF, 2015; Ministry of Health, 2022), which works for mental health awareness and it facilitates training on mental health to the doctors, social workers, and nurses in Maldives. The "*Central and Regional Mental Health Services Development Plan 2022–2025*" developed by the Ministry of Health, Maldives, has developed a strategic action framework on a yearly basis from

2022 to 2025 (Ministry of Health, 2022). This document discusses about the teaching and training related to mental health under the "item *4.2 Strengthen the capacity of health care workers to deliver services (prevention, diagnosis, treatment and care), capacity building—whole team approach*" (Ministry of Health, 2022). However, these teachings and trainings are unrelated to undergraduate or postgraduate medical teaching. It is aiming at training individuals, existing doctors, volunteers, non-government organizations, clubs, healthcare workers about prevention of mental illness, promotion of mental health, forensic mental health, community mental health, psychosocial interventions for mental illnesses and case management (Ministry of Health, 2022). The national mental health policy (2015–2025) document developed by the Health Protection Agency, the Ministry of Health, Maldives, in collaboration with the World Health Organization, also emphasizes on human resources and training (capacity building) (WHO Country Office for Maldives, 2017). For mental health capacity building in the Maldives, the focus is on (WHO Country Office for Maldives, 2017):

- *Bridging the human resource gap by training the personals working at the primary healthcare level and those who are providing informal mental healthcare.*
- *Strengthening the teaching at the mental health training institutions.*
- *Initiating new mental health-related courses.*
- *Facilitating overseas training on mental health.*

As there is no scope of medical teaching and training at the Maldives at this moment, the Government of Maldives is largely relying on overseas training for the psychiatrists, clinical psychologists, psychiatric nurses, and psychiatric social workers (Arafat et al., 2021; Kallivayalil & Enara, 2021; WHO Country Office for Maldives, 2017). As there is no facility for formal medical teaching and training of psychiatry at the undergraduate and postgraduate level, the country needs to develop a scheme or program for the skill enhancement of mental health professionals. Digital psychiatry can be a solution to bridge the gap in psychiatry education (Orsolini et al., 2021).

## 4 Conclusion

Bhutan and the Maldives are two small yet vibrant nations located in South Asia, both facing significant challenges in their mental health sectors due to limited resources. In order to significantly enhance the quality and accessibility of mental healthcare services in these countries, it is crucial to focus on developing a robust framework for training mental health professionals. This involves not only investing in essential infrastructure, such as healthcare facilities and support systems, but also creating a well-organized and comprehensive curriculum in psychiatry that meets international standards. Furthermore, attracting and retaining qualified educators in psychiatry is vital for ensuring the next generation of mental health practitioners is well-trained. Both these countries must engage in a thorough evaluation of their unique mental healthcare needs to effectively tailor training programs. By prioritizing investments in psychiatry education and professional development, Bhutan and the Maldives can build a sustainable foundation for improving mental health services and ultimately enhance the well-being of their populations.

## References


Arafat, S. M. Y., Kar, S. K., Sharma, P., Marahatta, K., & Baminiwatta, A. K. A. B. (2021). A comparative analysis of psychiatry curriculum at undergraduate level of Bangladesh, India, Nepal, and Sri Lanka. *Indian Journal of Psychiatry, 63*(2), 184–188. https://doi.org/10.4103/psychiatry.IndianJPsychiatry_615_20

Dorji, C. (2004). *Achieving gross national happiness through community-based mental health services in Bhutan*. Centre for Bhutan Studies. https://fid4sa-repository.ub.uni-heidelberg.de/1358/

Dorji, J. (2016). International influence and support for educational development in Bhutan. In M. J. Schuelka & T. W. Maxwell (Eds.), *Education in Bhutan* (Vol. 36, pp. 109–124). Springer Singapore. https://doi.org/10.1007/978-981-10-1649-3_7

Dorji, G., Choki, S., Jamphel, K., Wangdi, Y., Chogyel, T., Dorji, C., & Nirola, D. K. (2017). Policy and governance to address depression and suicide in Bhutan: The national suicide-prevention strategy. *WHO South-East Asia Journal of Public Health, 6*(1), 39–44. https://doi.org/10.4103/2224-3151.206163

Gupta, S., & Menon, V. (2022). Psychiatry training for medical students: A global perspective and implications for India's competency-based medical education curriculum. *Indian Journal of Psychiatry, 64*(3), 240–251. https://doi.org/10.4103/indianjpsychiatry.indianjpsychiatry_187_22

Gyeltshen, K., Chhetri, B., & Gyeltshen, D. (2024). Delivery of mental health services in Bhutan: Challenges and way forward. *Public Health Challenges, 3*(3), e211. https://doi.org/10.1002/puh2.211

Gyeltshen, K., & Dorji, R. (2020). Higher education in Bhutan: Policy, current status, and challenges. In P. M. Sarangapani & R. Pappu (Eds.), *Handbook of education systems in South Asia* (pp. 1–28). Springer Singapore. https://doi.org/10.1007/978-981-13-3309-5_58-1

Kallivayalil, R. A. (2012). The importance of psychiatry in undergraduate medical education in India. *Indian Journal of Psychiatry, 54*(3), 208. https://doi.org/10.4103/0019-5545.102336

Kallivayalil, R. A., & Enara, A. (2021). Education and training in psychiatry in South Asian countries. *Asia-Pacific Psychiatry, 13*(4), e12494. https://doi.org/10.1111/appy.12494

Kar, S. K. (2022). Post-graduate psychiatry teaching and training in India. *Indian Journal of Behavioural Sciences, 25*(02), Article 02. https://doi.org/10.55229/ijbs.v25i2.11

MHAF. (2015). *MHAF Maldives*. chrome-extension://efaidnbmnnnibpcajpcglclefindmkaj/https://www.rcpsych.ac.uk/docs/default-source/members/sigs/volunteering-and-international-vipsig/vipsig-resources/mhaf-maldives-project.pdf?sfvrsn=e51f1dee_2#:~:text=There%20is%20extremely%20limited%20research,within%20their%20own%20related%20field.

Ministry of Health. (2022, March). *Central and Regional Mental Health Services Development Plan 2022–2025*. Republic of Maldives. chrome-extension://efaidnbmnnnibpcajpcglclefindmkaj/https://health.gov.mv/storage/uploads/NAq7Loeg/opbcrit8.pdf

Mohamed, A., & Mansoor, S. (2025). Challenges and opportunities in the mental health landscape of the Maldives. *Australasian Psychiatry, 33*, 195–196. https://doi.org/10.1177/10398562241289879

Nirola, D. K. (2010). Where psychiatrists are scarce: Bhutan. *Asia-Pacific Psychiatry, 2*(3), 126. https://doi.org/10.1111/j.1758-5872.2010.00073.x

Nirola, D. K., Durham, J. C., & Kraus, K. L. (2015). Balancing traditional beliefs and medical science: Mental health care in Bhutan. *Bhutan Health Journal, 1*(1), 66–69.

Orsolini, L., Jatchavala, C., Noor, I. M., Ransing, R., Satake, Y., Shoib, S., Shah, B., Ullah, I., & Volpe, U. (2021). Training and education in digital psychiatry: A perspective from Asia-Pacific region. *Asia-Pacific Psychiatry, 13*(4), e12501. https://doi.org/10.1111/appy.12501

Pradhan, S., & Lhamo, U. S. (2023). Global crisis, national commitment: Overcoming challenges to inclusive mental health in Bhutan. *The Druk Journal, 9*(1), 71–76.

Sharma, P., & Joshi, D. (2024). Access to mental health care in Bhutan: Current status, potential challenges, and ways out. In S. M. Y. Arafat & S. K. Kar (Eds.), *Access to mental health care in South Asia* (pp. 57–69). Springer Nature Singapore. https://doi.org/10.1007/978-981-99-9153-2_4

Singh, B., & Ng, C. H. (2008). Psychiatric education and training in Asia. *International Review of Psychiatry, 20*(5), 413–418. https://doi.org/10.1080/09540260802397362

Tenzin, K., Dorji, T., Sherub, K., Chhezom, K., Dorji, G., Tshering, K., Choden, R. S., Mukhia, S., Choeda, T., & Galey, K. (2023). An integrated competency-based curriculum for undergraduate medical education programme in Bhutan. *South-East Asian Journal of Medical Education, 17*(2) https://seajme.sljol.info/articles/576

Tenzin, K., Tenzin, T., Dorji, T., & Tshering, K. P. (2018). Curriculum for postgraduate medicine in Bhutan's only medical university: Time for need-based curricula, review, development and implementation. *South-East Asian Journal of Medical Education, 12*(2), 3. https://doi.org/10.4038/seajme.v12i2.46

Tobgay, T., Dophu, U., Torres, C. E., & Na-Bangchang, K. (2011). Health and gross national happiness: Review of current status in Bhutan. *Journal of Multidisciplinary Healthcare, 4*, 293. https://doi.org/10.2147/JMDH.S21095

Trivedi, J. K., & Dhyani, M. (2007). Undergraduate psychiatric education in South Asian countries. *Indian Journal of Psychiatry, 49*(3), 163. https://doi.org/10.4103/0019-5545.37314

WHO. (2006). *WHO-AIMS report on mental health system in Maldives* (pp. 1–19). WHO Regional Office for South-East Asia. https://apps.who.int/iris/bitstream/handle/10665/206158/B0768.pdf

WHO. (2016). *WHO-AIMS report on Mental Health System in Maldives. 2006*. chrome-extension://efaidnbmnnnibpcajpcglclefindmkaj/https://iris.who.int/bitstream/handle/10665/312323/9789290223030-eng.pdf?sequence=1&isAllowed=y

WHO. (2022). *Addressing mental health in Maldives* [World Health Organization; Regional office for South-East Asia]. chrome-extension://efaidnbmnnnibpcajpcglclefindmkaj/https://iris.who.int/bitstream/handle/10665/364879/9789290210191-eng.pdf?sequence=1

WHO Country Office for Maldives. (2017). *National Mental Health Policy 2015–2025*. chrome-extension://efaidnbmnnnibpcajpcglclefindmkaj/https://health.gov.mv/storage/uploads/EoAjylw9/zae5c6sf.pdf

Williams, S. S. (2024). Fine-tuning postgraduate psychiatry training in South Asia. *Indian Journal of Psychological Medicine, 46*(5), 380–381. https://doi.org/10.1177/02537176241280284

# Chapter 11
# Competency-Based Medical Education in Psychiatry Teaching: A Conceptual Overview and Application

**H. R. Vinay, H. K. Tejaswi Prithviraj, P. S. Vaibhavi, and Shreekara**

**Abstract** Competency-Based Medical Education (CBME) is a transformative approach in medical training, which emphasizes achieving defined clinical competencies, patient-centred outcomes, continuous assessment, and individualized learning progressions. In psychiatry, CBME is particularly relevant as it fosters critical skills in communication, ethics, cultural sensitivity, and community-oriented care. Across South Asia, the implementation of CBME in psychiatry is varied and evolving. India introduced CBME nationally in 2019, with structured reforms like early clinical exposure and skill labs, though psychiatry-specific implementation remains uneven due to faculty shortages. Sri Lanka, Bangladesh, and Nepal have made gradual progress but continue to face significant challenges in standardization, faculty capacity, and infrastructure. Pakistan has pioneered innovative CBME models in psychiatry through leading institutions like Aga Khan University. Bhutan has embraced CBME fully, aligning it with the country's Gross National Happiness philosophy, while Maldives and Afghanistan are in the early stages of integration. Regional barriers also include inadequate simulation facilities and persistent cultural stigma surrounding mental health. However, there are significant opportunities for regional collaboration, technology-driven teaching, and shared curriculum development. Moving forward, South Asian psychiatry education must focus on faculty training, policy support, telepsychiatry, and integrating disaster psychiatry, migration stress to address the region's evolving psychiatric care needs.

**Keywords** Psychiatry · Competency · Medical education · Curriculum · Assessment · Feedback · Knowledge · Skill · Attitudes

---

H. R. Vinay (✉)
Siddaganga Medical College and Research Institute, Tumakuru, Karnataka, India
e-mail: drvinayhr@gmail.com

H. K. T. Prithviraj · P. S. Vaibhavi
Adichunchanagiri Institute of Medical Sciences, Mandya District, Karnataka, India

Shreekara
Koppal Institute of Medical Sciences, Bhagyanagar, Karnataka, India



S. K. Kar et al. (eds.), *Teaching and Training in Psychiatry in South Asia*, South Asian Perspectives in Mental Health and Psychology,
https://doi.org/10.1007/978-981-95-1845-6_11

# 1 Introduction

## 1.1 Definition of Competency-Based Medical Education (CBME)

CBME is a learner-centred, outcomes-based approach to medical education, which emphasizes the attainment of predefined competencies (knowledge, skills, values, and attitudes) essential for the practice of medicine, ensuring that graduates are adequately prepared to meet the needs of patients and society.

## 1.2 Milestones and Implementation in Other Countries

Introduction of Competency-Based Medical Education (CBME) concepts happened in the 1980s to start with in the USA (McGaghie et al., 1978). There was emergence of CBME frameworks in Canada in the 1990s followed by the United Kingdom in the 2000s (Carraccio & Englander, 2013; Dagnone et al., 2019). A widespread global shift to CBME in undergraduate and postgraduate education occurred in Australia, Europe, and South America in the 2010s (Carraccio et al., 2002; Harris et al., 2010).

## 1.3 Rationale for CBME in Psychiatry Education

CBME equips medical graduates with the necessary clinical, communication, and attitudinal competencies to provide basic mental health care at all levels of the health system, helping to bridge this gap. CBME fosters attitudinal competencies like empathy, ethical sensitivity, and cultural competence, which are essential in psychiatry. CBME prepares all medical graduates—not just psychiatrists—to recognize and manage common psychiatric disorders and to provide appropriate referrals, reducing the mental health care burden on tertiary centres. CBME uses workplace-based assessments, objective structured clinical examinations (OSCEs), and longitudinal performance tracking, which provide a more authentic assessment of competence (Frank et al., 2010).

## 2 Conceptual Framework of CBME

### *2.1 Core Principles of CBME (Bhattacharya, 2023)*

Competency Focused: Centres on the development of clearly defined competencies rather than time spent in training.
Outcome-Based: Prioritizes the achievement of desired outcomes in patient care and professional behaviour.
Learner-Centric: Allows flexible, individualized learning paths based on the learner's progress.
Progression Based on Competence: Advancement occurs when competencies are achieved, not merely based on time or completion of courses.
Continuous Feedback and Assessment: Regular, formative assessments guide learners towards competence.

### *2.2 Comparison of CBME with Traditional Medical Education*

Table 11.1 mentions about the differences between CBME and traditional medical education for simplifying the concepts.

### *2.3 Competency Domains Relevant to Psychiatry (National Medical Commission, India, 2019, 2022)*

1. Knowledge (Cognitive Domain)

   - Understanding of major psychiatric disorders: mood, psychotic, anxiety, personality, and substance use disorders.
   - Knowledge of psychiatric classifications (ICD, DSM).
   - Awareness of psychopharmacology: indications, mechanisms, side effects.
   - Knowledge of psychotherapeutic principles: CBT, psychoanalysis, supportive therapy.
   - Understanding biological, psychological, and social determinants of mental illness.
   - Concepts of child, adolescent, geriatric, and forensic psychiatry.
   - Legal and ethical aspects: Mental Health Acts, informed consent, confidentiality.
   - Principles of crisis intervention, suicide prevention, and psychiatric emergencies.
   - Awareness of comorbidities between physical and mental health.

**Table 11.1** Comparison of CBME with traditional medical education

| Feature | Traditional medical education | Competency-based medical education (CBME) |
|---|---|---|
| Focus | Time-based learning; completion of courses and rotations | Competency/outcome-based learning; mastery of specific skills and attitudes |
| Curriculum design | Discipline-specific, subject-centred | Integrated, competency-focused, aligned with patient care outcomes |
| Progression criteria | Time-dependent; advancement based on academic years | Competency-dependent; advancement based on skill mastery |
| Assessment approach | Summative, largely knowledge-based exams | Continuous, formative, and workplace-based assessments (OSCEs, direct observation) |
| Teaching method | Teacher-centred (lectures, didactic sessions) | Learner-centred (problem-based learning, self-directed learning, active participation) |
| Learning pace | Fixed; all students progress together | Flexible; progression can vary based on individual achievement |
| Role of feedback | Limited, often at the end of rotations or exams | Frequent, structured feedback to guide ongoing improvement |
| Clinical skills emphasis | Sometimes fragmented, late exposure to clinical practice | Early and repeated clinical exposure, integrated skills training |
| Graduate readiness | May produce knowledge-rich but skill-variable graduates | Ensures readiness for independent practice with demonstrated competencies |
| Assessment tools | Traditional exams (written, oral, practical) | Entrustable Professional Activities (EPAs), milestone assessments, portfolios |
| Outcome measurement | Knowledge acquisition and exam scores | Real-world competence, performance, professionalism, and patient outcomes |
| Student autonomy | Passive learning, limited individualization | Active learning: self-assessment, reflection, and individualized learning paths |
| Interdisciplinary learning | Often compartmentalized by subjects | Emphasizes team-based and interprofessional education |

(Adapted from multiple sources—McGaghie et al., 1978; Carraccio & Englander, 2013; Harris et al., 2010; Gehlawat et al., 2024)

2. Skills (Psychomotor Domain)

    - Conducting comprehensive psychiatric history and mental status examination (MSE).
    - Basic proficiency in psychotherapeutic techniques (e.g. supportive therapy, motivational interviewing).
    - Administration of Electro Convulsive Therapy (ECT), Repetitive Transcranial Magnetic Stimulation (RTMS), biofeedback to patients.

**Table 11.2** Alignment of domain specific objectives to TL methods and assessment strategies

| Domain | Learning objectives | Teaching-learning methods | Assessment strategies |
|---|---|---|---|
| Knowledge | Describe common psychiatric disorders, basic psychopharmacology, and mental health laws | Lectures, Small Group Discussions (SGDs), Case-Based Learning (CBL), E-learning modules | Written exams (MCQs, SAQs), Viva Voce |
| Skills | Perform basic psychiatric history and MSE, identify psychiatric emergencies, provide psychoeducation, and initiate referral | Bedside clinics, role-plays, simulated patients, supervised OPD/IPD exposure, skill labs | Direct observation, OSCE, case presentation, Mini-CEX |
| Attitudes | Demonstrate empathy, reduce stigma, respect confidentiality, and work collaboratively | Reflective writing, group discussions, patient interviews, Role modelling by faculty | Reflective portfolio, faculty feedback, 360-degree assessment, peer assessment |

(Adapted from—National Medical Commission, India, 2019)

- Risk assessment and management of psychiatric emergencies (e.g. suicide risk, acute agitation) including physical restraint.
- Safe and appropriate prescription of psychotropic medications.

3. Attitudes (Affective Domain)

- Demonstrating empathy, respect, and compassion towards patients upholding confidentiality and ethical principles.
- Non-judgmental approach to all psychiatric conditions, including substance use.
- Advocacy for mental health awareness and community engagement.
- Commitment to professional integrity, accountability, and teamwork.

In Competency-Based Medical Education and all modern educational frameworks, alignment of learning objectives, teaching-learning (TL) methods, and assessment strategies is critical for ensuring effective, meaningful, and measurable learning. Table 11.2 highlights the importance of this alignment with examples:

## 2.4 *Role of Feedback and Reflection in Learning (Nousiainen et al., 2017; Isaacson et al., 2008)*

*What is Feedback in CBME?*

Feedback is a timely, and specific information provided to learners about their performance with the goal of helping them improve.

CBME is not time-based but performance-based.
Learners need continuous formative feedback to identify gaps and make real-time improvements.
Feedback helps learners understand whether they are meeting the competency milestones.

*What is Reflection in CBME?*
Reflection is the intentional process of critically analysing one's own experiences to gain insights for future improvement.
Key Roles of Reflection in CBME:
Promotes Self-Awareness: Learners become conscious of their clinical reasoning, communication, and decision-making.
Facilitates Personal Growth: Encourages accountability and ethical practice.
Reinforces Competency: Learners can connect theory to practice through reflective analysis.
Supports Emotional Processing: Especially important in psychiatry and clinical settings that involve complex human emotions.

Feedback provides direction. Reflection creates depth.

Both are essential for competency acquisition, lifelong learning, and professional growth.

## 2.5 *Standardized Patient Assessment and Simulation-Based Training (Doolen et al., 2014; Piot et al., 2021)*

A Standardized Patient (SP) is a person trained to consistently simulate a real patient's medical, psychological, or social condition for teaching and assessing clinical skills. Key roles include:

- Assessment of Communication Skills: Psychiatry heavily depends on evaluating rapport, empathy, and interview techniques, which can be effectively tested using SPs.
- Evaluation of Clinical Reasoning: SPs allow the assessment of history-taking, mental status examination, and diagnostic formulation in a structured way.
- Immediate Feedback Opportunities: SPs can give learners direct feedback from the patient's perspective.
- Safe Testing of Professionalism and Ethics: Learners can be assessed on handling difficult scenarios (breaking bad news, suicidal ideation) without real-life consequences.
- Objective Structured Clinical Examinations (OSCEs): SPs are frequently used in OSCEs to standardize and fairly assess clinical competencies.

Simulation involves the use of mannequins, virtual reality, role-plays, or standardized scenarios to replicate clinical situations in a risk-free environment.

Importance of simulation in CBME:

- Provides hands-on practice in complex or rare clinical scenarios.
- Offers opportunities to make mistakes safely and learn from them.
- Facilitates immediate debriefing and reflection.

**Interdisciplinary and Team-Based Learning Approaches**

- Teamwork is not optional in modern healthcare—it is essential.
- Interdisciplinary and team-based learning mirror real clinical practice. Promotes interprofessional communication, role clarity, and mutual respect.
- These approaches build competencies in communication, collaboration, leadership, and holistic care.
- Particularly relevant in psychiatry for handling substance use, suicide prevention, child abuse, forensic issues, and psychosocial rehabilitation.

**Use of Technology and E-Learning Platforms in CBME**

- Technology in Psychiatry CBME enhances realism, flexibility, and safety in learning.
- It supports competency tracking, skill development, communication training, and reflection, all crucial in psychiatric practice.
- Telepsychiatry and psychiatry-specific apps for suicide risk assessment tools, mental status examination checklists, psychotropic medication references.
- E-portfolios for reflection and feedback.
- Simulation and virtual learning can complement but not replace real patient interaction; balance is key.

# 3 Implementation of CBME in Psychiatry Teaching—Status in South Asia (Country Wise—Afghanistan, Bangladesh, Bhutan, India, Maldives, Nepal, Pakistan, and Sri Lanka)

**Afghanistan**

In countries with limited financial resources like Afghanistan, most individuals with psychiatric conditions primarily benefit from psychosocial interventions, as they are unlikely to ever consult a psychiatrist. In such settings, it is equally important to focus on avoiding unnecessary medications and polypharmacy to prevent treatment-related harm, alongside providing essential training in effective medical practices (Missmahl et al., 2012).

When it comes to psychosocial interventions, simply acquiring counselling skills is not sufficient. There is a significant need to ensure that counsellors do not unconsciously impose their own personal or cultural beliefs on clients, disregarding the clients' own perspectives.

In Afghanistan, person-centred counselling has now been introduced in several provinces and is currently being evaluated. Such research is crucial to build evidence-based knowledge on psychosocial counselling, which can be a valuable and much-needed treatment option, especially in regions where psychiatrists and specialized mental health professionals are extremely scarce (Stanikzai et al., 2025).

**Bangladesh**

Bangladesh has taken strides to include psychiatry more meaningfully in the MBBS curriculum through the introduction of CBME elements by the Bangladesh Medical & Dental Council (BMDC) (Arafat, 2019). The 2019 MBBS curriculum includes specific learning outcomes related to psychiatric disorders, emphasizing clinical competence, ethical practice, and communication skills (Bangladesh Medical and Dental Council, 2019).

Medical colleges in Bangladesh now conduct OSCEs (Objective Structured Clinical Examinations) and case-based discussions as part of psychiatry assessment. However, challenges include large student numbers, insufficient clinical training facilities, and a lack of full-time psychiatric faculty in many institutions (Arafat et al., 2021; Rahman et al., 2022).

**Challenges:**

- Limited trained faculty in psychiatry and CBME.
- Infrastructure limitations for skills-based teaching.
- Cultural stigma around mental health.
- Inconsistent implementation across institutions.

**Bhutan**

Bhutan's medical education is largely centralized under the Khesar Gyalpo University of Medical Sciences of Bhutan (KGUMSB), established in 2012. KGUMSB offers postgraduate programmes, including MD Psychiatry, and launched a competency-based MBBS programme in 2023. Regulation falls under the Ministry of Health and the Bhutan Qualifications and Professional Certification Authority (BQPCA).

Bhutan has explicitly embraced CBME. KGUMSB revised its postgraduate curricula around 2018 to incorporate competency frameworks (adapted from ACGME), constructive alignment, medical humanities, and a strong emphasis on WPBA (Mini-CEX, DOPS, CbD, MSF). Initial evaluations suggest these WPBA tools are perceived positively by faculty and trainees regarding feasibility, acceptability, and educational impact. Competency frameworks are also being developed for other health professionals.

Despite this clear commitment, challenges exist. Bhutan's medical education system is relatively nascent, facing faculty capacity limitations and the need for ongoing development in CBME methods. Significant health workforce shortages and high attrition rates, particularly among nurses and doctors, strain the system and create challenges for supervision and assessment. Opportunities arise from the centralized KGUMSB structure enabling coordinated implementation, the strong institutional commitment to CBME, positive early feedback on WPBA, and the potential for innovation within a newer system.

A unique dimension in Bhutan is the national philosophy of Gross National Happiness (GNH), which prioritizes holistic well-being across domains including psychological health, education, culture, and community vitality. CBME aligns naturally with the GNH health domain. Furthermore, competencies like professionalism, communication, ethics, and patient-centredness resonate with GNH values. KGUMSB's inclusion of medical humanities offers a vehicle for integrating GNH. Bhutan has a distinct opportunity to enrich its CBME framework by explicitly incorporating GNH principles into competency definitions and assessments, creating a model deeply aligned with its national identity and goals, potentially serving as an example of culturally resonant medical education (Tenzin et al., 2023).

**India**

Introduced by the National Medical Commission (NMC) (formerly Medical Council of India) in 2019, the first batch of MBBS students under the CBME curriculum started in August 2019 (National Medical Commission, India, 2019).

Objectives of CBME in India are to produce Indian Medical Graduates (IMGs) who are:

- Clinically competent.
- Ethical and compassionate.
- Lifelong learners.
- Able to work in a multi-disciplinary healthcare team.
- Responsive to societal needs.

Core Components:
Foundation Course (1 month).
Early Clinical Exposure (ECE).
AETCOM Module (across phases).
Electives (2 months).
Skill Labs for clinical competence.
Competency Logbooks.

**Progress Made So Far**

- Foundation Courses and ECE have been implemented across medical colleges.
- Skill labs have been established in many institutions.
- Faculty Development Programmes (FDPs) like CISP (Curriculum Implementation Support Programme) have trained thousands of medical teachers.
- AETCOM modules are integrated into assessments.

- Institutions have started using portfolios and workplace-based assessments.
- Curriculum revision has happened based on stakeholders' feedback (Sethi et al., 2024).

**Maldives**

In the Maldives, faith healers traditionally managed mental health care. Over time, this began to shift with the introduction of medical treatments and growing public awareness. Today, mental health is increasingly acknowledged as an important health concern. However, the mental health system still faces significant challenges, including issues related to governance, limited access to services, shortages of trained professionals, inadequate prevention strategies, and a lack of research in the field (Mohamed & Mansoor, 2025).

**Nepal**

Postgraduate psychiatry training (MD Psychiatry, 3 years) in Nepal is offered by several institutions, including Tribhuvan University's Institute of Medicine (IOM), B.P. Koirala Institute of Health Sciences (BPKIHS), Kathmandu University School of Medical Sciences (KUSMS) affiliates, and Patan Academy of Health Sciences (PAHS). Regulation involves the Nepal Medical Council (NMC) and the newer Medical Education Commission (MEC) (Singh et al., 2022).

While national bodies signal a move towards CBME, implementation appears varied. PAHS stands out for explicitly adopting a competency-based postgraduate programme, defining core competencies (including "Community orientation") and utilizing EPAs. Evidence for similar systematic CBME adoption in psychiatry at other major institutions is less clear from available data, suggesting curricula may be transitional or retain traditional elements. This indicates a fragmented landscape where national intent may precede widespread, uniform implementation.

Challenges to implementing CBME in Nepal include resource constraints (funding, infrastructure, faculty time), the critical need for extensive faculty development in CBME principles and assessment, difficulties in establishing consistent and valid assessment systems across institutions, and the impact of high clinician turnover, particularly in rural areas. Aligning training with the significant need for mental health services in underserved rural communities is paramount. Opportunities lie in leveraging the national regulatory framework (MEC/NMC), learning from pioneers like PAHS, utilizing the growing number of psychiatrists, and potentially enhancing international collaborations for support. The key opportunity involves using the national push and local experience to standardize quality CBME tailored to Nepal's specific health needs, especially rural mental healthcare (Gupta et al., 2021).

**Pakistan**

Psychiatric training in Pakistan is at the very early stages, at both the undergraduate and postgraduate levels. The country has fewer than 500 psychiatrists and negligible mental health facilities, with only four major psychiatric hospitals. There are a small number of psychiatric units in teaching and general hospitals (Gilani et al., 2005).

Since there is a deficit of psychiatrists, the focus was more on community psychiatry rather than psychiatry education. Competency-Based Medical Education (CBME) in psychiatry is progressively shaping medical training in Pakistan, aligning with global trends towards outcome-focused, learner-centred education. Here is an overview of its implementation across undergraduate and postgraduate psychiatry programmes in the country:

Aga Khan University (AKU), Karachi, has pioneered CBME in undergraduate psychiatry education. In 2017, AKU redesigned its one-month mandatory psychiatry rotation into a competency-based, blended curriculum integrating virtual learning, classroom sessions, and patient-skills training. This approach enhanced student engagement, critical thinking, and alignment of assessments with learning outcomes. Psychiatry has been taught to the undergraduates as a mandatory one-month clinical rotation since 1987 (Chachar et al., 2020).

In King Edward Medical University (KEMU), College of Physicians & Surgeons of Pakistan (CPSP) offers Membership of the College of Physicians & Surgeons of Pakistan (MCPS) program, a2 years PG training in psychiatry which serves as a crucial link between the primary health care facilities and the tertiary care mental health facilities. It covers basic sciences, psychometry, behavioural sciences, and ethics.

In summary, Pakistan is making significant strides in integrating CBME into psychiatry education, with institutions like AKU, RMU, and CPSP leading the way. These efforts aim to enhance the quality of psychiatric training and address the growing mental health needs of the countries.

**Sri Lanka**

Sri Lanka's undergraduate psychiatry education has traditionally been limited in duration and scope. However, recent curriculum reforms have introduced CBME principles. The Sri Lanka Medical Council (SLMC) has encouraged medical faculties to adopt CBME frameworks that integrate psychiatry more holistically into undergraduate training (Sri Lanka Medical Council, 2022).

Some medical faculties now include early clinical exposure to psychiatry, assessment of communication skills, and modules on suicide prevention, community psychiatry, and addiction medicine. However, challenges remain in standardization across institutions and availability of faculty trained in CBME methodology (Perera et al., 2023; Hanwella & De Silva, 2024).

# 4 Evaluation of CBME Programme

## 4.1 *Effectiveness of the Programme*

Since its 2019 launch, India's CBME has been broadly accepted but unevenly implemented. Surveys report high faculty awareness and widespread training. Almost all institutions held CBME sensitization workshops. However, many teachers still report feeling unprepared. Psychiatry departments face unique staffing pressures. Unlike major subjects, psychiatry often has only 2–3 faculty members per college (Gupta & Menon 2022).

## 4.2 *Stakeholder Perceptions (Salazar et al., 2022; Kumar et al., 2024; Sethuraman et al., 2024; Kar & Singh, 2024; Deshpande et al., 2024; Perugu et al., 2024)*

Recent studies of CBME psychiatry postings report strong student engagement and positive learning outcomes. Learners especially valued hands-on experiences and communication skill practice. They reported better OPD exposure (observing and presenting cases), enhanced knowledge of non-pharmacological therapies, and improvements in interviewing and ethical skills.

Many noted that structured case-based discussions and feedback sessions helped clarify psychiatric concepts. One evalúation concluded the CBME-informed psychiatry rotation was "instrumental in improving psychiatry training and promoting mental health awareness" among future doctors. Psychiatry CBME employs multiple assessment methods. Examinations typically include MCQs and OSCE stations focused on history-taking or mental status exams. The new AETCOM modules are integral to psychiatry training, too, often taught through role-play and patient interviews to emphasize communication and ethics.

# 5 Challenges and Opportunities in South Asia

## 5.1 *Infrastructure and Resource Constraints*

There is a significant shortage of trained psychiatry faculty across most South Asian countries. Limited numbers of teachers make it difficult to implement small group teaching, workplace-based assessments (WBAs), and adequate student supervision. This is especially problematic in low-resource settings like rural India, Bangladesh, Nepal, and Afghanistan.

Many medical colleges lack simulation labs, dedicated psychiatry skill centres, and technology support to conduct OSCEs and formative assessments effectively. Infrastructure to support small group sessions, early clinical exposure, and integrated teaching is often insufficient (Orsolini et al., 2021).

## 5.2 *Faculty Training and Capacity Building*

Assessment complexity is another major issue—CBME calls for multiple exams (MCQs, OSCEs, portfolios, etc.) and formative feedback, imposing a heavy workload on busy faculty (Hawkins et al., 2015). Other problems are logistical (scheduling integrated classes, low attendance in non-major subjects) and the COVID-era disruptions to early CBME training. Yet many still feel underprepared to design and deliver the new curriculum: roughly three-quarters of faculty (across disciplines) admitted difficulty in writing specific learning objectives for CBME (Kishor et al., 2020). In response, specialty groups are stepping up: for example, the Indian Teachers of Psychiatry programme now offers targeted training scholarships to enhance CBME teaching skills (Kishor et al., 2023). In addition, creating digital platforms and appropriate faculty training can bridge infrastructural gap. (Sahadevan et al., 2021)

## 5.3 *Cultural and Societal Influences on Psychiatric Education*

In psychiatry, cultural competence is especially critical, as mental health beliefs, stigma, and help-seeking behaviours vary widely across societies. Diverse Belief Systems: In many cultures, mental illness is linked to supernatural or religious explanations, which may conflict with the biomedical model taught in CBME. Expression of Psychiatric Symptoms: Cultural factors influence how symptoms manifest (somatization in some Asian cultures, for example) and how they are interpreted by both patients and healthcare providers.

In many societies, including South Asia, families play a pivotal role in psychiatric decision-making. Training must prepare students to work within these family dynamics. Hence, the training imparted to the budding psychiatrists has to make them culturally competent and socially responsible.

## 5.4 *Opportunities for Collaboration and Innovation*

South Asian countries can collaborate to develop context-sensitive, regionally relevant curricula in psychiatry, focusing on common psychiatric issues, cultural practices, and health system limitations. The shared cultural, economic, and healthcare challenges of the region create a fertile ground for collective progress in psychiatric education. Encourage student exchange programmes, psychiatry interest groups, and cross-border case conferences to build cultural competence and mutual learning.

## 6 Future Directions and Policy Recommendations

- Strengthening CBME Implementation in Psychiatry Education.

  Regular workshops on CBME principles, competency mapping, and innovative teaching methods. Training in formative and summative assessment techniques specific to psychiatry, including Mini-CEX, DOPS, and OSCE (Ten Cate, 2017).

- Role of National and Regional Medical Education Bodies.

  Ensure national regulatory bodies actively support the CBME psychiatry framework with adequate funding and policy backing. Implement systems for regular internal and external audits of CBME implementation.

- Research and Innovation in Psychiatric Education Methodologies.

  Development of regional centres of excellence for simulation-based psychiatric training to standardize skills like communication, crisis management, and suicide risk assessment.
  Technology-Driven Learning: Telepsychiatry-based Teaching: Leverage telepsychiatry for cross-border case discussions, webinars, and virtual clinical exposure.
  E-learning Modules: Develop interactive, competency-aligned e-learning resources accessible across South Asia, accommodating language and cultural differences.
  Virtual Reality (VR) and Augmented Reality (AR): Introduce VR/AR simulations for psychiatric interviewing, managing challenging behaviours, and understanding hallucinations (Sharma et al., 2024).
  Establish South Asian research networks focusing on CBME implementation outcomes, psychiatric epidemiology, cultural psychiatry, stigma reduction, and innovative teaching methods (Chauhan et al., 2022).
  Shared data can help develop evidence-based region-specific competencies.

### *6.1 Adapting CBME to Evolving Mental Health Needs in South Asia*

Disaster Psychiatry: Teach crisis intervention and disaster response in the context of frequent natural calamities and humanitarian emergencies in the region (Groom et al., 2015).

Migration and Urbanization: Equip students to understand migration stress, acculturation issues, and urban mental health dynamics.

## 7 Conclusion

### *7.1 Summary of Conceptual Framework and Status of Implementation*

Competency-Based Medical Education (CBME) represents a significant paradigm shift in medical education. Its core principles emphasize:

- Competency-Focused Learning: Prioritizing the achievement of well-defined, observable competencies rather than time spent in training.
- Outcome-Based Approach: Focusing on preparing learners to deliver effective, ethical, and patient-centred care.
- Learner-Centric Progression: Allowing flexibility and individualized learning paths based on demonstrated competence, not just course completion.
- Continuous Assessment: Employing regular formative assessments, workplace-based evaluations, and constructive feedback to guide learner development.
- Alignment of Educational Components: Ensuring that learning objectives, teaching methods, and assessment strategies are cohesively integrated.

CBME is particularly relevant in psychiatry, where clinical skills, communication, ethics, and cultural sensitivity are as critical as theoretical knowledge. t. CBME implementation in psychiatry across South Asia is heterogeneous, evolving, and context-dependent.

Afghanistan: Psychiatry education focuses on person-centred psychosocial interventions due to limited resources and workforce, with early efforts in competency-based counselling.

Bangladesh: The 2019 MBBS curriculum introduced CBME elements, including OSCEs and case-based assessments in psychiatry. However, faculty shortages and infrastructure limitations are major barriers.

Bhutan: KGUMSB has fully embraced CBME, aligning with the country's Gross National Happiness (GNH) philosophy and incorporating structured workplace-based assessments.

India: National Medical Commission (NMC) introduced CBME in 2019 with structured reforms like the foundation course, early clinical exposure (ECE), AETCOM modules, and skill labs. Faculty development programmes (FDPs) have been widely conducted, but implementation remains uneven, particularly in psychiatry departments with limited faculty.

Maldives: Mental health services are developing, but CBME integration in psychiatry is at an early stage.

Pakistan: Institutions like Aga Khan University (AKU) and Rawalpindi Medical University (RMU) are leading CBME adoption in psychiatry, using blended learning and workplace-based assessments. Broader national implementation is still emerging.

Nepal: Postgraduate CBME in psychiatry is progressing, notably at PAHS, but national implementation remains fragmented.

Sri Lanka: CBME principles are gradually being integrated with early psychiatry exposure and community-oriented modules, though challenges in standardization and faculty training persist.

## 7.2 Way Forward for CBME in Psychiatry Teaching

Psychiatry education in South Asia faces several challenges in implementing Competency-Based Medical Education (CBME). A major issue is the shortage of trained psychiatry faculty, especially in rural and low-resource settings like Bangladesh, Nepal, and Afghanistan. Many medical colleges lack essential infrastructure such as simulation labs, skill centres, and technological support for conducting OSCEs and workplace-based assessments. Faculty often struggle with the complex demands of CBME assessments and feel underprepared to design and deliver the new curriculum. Cultural and societal influences further complicate psychiatric education, as mental health stigma, supernatural beliefs, and family-centric care models shape patient attitudes and symptom presentation.

Despite these challenges, South Asia has significant opportunities for collaboration and innovation. The region can develop shared, culturally sensitive curricula, promote cross-border training, and build regional psychiatry networks. Future strategies should focus on strengthening faculty through targeted training and regular

CBME workshops. National bodies must actively support CBME psychiatry with policy backing and regular audits. Embracing technology such as telepsychiatry, e-learning, and VR-based simulations can revolutionize psychiatric training. Additionally, disaster psychiatry, migration-related stress, and urban mental health should be integrated into evolving curricula to better address the region's emerging mental health needs.

## References


Arafat, S. M. Y. (2019). History of psychiatry in Bangladesh. *Asian Journal of Psychiatry, 46*, 11–12. https://doi.org/10.1016/j.ajp.2019.09.024

Arafat, S. M. Y., Kar, S. K., Sharma, P., Marahatta, K., & Baminiwatta, A. K. A. B. (2021). A comparative analysis of psychiatry curriculum at undergraduate level of Bangladesh, India, Nepal, and Sri Lanka. *Indian Journal of Psychiatry, 63*(2), 184–188. https://doi.org/10.4103/psychiatry.IndianJPsychiatry_615_20

Bangladesh Medical and Dental Council. (2019). Revised MBBS Curriculum. http://www.bmdc.org.bd

Bhattacharya, S. (2023). Competency-based medical education: An overview. *Annals of Medical Science and Research, 2*(3), 132–138. https://doi.org/10.4103/amsr.amsr_27_23

Carraccio, C. L., & Englander, R. (2013). From Flexner to competencies: Reflections on a decade and the journey ahead. *Academic Medicine: Journal of the Association of American Medical Colleges, 88*(8), 1067–1073. https://doi.org/10.1097/ACM.0b013e318299396f

Carraccio, C., Wolfsthal, S. D., Englander, R., Ferentz, K., & Martin, C. (2002). Shifting paradigms: From Flexner to competencies. *Academic Medicine: Journal of the Association of American Medical Colleges, 77*(5), 361–367. https://doi.org/10.1097/00001888-200205000-00003

Chachar, A. S., Siddiqui, S. A., Saeed, H., Naseem, A., & Mian, A. I. (2020). Designing a competency-based, blended curriculum using Kern's model for undergraduate psychiatry clerkship in Pakistan. *SOTL in the South, 4*(2), 100–117. https://doi.org/10.36615/sotls.v4i2.111

Chatterjee, S., & Kar, S. K. (2023). Undergraduate research elective under Competency-Based Medical Education (CBME) in India: Challenges and directions. *Indian Journal of Psychological Medicine, 45*(5), 548–551. https://doi.org/10.1177/02537176231165219

Chauhan, V. S., Chatterjee, K., Prakash, J., Singh, Y. M., Dangi, A., Dubey, A., Chail, A., & Sharma, R. (2022). Identifying entrustable professional activities for postgraduation in psychiatry: What should a psychiatrist be able to do? *Industrial Psychiatry Journal, 31*(1), 49–55. https://doi.org/10.4103/ipj.ipj_124_21

Dagnone, D., Stockley, D., Flynn, L., Egan, R., van Wylick, R., McEwan, L., Walker, R., & Reznick, R. (2019). Delivering on the promise of competency based medical education – An institutional approach. *Canadian Medical Education Journal, 10*(1), e28–e38.

Deshpande, S., Agawane, S., Zachariah, A., Innamuri, R., & Menon, V. (2024). Focus group discussion with the medical interns regarding psychiatry posting. *Indian Journal of Psychiatry, 66*(9), 859–862. https://doi.org/10.4103/indianjpsychiatry.indianjpsychiatry_698_22

Doolen, J., Giddings, M., Johnson, M., Guizado de Nathan, G., & Badia, L. O. (2014). An evaluation of mental health simulation with standardized patients. *International Journal of Nursing Education Scholarship, 11*, /j/ijnes.2014.11.issue-1/ijnes-2013-0075/ijnes-2013-0075.xml. https://doi.org/10.1515/ijnes-2013-0075

Frank, J. R., Snell, L. S., Cate, O. T., Holmboe, E. S., Carraccio, C., Swing, S. R., Harris, P., Glasgow, N. J., Campbell, C., Dath, D., Harden, R. M., Iobst, W., Long, D. M., Mungroo, R., Richardson, D. L., Sherbino, J., Silver, I., Taber, S., Talbot, M., & Harris, K. A. (2010). Competency-based medical education: Theory to practice. *Medical Teacher, 32*(8), 638–645. https://doi.org/10.3109/0142159X.2010.501190

Gehlawat, M., Thumati, G., Samala, P., Alekhya, C. L., Shailaja, A., & Sharma, A. (2024). Competency-based medical education for Indian undergraduates: Where do we stand?. APIK. *Journal of Internal Medicine, 12*(1), 7–12. https://doi.org/10.4103/ajim.ajim_161_22

Gilani, A. I., Gilani, U. I., Kasi, P. M., & Khan, M. M. (2005). Psychiatric health laws in Pakistan: From lunacy to mental health. *PLoS Medicine, 2*(11), e317. https://doi.org/10.1371/journal.pmed.0020317

Groom, R. M., Carr, R. B., Leong, S. L., & Hornbaker-Park, M. B. (2015). Impact of an enduring war on two military psychiatry residency programs. *Academic Psychiatry: The Journal of the American Association of Directors of Psychiatric Residency Training and the Association for Academic Psychiatry, 39*(4), 354–359. https://doi.org/10.1007/s40596-015-0284-2

Gupta, S., & Menon, V. (2022). Psychiatry training for medical students: A global perspective and implications for India's competency-based medical education curriculum. *Indian Journal of Psychiatry, 64*(3), 240–251. https://doi.org/10.4103/indianjpsychiatry.indianjpsychiatry_187_22

Gupta, A. K., Joshi, S., Kafle, B., Thapa, R., Chapagai, M., Nepal, S., Niraula, A., Paudyal, S., Sapkota, P., Poudel, R., Gurung, B. S., Pokhrel, P., Jha, R., Pandit, S., Thapaliya, S., Shrestha, S., Volpe, U., & Sartorius, N. (2021). Pathways to mental health care in Nepal: A 14-center nationwide study. *International Journal of Mental Health Systems, 15*(1), 85. https://doi.org/10.1186/s13033-021-00509-4

Hanwella, R., & De Silva, V. (2024). Undergraduate psychiatry education in Sri Lanka: The current situation and the way forward. *Sri Lanka Journal of Psychiatry, 15*(1), 1–4. https://doi.org/10.4038/sljpsyc.v15i1.8565

Harris, P., Snell, L., Talbot, M., & Harden, R. M. (2010). Competency-based medical education: Implications for undergraduate programs. *Medical Teacher, 32*(8), 646–650. https://doi.org/10.3109/0142159X.2010.500703

Hawkins, R. E., Welcher, C. M., Holmboe, E. S., Kirk, L. M., Norcini, J. J., Simons, K. B., & Skochelak, S. E. (2015). Implementation of competency-based medical education: Are we addressing the concerns and challenges? *Medical Education, 49*(11), 1086–1102. https://doi.org/10.1111/medu.12831

Isaacson, J. H., Salas, R., Koch, C., & McKenzie, M. (2008). Reflective writing in the competency-based curriculum at the Cleveland Clinic Lerner College of Medicine. *The Permanente Journal, 12*(2), 82–88. https://doi.org/10.7812/TPP/07-136

Kishor, M., Gupta, R., Ashok, M. V., Isaac, M., Chaddha, R. K., Singh, O. P., Shah, H., Nishchal, A., Dave, M., Vinay Kumar, H. R., Das, A., Rohilla, J. K., Singh, P. K., Kumar, P., Swami, M., Solanki, R. K., Sahadevan, S., Pal, A., Ray, R., Garg, S., et al. (2020). Competency-based medical curriculum: Psychiatry, training of faculty, and Indian Psychiatric Society. *Indian Journal of Psychiatry, 62*(2), 207–208. https://doi.org/10.4103/psychiatry.IndianJPsychiatry_81_20

Kishor, M., Menon, V., Vinay, H. R., Shah, H., Isaac, M., & Arun, M. (2023). The IToP-STEPS: A unique scholarship program to upskill teachers of psychiatry. *Indian Journal of Psychiatry, 65*(3), 381–384. https://doi.org/10.4103/indianjpsychiatry.indianjpsychiatry_428_22

Kumar, A., Gupta, S., Jain, J., Ghosh, S., Basera, D., Pakhre, A., & Modak, T. (2024). Perceived learning and feedback of students following the competency-based clinical rotation in psychiatry: A retrospective review from tertiary-care Teaching Institute in Central India. *Indian Journal of Psychological Medicine, 46*(5), 429–438. https://doi.org/10.1177/02537176241277518

McGaghie, W. C., Miller, G. E., Sajid, A. W., & Telder, T. W. (1978). *Competency-based curriculum development in medical education – An introduction.* http://whqlibdoc.who.int/php/WHO_PHP_68.pdf. [Accessed 19 June 2025.]

Missmahl, I., Kluge, U., Bromand, Z., & Heinz, A. (2012). Teaching psychiatry and establishing psychosocial services – lessons from Afghanistan. *European Psychiatry: The Journal of the Association of European Psychiatrists, 27*(Suppl 2), S76–S80. https://doi.org/10.1016/S0924-9338(12)75712-7

Mohamed, A., & Mansoor, S. (2025). Challenges and opportunities in the mental health landscape of the Maldives. *Australasian Psychiatry: Bulletin of Royal Australian and New Zealand College of Psychiatrists, 33*(2), 195–196. https://doi.org/10.1177/10398562241289879

National Medical Commission, India, 2019. Available from: www.nmc.org.in/wp-content/uploads/2020/01/UG-Curriculum-Vol-II.pdf

National Medical Commission, India, 2022. Available from www.nmc.org.in/wp-content/uploads/2022/revised/MD_Psychiatry_(%20revised%20).pdf

Nousiainen, M. T., Caverzagie, K. J., Ferguson, P. C., Frank, J. R., & ICBME Collaborators. (2017). Implementing competency-based medical education: What changes in curricular structure and processes are needed? *Medical Teacher, 39*(6), 594–598. https://doi.org/10.1080/0142159X.2017.1315077

Orsolini, L., Jatchavala, C., Noor, I. M., Ransing, R., Satake, Y., Shoib, S., Shah, B., Ullah, I., & Volpe, U. (2021). Training and education in digital psychiatry: A perspective from Asia-Pacific region. *Asia-Pacific Psychiatry: Official Journal of the Pacific Rim College of Psychiatrists, 13*(4), e12501. https://doi.org/10.1111/appy.12501

Perera, H., et al. (2023). Implementing competency-based psychiatry training in undergraduate medical education: Sri Lankan perspective. *Sri Lanka Journal of Psychiatry, 14*(1).

Perugu, S., Sreedaran, P., Chari, U., Sethuraman, B., & Salazar, L. J. (2024). An evaluation of the first clinical posting in psychiatry of the Competency-Based Medical Education (CBME) curriculum for undergraduate medical students in India. *Indian Journal of Psychological Medicine, 46*(5), 452–458. https://doi.org/10.1177/02537176241284358

Piot, M. A., Attoe, C., Billon, G., Cross, S., Rethans, J. J., & Falissard, B. (2021). Simulation training in psychiatry for medical education: A review. *Frontiers in Psychiatry, 12*, 658967. https://doi.org/10.3389/fpsyt.2021.658967

Rahman, M. M., et al. (2022). Evaluation of CBME framework in psychiatry teaching in Bangladesh. *Bangladesh Journal of Medical Education, 13*(2), 45–52.

Sahadevan, S., Kurian, N., Mani, A. M., Kishor, M. R., & Menon, V. (2021). Implementing competency-based medical education curriculum in undergraduate psychiatric training in India: Opportunities and challenges. *Asia-Pacific Psychiatry: Official Journal of the Pacific Rim College of Psychiatrists, 13*(4), e12491. https://doi.org/10.1111/appy.12491

Salazar, L. J., Chari, U., Sharma, P., & Sreedaran, P. (2022). Facilitators and barriers to student learning and impact of an undergraduate clinical posting in psychiatry: A thematic analysis. *Indian Journal of Psychological Medicine, 44*(4), 392–398. https://doi.org/10.1177/02537176211056366

Sethi, S., Tekkalaki, B., Shah, N., Smitha, C. A., & Kumar, R. (2024). Undergraduate psychiatry CBME curriculum revision: The process and the way ahead. *Indian Journal of Psychiatry, 66*(11), 1066–1069. https://doi.org/10.4103/indianjpsychiatry.indianjpsychiatry_821_24

Sethuraman, B., Chari, U., Perugu, S., Salazar, L. J., & Sreedaran, P. (2024). Students' perspectives of competency-based medical education in undergraduate psychiatry clinical training: A qualitative evaluation. *Indian Journal of Psychological Medicine, 46*(5), 400–407. https://doi.org/10.1177/02537176241265484

Sharma, N., Sharma, M., Tailor, J., Chaudhari, A., Joshi, D., & Acharya, U. R. (2024). Automated detection of depression using wavelet scattering networks. *Medical Engineering & Physics, 124*, 104107. https://doi.org/10.1016/j.medengphy.2024.104107

Singh, R., Gupta, A. K., Singh, B., Basnet, P., & Arafat, S. M. Y. (2022). History of psychiatry in Nepal. *BJPsych International, 19*(1), 7–9. https://doi.org/10.1192/bji.2021.51

Sri Lanka Medical Council. (2022). Standards for Accreditation of Medical Education Programs in Sri Lanka.

Stanikzai, M. H., Shanawa, S., Karimkhil, A. T., & Dadras, O. (2025). Medical education in Afghanistan: Challenges and policy implications. *Advances in Medical Education and Practice, 16*, 477–482. https://doi.org/10.2147/AMEP.S510309

Ten Cate, O. (2017). Competency-based postgraduate medical education: Past, present and future. *GMS Journal for Medical Education, 34*(5), Doc69. https://doi.org/10.3205/zma001146

Tenzin, K., Dorji, T., Sherub, K., Chhezom, K., Dorji, G., Tshering, K., Choden, R. S., Mukhia, S., Choeda, T., Galey, K., Gyamtsho, S., Tshering, P., Siebeck, M., Jayasinghe, S., & Dhakal, G. P. (2023). An integrated competency-based curriculum for undergraduate medical education programme in Bhutan. *South-East Asian Journal of Medical Education, 17*(2), 3–9. https://doi.org/10.4038/seajme.v17i2.576

# Chapter 12
# Attitudes, Ethics, and Communication Skills in Psychiatry Teaching

**Priya Sreedaran, Bhuvaneshwari Sethuraman, and Shalini Perugu**

**Abstract** It is essential for a medical professional to inculcate qualities like a compassionate attitude, professionalism, empathy for patients and caregivers, an ethical core, and effective communication skills. Medical education plays an important role in instilling these qualities. In certain South Asian countries, achieving competency in skills that reflect the appropriate attitudes, ethics, and communication (AETCOM), has been formally included as part of the mandated medical curriculum. The psychiatrist would be an ideal medical teacher to impart these skills to the budding medical professional. This role is especially important in South Asian countries due to their cultural diversity and resource constraints. This chapter discusses the history of AETCOM and the potential role of the psychiatrist in imparting AETCOM skills to undergraduate and postgraduate medical students.

**Keywords** Communication skills · Ethics · Empathy · Professional behaviors · Psychiatrist · Psychiatry training

## 1 Introduction

A compassionate attitude, a sense of professional duty, and empathetic communication skills are essential attributes for the budding young doctor and healthcare worker. This necessity—has led to the inclusion of training in medical ethics and communication skills in medical curricula across the world (Wong et al., 2022). Over the last decade, South Asian countries like Sri Lanka, Bangladesh, and Nepal have integrated medical ethics and communication skills in their medical training. In India, the National Medical Commission has mandated the inclusion of medical

P. Sreedaran (✉) · B. Sethuraman · S. Perugu
Department of psychiatry, St. John's Medical College, Bengaluru, Karnataka, India



S. K. Kar et al. (eds.), *Teaching and Training in Psychiatry in South Asia*, South Asian Perspectives in Mental Health and Psychology,
https://doi.org/10.1007/978-981-95-1845-6_12

ethics, communication skills, and attitudes or AETCOM (Attitudes, Ethics, Communication) in the undergraduate medical curriculum (National Medical Commission, 2018). While these changes are welcome, it is important to prepare medical teachers accordingly.

The specialty of psychiatry deals with chronic behavioral and emotional disorders. It is necessary for psychiatrists to possess communication skills that enable engaging and empathizing with patients with persistent suffering. The psychiatry teacher is thus uniquely positioned to play an important role in inculcating adequate competencies in medical ethics and communication in the medical student (Sahadevan et al., 2021). In this background, this chapter examines AETCOM in psychiatry teaching. To maintain uniformity, we will use the term AETCOM to refer to bioethics, communication skills, the development of empathy, and related attitudes and behaviors across this chapter.

## 2 History of AETCOM in Medical Education in South Asia

In 1975, there were three separate documented endeavors that described how medical ethics training was included in the medical curricula in Sweden, the United Kingdom, and United States of America (Blomquist, 1975; Jones, 1975; Veatch & Fenner, 1975). The ethics training occurred informally, using teaching-learning methods like lectures and case discussions, with religious and philosophical principles playing a key role in the deliberations. In 1999, a survey of medical colleges in Southeast Asia showed that most colleges had some kind of formal training in medical ethics with an emphasis on the obligations of the physician to the patient and patient rights (Miyasaka et al., 1999). That survey did not include any colleges from South Asia. There was no mention of the role of the psychiatrist in any of these undertakings.

The South Asian region comprises Afghanistan, Bangladesh, Bhutan, India, Maldives, Nepal, Pakistan, and Sri Lanka. This region is characterized by diversity in language, religion, customs, political instability, and shortage of medical doctors. There is a wide variation in the incorporation of AETCOM in medical education in South Asia. While the first medical college in Afghanistan was established in 1932, the subsequent unrest and wars have led to unpredictable standards in medical education with low priority to AETCOM (Stanikzai et al., 2025). The history of AETCOM in medical education in Bhutan and Maldives is unclear.

In 2002, in Pakistan, the national accreditation body for medical education recommended the introduction of bioethics in the undergraduate medical curriculum (Shirazi et al., 2024). Training in medical ethics was mentioned in the medical curricula in Bangladesh and Nepal around 2010 (Adhikari, 2014; Jahan & Flora, 2022). In Sri Lanka, AETCOM training was restricted to the knowledge of medical ethics around professional conduct, doctor–patient relationships, confidentiality, and medical negligence (Babapulle, 1992). In all these countries, the AETCOM teaching was intended to be conducted by forensic or community medicine departments.

In 1955, in India, a key medical conference documented the first formal attempt to include ethics into medical education (Tom Mishael et al., 2019). However, this did not result in an official recommendation for the inclusion of medical ethics in the medicine curriculum. From 1985 onward, St. John's Medical College in Bengaluru (India) instituted formal and structured training in medical ethics. This training was conducted by expert teachers and included psychiatrists and psychologists (Tom Mishael et al., 2019).

While there are multiple instances from South Asia on the inclusion of bioethics in the medicine curriculum, there is limited information on teaching communication skills. The history of medical education shows the low priority given to AETCOM. The role of the psychiatry teacher was non-existent. The possible reasons for this lack of importance to AETCOM in South Asia, could be the resource constraints for psychiatry and medicine overall in the region.

In 2009, the World Health Organization (WHO) recommended the teaching of medical ethics to medical students as part of their education (World Health Organization, 2009). The expected learning outcome of this recommendation was the increased proficiency of students with concepts like doctor–patient relationships, patient confidentiality, patient autonomy, medical negligence, bioethics, and informed consent. The WHO module reiterated the need to instill an awareness of cultural sensitivities and local ethical codes in undergraduate medical students. Medical teachers would serve as positive role models for demonstration of ethical practices. The module recommended seeking continuous feedback from all stakeholders for program improvement. While this module discussed the ethical issues in treating those with psychiatric disorders, there was no specific mention on the role of the psychiatrist in teaching medical ethics to undergraduate students.

## 3 Is There a Perceived Need for Formal AETCOM in Medical Education?

The young doctor is influenced to a significant degree by the medical education and curriculum that they receive. The components of the medical curriculum include the explicit and hidden curriculum (Pourbairamian et al., 2022). While the explicit curriculum specifies the goals, outcomes, and objectives to be attained by the medical student in training, the hidden curriculum reflects what the medical student learns through their experiences and interactions. AETCOM related skills are implied to be absorbed by the medical student through the hidden curriculum. However, there is a perceived need of medical students for the incorporation of formal training in AETCOM as a part of the explicit curriculum.

In Nepal, medical students wanted training in communication skills with an emphasis on communication styles with patients that was reflective of local sensitivities (Moore, 2009). In Pakistan, a systematic needs assessment showed that it was essential to bring in courses on medical ethics, time management, and communication skills in undergraduate medical education (Javaeed, 2019).

In Sri Lanka, the knowledge of medical ethics among doctors was low, and the majority were keen on acquiring more information (Ranasinghe et al., 2020). In another study from the same country, medical students believed that training in communication skills was important (Marambe et al., 2012). In Bangladesh, recent medical graduates favored the addition of a separate module for medical ethics and professionalism in the medical education curriculum (Jahan & Flora, 2022). In India, a rapid rise in medical negligence cases against doctors and violence toward healthcare workers were factors that contributed to the inclusion of medical ethics as part of the explicit medical curriculum (Ambesh, 2016). Overall, the addition of courses on medical ethics and professionalism in medical education is a beneficial change that addresses the perceived needs of medical students.

## 4 Initiatives for Implementation of AETCOM Across South Asia

### *4.1 Afghanistan*

The published literature on medical education in Afghanistan is sparse. It focuses on the infrastructure and resource challenges, lack of capacity building, restriction of women for higher medical education, teaching-learning methods among others with an absence of clarity on the formal role of AETCOM in medical education (Stanikzai et al., 2025).

### *4.2 Bangladesh*

In 2012, the Bangladesh Academic Council was at the forefront in South Asia with its recommendation of the inclusion of ethics, attitude, and communication in the MBBS curriculum (Talukder et al., 2021). The departments of medical education, forensic medicine, and community medicine were to take the lead in teaching medical ethics to students across all phases of the undergraduate medical course (Nurunnabi et al., 2022).

### 4.3 Bhutan

After discussion with experts from Germany, India, Nepal, and Sri Lanka the undergraduate medical curriculum has mandated subjects, including medical humanities, from the first year to the fourth year. Ethics, professionalism, and communication skills are featured in the list of core competencies for the medical student. The role of the Psychiatrist is unclear.

Bhutan has defined skills training in the domains of effective communication with patients and families for the general practice residents. These include breaking bad news and dealing with agitated families. Professional and ethical behaviors, including ethical dilemmas and a code of conduct, have also been defined (Adhikari, 2021; Tenzin et al., 2023).

### 4.4 Maldives

The Maldives Medical Council has given a framework for specialist medical education providers for the inclusion of topics on attitudes and professional behaviors, communication skills, professionalism, leadership qualities, and medical ethics (Maldives Medical and Dental Council, 2021). These topics are integrated with mainstream clinical sciences. The role of the psychiatrist is not specified in this framework.

### 4.5 Nepal

Nepal has led the way in the implementation of medical humanities with the use of a module for the same as early as 2009 (Shankar, 2009). This module contains sections on empathy, doctor–patient relationships, breaking bad news, ethical issues in treating the mentally ill, informed consent, and research ethics. The Tribhuvan University Institute of Medicine has integrated the study of medical ethics in their medical education curriculum and the subject is learnt across the duration of the entire course (Khanal, 2011). In 2018, the Patan Academy of Health Sciences has included a module on medical humanities for the undergraduate medical course. This module covers topics on doctor–patient relationships and compassion using literature and audio-visual media as teaching-learning methods (Krishna Bahadur et al., 2022). The Patan Academy has also initiated a communication skills course in pre-clinical years of undergraduate medicine (Douglas et al., 2020).

### 4.6 Pakistan

The Pakistan Medical and Dental Council (PMDC) recommended the introduction of bioethics education as a part of undergraduate medical curricula as early as 2002. There is a prescribed syllabus for medical ethics, which is covered by the departments of Forensic and Community Medicine and is taught in the 3rd and 4th years of the MBBS. The Aga Khan University in Karachi had initiated a course in humanities and social sciences as part of the medical curriculum (Ghias et al., 2016).

### 4.7 Sri Lanka

The University of Colombo has established a department of medical humanities with the aim of fostering a sense of compassionate care, professionalism, and ethics in medical students (Department of Medical Humanities, n.d.). This marks a formal inclusion of AETCOM in undergraduate medicine at that university.

### 4.8 India

In 2018, in India, the National Medical Commission announced the implementation of a uniform standardized competency-based medical education (CBME) curriculum for the undergraduate medical degree (National Medical Commission, 2018). The CBME has been in operation for undergraduate medical education since 2018 and is expected to be implemented for postgraduate medical education soon. The CBME has placed AETCOM in the explicit curriculum with its emphasis on the medical student achieving competency in medical ethics, developing the right professional attitudes and communication skills.

## 5 The Formal Inclusion of AETCOM in Medical Education

In India, the CBME is a paradigm shift aimed to ensure that the budding medical doctor—irrespective of the university that they had graduated from—had the knowledge, the skills, values, and attitudes to work as a primary care physician. The CBME uses the principle of building competencies in the medical student to confirm a standard skill level. The skills are classified into three domains: cognitive, psychomotor, and affective. AETCOM figures prominently in the CBME, especially in the affective domain.

The following are some AETCOM definitions with examples from psychiatry.

- **Goal**: This refers to the broad purpose of the curriculum. For example: *the goal of the psychiatry clinical posting is to ensure that the medical student can treat people with mental health problems.*
- **Competency**: This refers to the ability to demonstrate a skill. This is more focused in comparison to a goal. For example: *the medical student should have the competency to be able to diagnose alcohol use disorders in an affected individual.*
- **Cognitive skills**: This refers to mental skills and knowledge. The student should know specific information. For example: *the medical student should be able to name indications and adverse effects of Lithium*
- **Psychomotor skills**: Thie refers to manual or physical skills. The student should be able to perform specific procedures. For example: *the psychiatry resident should be able to administer electroconvulsive therapy (ECT)*
- **Affective skills**: This refers to attitudes, ethics, professional behaviors, and communication skills. The student should be able to perform specific tasks related to behaviors. For example: *the medical student should be able to communicate and educate the caregivers of persons with depression about the disorder and treatment.*
- **Certifiable skills**: These are mandatory skills that the medical student (under evaluation) needs to demonstrate independently and be certified accordingly by a trained faculty. For example: *the medical student should be able to identify depression in an individual in the community clinic. Typically, a psychiatry teacher with a qualified specialized degree in psychiatry should evaluate and certify this skill.*
- **Teaching-Learning Methods**: This refers to the methods to inculcate the skill in the learner. For example: *lectures on psychopharmacology, role-play techniques for family caregiver education*
- **Evaluation methods**: This refers to the methods to demonstrate whether the learner has attained proficiency in the skills under assessment. For example: *Multiple Choice Questions for neuroanatomy, Observed Structure Clinical Examination (OSCE) for demonstration of ability to take informed consent.*
- **Integration**: This refers to the interlinking of skill building across subjects to ensure proficiency. This means that skill development in the budding doctor will occur in an interdisciplinary fashion and not in silos.
- **Vertical or longitudinal integration**: This refers to the interlinking of skill building across subjects to ensure proficiency across the years. For example: *the medical student must learn the principles of bioethics. This is facilitated by the collaborative efforts of the physiology (basic science subject) and psychiatry (clinical subject) teacher.*
- **Lateral integration:** This refers to the interlinking of skill building across subjects to ensure proficiency within the same year. For example: *the medical student must learn to break bad news to a caregiver of a patient with terminal illness. This is facilitated by the collaborative efforts of the medicine and psychiatry teacher.*

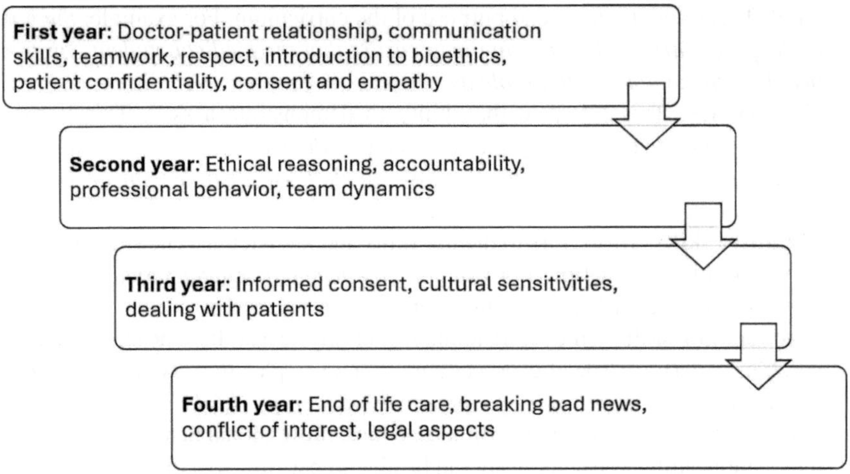


**Fig. 12.1** Flow chart illustrating a four-year medical education curriculum in AETCOM

The AETCOM module is designed to inculcate professional behaviors, ethical ways of thinking, and empathetic and compassionate communication skills in the medical graduate. The AETCOM is to be conducted throughout the entire duration of the undergraduate medical course with explicit specifications for the same including core competencies and certifiable skills (National Medical Commission, 2018). The assessment methods for AETCOM include formative methods like reflective writing and summative measures like short note answer in theory papers and Viva Voce and OSCE demonstrations in the practical examinations. Figure 12.1 shows a tentative rollout of AETCOM across the undergraduate course in India.

## 6 Implications of AETCOM in Undergraduate Medical Education and the Role of the Psychiatry Teacher

As described above, in South Asia, the implementation of AETCOM is throughout the undergraduate medical course. This gives an opportunity to the psychiatry teacher to build collaborations with medical teachers from other specialties (Sarkhel, 2024). The following are some indications of the role of the psychiatry teacher in AETCOM in medical training:

- A good doctor–patient relationship is built on the pillars of communication skills, empathy, professionalism, attitude, and ethics (Fathima et al., 2022). *In the first year, the psychiatry teacher with their knowledge of forming therapeutic alliances while maintaining boundaries could take the start for teaching doctor–patient relationships to medical students.*

- Most psychiatric disorders are treated using biopsychosocial formulations. *In the second year, where the medical students get their first clinical exposure, the psychiatry teacher—with their experience in working with clinical psychologists, social workers, and other stakeholders like schools and similar organizations—could provide guidance for teamwork and dynamics.*
- Psychiatrists are responsible for the care of people with chronic disorders like schizophrenia which are characterized by impaired insight and diminished capacity during acute episodes. *In the third year, when medical students have active clinical training, the psychiatry teacher—with their learning from working with such patients who need supported inpatient treatment—could play a key role in emphasizing the importance and nuances of informed consent.*
- Due to the chronicity of psychiatric conditions, psychiatrists are obligated to work with patient caregivers in ensuring continuity of care. *In the fourth year, when the medical students are fully focused on clinical skill building, the psychiatry teacher could take the lead in teaching the medical student the skill of empathetic listening and sensitive communication in competencies like breaking bad news.*

Table 12.1 shows examples of the role of psychiatry teachers in AETCOM competencies.

The psychiatry teacher could take advantage of the vertical and lateral integration of AETCOM in medical education.

- The collaboration of the psychiatry teacher with the anatomy teacher for a class on genetics could serve as an introduction to bioethics. This is an example of vertical integration.
- The partnership of the psychiatry teacher with the pediatrics teacher for a demonstration on how to address the grief of a parent of a child admitted to the intensive care unit is an illustration of lateral integration in AETCOM. The use of simulated patients with debriefing afterward is a potential teaching method for this competency.

Table 12.2 shows the potential role of the psychiatry teacher as a facilitator for AETCOM across the entire duration of the undergraduate medical course.

**Table 12.1** AETCOM competencies and the role of the psychiatry teacher

| | AETCOM competency | Role of a psychiatry teacher |
|---|---|---|
| 1 | Doctor–patient relationships | Therapeutic alliance, boundaries |
| 2 | Empathy | Empathetic listening |
| 3 | Communication skills | Breaking bad news |
| 4 | Ethics | Confidentiality, consent, involuntary treatment |
| 5 | Professional behavior | Addressing the burnout |
| 6 | Cultural sensitivity | Combating stigma |
| 7 | Palliative ethics | Addressing grief |
| 8 | Teamwork | Interdisciplinary collaboration |

**Table 12.2** Psychiatry teacher facilitating AETCOM across the medical course

| | AETCOM competency | Year of course | Teaching method |
|---|---|---|---|
| 1 | Empathy for the patient | First year | Audio-visual content of patients with chronic suffering and subsequent small group discussions |
| 2 | Professional behavior | Second year | Observation of expert consultants in clinics |
| 3 | Developing awareness of cultural sensitivities | Third year | Community psychiatry posting and clinics |
| 4 | Conflict of interest | Fourth year | Role-plays with subsequent discussions |

Benefits of involvement of the psychiatry teacher in AETCOM in undergraduate medical training include the following:

- Medical students observe the simulated and real-world skills involved in communicating with patients with prolonged suffering and their caregivers
- These observations help develop empathy in these students who might otherwise have not had the exposure to these scenarios
- The development of empathy and communication skills could lead to attitudinal shifts in the young doctor
- These attitudinal shifts could lead to a strong foundation for using bioethics in clinical practice
- This could also lead to a secondary consequence in the reduction of negative attitudes of medical students toward psychiatry (Wang et al., 2016)

## 7 Implications of AETCOM in Postgraduate Medical Education and the Role of the Psychiatry Teacher

While the role of AETCOM in undergraduate medical education is evident, there is no explicit mention of it in most postgraduate curricula across South Asia. In India, the National Medical Commission has proposed the rollout of the CBME for postgraduate medical training soon. It is yet to be seen whether AETCOM will have the same level of structured inclusion as mandated in the undergraduate medical training.

It is generally accepted that irrespective of the type of specialty, postgraduate residents are expected to demonstrate much higher levels of professionalism, ethical behaviors, and communication skills in comparison to the undergraduate medical student. In specialties like psychiatry, it is understood that AETCOM learning will happen simultaneously along with learning core skills and is a prominent aspect in the hidden curriculum. An example of this is suicide prevention.

Suicide prevention is a topic of fundamental importance for the psychiatry resident and teacher. However, psychiatry residents have reported a sense of inadequacy in their skills in this topic (Melton & Coverdale, 2009). For achieving proficiency in the domain of suicide prevention, the psychiatry resident must possess the knowledge of risk factors for suicide, the communication skills to perform risk assessment and show sound judgment on the balance between maintaining patient confidentiality and preventing death by suicide. This proficiency cannot be achieved without the psychiatry residents having made significant strides in their AETCOM skills.

- **Knowledge of risk factors**: In addition to theoretical knowledge, the psychiatry resident should be acquainted with and be aware of the cultural contributors to suicide risk. This will require a high level of cultural sensitivity in the psychiatry resident and teacher.
- **Risk assessment:** The psychiatry resident should be able to establish rapport and have difficult discussions with the patient and their caregivers. This will require a high level of empathy within the residents and appropriate communication skills.
- **Patient confidentiality:** The psychiatry resident should be certain of maintaining confidentiality especially within the context of South Asian culture wherein the family is given greater importance over the individual. This will require the psychiatry resident to have a nonjudgmental attitude and be conversant of the stigma associated with suicidal behaviors within the community. The psychiatry resident should also be aware of the legal implications of suicidal behaviors which are considered against the law in some South Asian societies.

Thus, the psychiatry teacher must facilitate the proficiency in AETCOM in the psychiatry resident. This can be achieved through teaching methods like case studies, ward rounds, observation of consultants and evaluated through assessment strategies like directly observed procedural skills (Chuop et al., 2021).

## 8 Current State of AETCOM in South Asia and Evidence of Effectiveness

Despite the resource constraints, regional diversity, and political and economic instability, the South Asian countries have embarked on inclusion of AETCOM in undergraduate medicine.

In Pakistan, despite the recommendation for inclusion of bioethics in medical education curriculum, the actual implementation has not been optimal (Shirazi et al., 2024). In Karachi, medical students showed positive opinions toward the incorporation of humanities and social sciences in the medical curriculum (Ghias et al., 2016). An interventional study utilized workbook-based ethical skills teaching (Shamim et al., 2021). The total duration of the skills teaching was 30 h across the duration of undergraduate courses with the use of constructional learning material. The teaching involved culturally relevant contextual reading followed by interactive sessions, role-plays, and reflective writing. The study participants reported positive attitudes to this intervention.

In Nepal, a study evaluating the impact of a medical humanities module showed the improvement in empathy in medical students (Krishna Bahadur et al., 2022). Authors from Bangladesh have concluded that continuous curriculum revisions and faculty development are necessary to improve patient care and ethical practice (Khan et al., 2025). In India, the implementation of AETCOM has led to more positive attitudes toward patients in medical students (Amarantha et al., 2022). Some suggested teaching methods for AETCOM include existing methods like ward rounds, seminars and innovative methods like mock ethics meetings and village visits (Fathima et al., 2022).

While these AETCOM initiatives are laudable, the role of the psychiatrist is neither clear nor specified in these endeavors.

## 9 Challenges in the Implementation of AETCOM

The challenges in the implementation of AETCOM in South Asia are manifold. These challenges are at a systemic and logistical level. At a systemic level, persistent regional conflicts and other medical emergencies like COVID 19 pandemics shift the medical training priorities to addressing acute emergencies. The absence of inclusion of AETCOM in the explicit curriculum does not encourage the upskilling of medical teachers in these domains. The time constraints of the medical course could lead to diversion of time from AETCOM to other medical domains. The absence of the requirement of assessment of AETCOM skills could disincentivize the skill building in medical students.

The solutions to these challenges include active advocacy for the inclusion of AETCOM in the explicit curriculum. As part of the explicit curriculum, there should be strong encouragement to involve medical teachers—including those from psychiatry—to obtain continuous training in AETCOM like the continuous medical education programs for other core skills. There should continuous feedback and monitoring from all stakeholders for AETCOM at institutional and university levels.

## 10 The Way Forward in AETCOM and Psychiatry Training

While the inclusion of AETCOM in South Asia in medical education is still emerging, the role of AETCOM in psychiatry training is not formalized. There is minimal research in this area. Neither does the psychiatry teacher figure in the training initiatives in AETCOM across most of South Asia, nor do the AETCOM components figure in the psychiatry curriculum in undergraduate medicine (Table 12.3) (Arafat et al., 2021).

**Table 12.3** Psychiatry training in undergraduate medicine and AETCOM.

| Country | Psychiatry clinics | Psychiatry theory | Psychiatry assessment | Psychiatry internship | AETCOM in psychiatry |
|---|---|---|---|---|---|
| Afghanistan | Not clear | Not clear | Not clear | Not clear | Not clear |
| Bangladesh | 3 weeks | 20 h | Not clear | Posting not mandatory | Present but not as part of psychiatry |
| Bhutan | Not clear | Not clear | Not clear | Not clear | Present but not as part of psychiatry |
| India | 6 weeks | 45 h | Formative and summative assessments with certifiable competencies mandated | 2 weeks mandatory posting | Present but not as part of psychiatry |
| Maldives | Not clear | Not clear | Not clear | Not clear | Present but not as part of psychiatry |
| Nepal | 2 weeks | Heterogenous across colleges | 1.1% of the total assessment marks in the medical council licensing Examination are allocated to mental health | 1–2 weeks of mandatory posting | Present but not as part of psychiatry |
| Pakistan | 3–6 weeks with 8–10 demonstrations | Not clear. Few lectures specified | Examined as part of General medicine paper | Not clear | Present but not as part of psychiatry |
| Sri Lanka | 8–12 weeks | 40–70 h | Final year exam—separate theory paper and practical exam | Posting not mandatory | Present but not as part of psychiatry |

Williams (2024) has averred that the South Asian psychiatrist should be more than just a clinician and should embrace the role of leadership and advocacy for their patients. This could be possible by welcoming opportunities to build bridges with the medical teachers from other basic and clinical sciences to facilitate learning in AETCOM. Matkar (2024) has reiterated the role of empathy in practice of medicine and the usefulness of AETCOM in psychiatry training to address this. There is a need for training initiatives to prepare young psychiatry faculty so that they can take their teaching role in AETCOM forward (Narasimha et al., 2024).

## 11 Conclusions

In South Asia, the psychiatry teacher should be cognizant of the truth that AETCOM in psychiatry training is essential and fundamental. The psychiatry teacher should also bear in mind that they will have to offer their expertise and advocate for their inclusion in AETCOM in medical education, as the current related initiatives do not prioritize psychiatrists.

## References

Adhikari, C. L. (2021). Curriculum for masters in general practice—Bhutan. *Journal of Family Medicine and Primary Care, 10*(6), 2061–2119. https://doi.org/10.4103/jfmpc.jfmpc_1727_20

Adhikari, R. (2014). Ethics in undergraduate medical courses in Nepal. *Kathmandu University Medical Journal, 11*(1), 1–3. https://doi.org/10.3126/kumj.v11i1.11014

Amarantha, D. R., Noor, T., & Swanand, S. P. (2022). Effect of education in AETCOM competencies in shaping the professional attitudes of medical students. *South-East Asian Journal of Medical Education, 16*(2). https://doi.org/10.4038/seajme.v16i2.429

Ambesh, P. (2016). Violence against doctors in the Indian subcontinent: A rising bane. *Indian Heart Journal, 68*(5), 749–750. https://doi.org/10.1016/j.ihj.2016.07.023

Arafat, S. Y., Kar, S. K., Sharma, P., Marahatta, K., & Baminiwatta, A. K. (2021). A comparative analysis of psychiatry curriculum at undergraduate level of Bangladesh, India, Nepal, and Sri Lanka. *Indian Journal of Psychiatry., 63*(2), 184–188. https://doi.org/10.4103/psychiatry.IndianJPsychiatry_615_20

Babapulle, C. J. (1992). Teaching of medical ethics in Sri Lanka. *Medical Education, 26*(3), 185–189. https://doi.org/10.1111/j.1365-2923.1992.tb00152.x

Blomquist, C. (1975). The teaching of medical ethics in Sweden. *Journal of Medical Ethics, 1*(2), 96–103. https://doi.org/10.1136/jme.1.2.96

Chuop, M., Michel, Z., Shah, R., Chen, J. I., & Black, W. (2021). From screening to interventions: Teaching clinical suicide prevention skills to medical students. *Academic Psychiatry, 45*(3), 292–296. https://doi.org/10.1007/s40596-020-01248-3

Department of Medical Humanities. (n.d.). Department of Medical Humanities. Faculty of Medicine, University of Colombo. Retrieved May 2, 2025, from https://med.cmb.ac.lk/medical-humanities/

Douglas, A. H., Acharya, S. P., & Allery, L. A. (2020). Communication skills teaching and learning in Nepal; what are medical students' perceptions and experiences? A qualitative study. *BMC Medical Education, 20*, 391. https://doi.org/10.1186/s12909-020-02330-y

Fathima, F. N., Shankar, N., & Lakshmi, T. A. (2022). Teaching and learning of attitudes, ethics and communication using the AETCOM module in India. *South-East Asian. Journal of Medical Education, 16*(2). https://doi.org/10.4038/seajme.v16i2.393

Ghias, K., Khan, K. S., Ali, R., Azfar, S., & Ahmed, R. (2016). Stretching the boundaries of medical education A case of medical college embracing humanities and social sciences in medical education. *Pakistan Journal of Medical Sciences, 32*(4), 911–916. https://doi.org/10.12669/pjms.324.10237

Jahan, S., & Flora, M. S. (2022). Mind-set of recent medical graduates: A channel for teaching medical ethics and professionalism in Bangladesh. *Bangladesh Medical Research Council Bulletin, 47*(1), 57–61. https://doi.org/10.3329/bmrcb.v47i1.55801

Javaeed, A. (2019). General needs assessment of the undergraduate medical students to integrate courses on medical ethics, time management and communication skills into the bachelor of medicine, bachelor of surgery curriculum of Pakistani medical colleges. *Cureus, 11*(4), e4433. https://doi.org/10.7759/cureus.4433

Jones, J. S. (1975). The Nottingham medical school. *British medical journal, 4*(5987), 29–31. https://doi.org/10.1136/bmj.4.5987.29

Khan, K. M., Ferdous, J., & Islam, M. (2025). Undergraduate medical education in Bangladesh: Current scenario and future challenges. *South-East Asian Journal of Medical Education, 18*(2). https://doi.org/10.4038/seajme.v18i2.622

Khanal, S. (2011, July 1). *Tribhuvan University (TU) Institute of Medicine (IOM) curriculum for MBBS*. Digital Medicine. https://digitalmedicine.com.np/tribhuvan-university-tu-curriculum-for-mbbs-cc70dae71f3.

Krishna Bahadur, G. C., Arjyal, A., Douglas, A. H., Subedi, M., & Gongal, R. (2022). A quantitative evaluation of empathy using JSE-S Tool, before and after a medical humanities module, amongst first-year medical students in Nepal. *BMC Medical Education, 22*(1), 159. https://doi.org/10.1186/s12909-022-03188-y

Maldives Medical and Dental Council. (2021). *Guide for accreditation assessment of specialty medical education programmes* (Report No. MMDC/DOC/2021/02-v01). https://health.gov.mv/storage/uploads/edYGjBwl/v1ivm6md.pdf.

Marambe, K. N., Edussuriya, D. H., & Dayaratne, K. M. (2012). Attitudes of Sri Lankan medical students toward learning communication skills. *Education for Health (Abingdon, England), 25*(3), 165–171. https://doi.org/10.4103/1357-6283.109796

Matkar, A. (2024). My journey with empathy. *Indian Journal of Psychological Medicine, 46*(5), 377–379. https://doi.org/10.1177/02537176241281994

Melton, B. B., & Coverdale, J. H. (2009). What do we teach psychiatric residents about suicide? A national survey of chief residents. *Academic Psychiatry, 33*(1), 47–50. https://doi.org/10.1176/appi.ap.33.1.47

Miyasaka, M., Akabayashi, A., Kai, I., & Ohi, G. (1999). An international survey of medical ethics curricula in Asia. *Journal of Medical Ethics, 25*(6), 514–521. https://doi.org/10.1136/jme.25.6.514

Moore, M. (2009). What do Nepalese medical students and doctors think about patient-centred communication? *Patient Education and Counseling, 76*(1), 38–43. https://doi.org/10.1016/j.pec.2008.11.018

Narasimha, V. L., Suhas, S., Kishor, M., Dixit, A., & Murthy, P. (2024). Advances in psychiatry training and faculty development in India. *Indian Journal of Psychological Medicine, 46*(5), 391–399. https://doi.org/10.1177/02537176241284348

National Medical Commission. (2018). *Attitude, ethics and communication (AETCOM) competencies for the Indian Medical Graduate [Internet]*. NMC. [cited 2025 Apr 29]. Available from: https://www.nmc.org.in/wp-content/uploads/2020/01/AETCOM_book.pdf

Nurunnabi, A. S. M., Hasan, M. J., Quddus, A. R., Khan, M. T. I., Sultan, M. T., Sharmin, S., Rahman, M. M., Tripura, K. K., & Alamgir, S. N. (2022). Teaching and learning medical ethics: how to bring positive change. *Community Based Medical Journal, 11*(2), 167–175. https://doi.org/10.3329/cbmj.v11i2.61290

Pourbairamian, G., Bigdeli, S., Arabshahi, S. K. S., Yamani, N., Sohrabi, Z., Ahmadi, F., & Sandars, J. (2022). Hidden curriculum in medical residency programs: a scoping review. *Journal of Advances in Medical Education & Professionalism, 10*(2), 69. https://doi.org/10.30476/JAMP.2021.92478.1486

Ranasinghe, A. W. I. P., Fernando, B., Sumathipala, A., & Gunathunga, W. (2020). Medical ethics: knowledge, attitude and practice among doctors in three teaching hospitals in Sri Lanka. *BMC Medical Ethics, 21*(1), 69. https://doi.org/10.1186/s12910-020-00511-4

Sahadevan, S., Kurian, N., Mani, A. M., Kishor, M. R., & Menon, V. (2021). Implementing competency-based medical education curriculum in undergraduate psychiatric training in India: Opportunities and challenges. *Asia-Pacific Psychiatry, 13*(4), e12491. https://doi.org/10.1111/appy.12491

Sarkhel, S. (2024). Teaching communication skills to Indian medical graduates: Time for psychiatrists to take the leading role! *Indian Journal of Psychiatry, 66*(7), 589–590. https://doi.org/10.4103/indianjpsychiatry.indianjpsychiatry_583_24

Shamim, M. S., Baig, L., Torda, A., & Balasooriya, C. (2021). Impact of a novel approach for undergraduate medical ethics education in the Middle East and South Asia. https://doi.org/10.21203/rs.3.rs-658417/v1.

Shankar, P. R. (2009). A voluntary medical humanities module in a medical college in Western Nepal: participant feedback. *Teaching and Learning in Medicine, 21*(3), 248–253. https://doi.org/10.1080/10401330903020605

Shirazi, B., Riaz, Q., Jafarey, A. M., Ahmed, R., & Shamim, M. S. (2024). The current status and challenges of bioethics education in undergraduate medical education in Karachi, Pakistan. *BMC Medical Education, 24*(1), 737. https://doi.org/10.1186/s12909-024-05599-5

Stanikzai, M. H., Shanawa, S., Karimkhil, A. T., & Dadras, O. (2025). Medical education in Afghanistan: Challenges and policy implications. *Advances in Medical Education and Practice, 16*, 477–482. https://doi.org/10.2147/AMEP.S510309

Talukder, M. H., Nazneen, R., Kabir, M. F., Nuruzzaman, M., Talukder, M. S., Tapu, T. T., Sa-Ad, S. A., & Faruque, T. B. (2021). Need assessment for updating the MBBS curriculum 2012 of Bangladesh. *Mymensingh Medical Journal: MMJ, 30*(3), 789–795. https://doi.org/10.3329/mmj.v30i3.53256

Tenzin, K., Dorji, T., Sherub, K., Chhezom, K., Dorji, G., Tshering, K., Choden, S., Mukhia, S., Choeda, T., Galey, K., Gyamtsho, S., Tshering, P., Siebeck, M., Jayasinghe, S., & Dhakal, G. P. (2023). An integrated competency-based curriculum for undergraduate medical education programme in Bhutan. *South-East Asian Journal of Medical Education, 17*(2). https://doi.org/10.4038/seajme.v17i2.576

Tom Mishael, J., Vaz, M., & Timms, O. (2019). Looking back–looking forward: ethics finds its place in the medical curriculum in India. *International Journal of Ethics Education, 4*, 97–107. https://link.springer.com/article/10.1007/s40889-019-00074-y

Veatch, R. M., & Fenner, D. (1975). The teaching of medical ethics in the United States of America. *Journal of Medical Ethics, 1*(2), 99–103. https://doi.org/10.1136/jme.1.2.99

Wang, P. W., Ko, C. H., Chen, C. S., Yang, Y. H., Lin, H. C., Cheng, C. C., Tsang, H. Y., Wu, C. K., & Yen, C. F. (2016). Changes of Explicit and Implicit Stigma in Medical Students during Psychiatric Clerkship. *Academic psychiatry, 40*(2), 224–228. https://doi.org/10.1007/s40596-015-0432-8

Williams, S. S. (2024). Fine-tuning postgraduate psychiatry training in South Asia. *Indian Journal of Psychological Medicine, 46*(5), 380–381. https://doi.org/10.1177/02537176241280284

Wong, M. K., Hong, D. Z. H., Wu, J., Ting, J. J. Q., Goh, J. L., Ong, Z. Y., Toh, R. Q. E., Chiang, C. L. L., Ng, C. W. H., Ng, J. C. K., Cheong, C. W. S., Tay, K. T., Tan, L. H. S., Ong, Y. T., Chiam, M., Chin, A. M. C., Mason, S., & Radha Krishna, L. K. (2022). A systematic scoping review of undergraduate medical ethics education programs from 1990 to 2020. *Medical Teacher, 44*(2), 167–186. https://doi.org/10.1080/0142159X.2021.1970729

World Health Organization. (2009). Module for teaching medical ethics to undergraduates. In *Module for teaching medical ethics to undergraduates*. https://apps.who.int/iris/bitstream/handle/10665/205534/B4401.pdf.

# Chapter 13
# Assessment in Psychiatry Teaching

**Henal Shah, Karishma Rupani, and Adnan Kadiani**

**Abstract** Assessment plays an important role in ensuring the quality of services and preparing students to achieve the defined requirements. Psychiatry is a field where students are required to achieve clinical competence, communication skills, and professional attitudes. This chapter describes the current landscape of psychiatry assessment in South Asia. It acknowledges the diversity of educational systems, the impact of contextual factors, and the increasingly important role of assessment in ensuring high-quality training. Drawing on examples from countries including India, Pakistan, Bangladesh, Sri Lanka, and Nepal, this chapter critically examines assessment methods and the evolving changes. This chapter highlights the challenges, such as resource constraints, stigma, variability in faculty training, and regulatory differences, while also mentioning the strengths and opportunities. Finally, a few recommendations for enhancing psychiatry assessment are suggested. This will ensure better training of future doctors and psychiatrists, capable of meeting the needs of the community.

**Keywords** Assessment · Undergraduate · Postgraduate · Psychiatry education · South Asia

H. Shah (✉)
Department of Psychiatry, TNMC and BYL Nair Ch. Hospital, Mumbai, Maharashtra, India

GSMC - FAIMER Regional Institute, Mumbai, Maharashtra, India

K. Rupani
Department of Psychiatry, Seth GSMC & KEMH, Mumbai, Maharashtra, India

A. Kadiani
Department of Psychiatry, TNMC and BYL Nair Ch. Hospital, Mumbai, Maharashtra, India



S. K. Kar et al. (eds.), *Teaching and Training in Psychiatry in South Asia*, South Asian Perspectives in Mental Health and Psychology,
https://doi.org/10.1007/978-981-95-1845-6_13

# 1 Introduction

Assessment is today's means of modifying tomorrow's instruction—Carol Ann Tomlinson.

Assessment is any systematic method of obtaining information from tests and other sources, used to draw inferences about characteristics of people, objects, or programmes (AERA, 1999). Assessment helps gauge a student's progress in learning, identify roadblocks, and provide direction and motivation for future learning, encompassing knowledge, skills, and professionalism. Assessment methods also encourage learning by providing feedback to the students and teachers. This facilitates refining their teaching-learning methods (TL) and improves learning outcomes in education. It ensures the standards of care are maintained.

An apt assessment involves defining outcomes based on a needs assessment and following Kern's cycle for designing a curriculum (Kern et al., 1998). Needs assessments are obtained from two sources: the burden of psychiatric disorders in the community, and the other involves an estimation of the strengths, weaknesses, knowledge, and skills of the students (Fig. 13.1). An effective assessment requires alignment between the objectives, teaching and learning methods, and assessment.

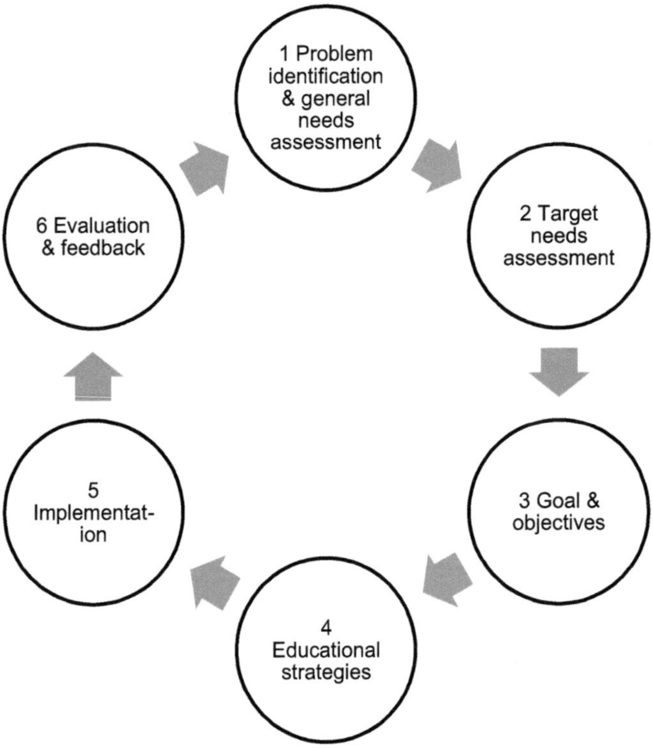


**Fig. 13.1** Kern's six-step approach to curriculum development

This chapter gives a broad outline of assessment methods and then takes a closer look at undergraduate and postgraduate assessment strategies. A closer look at Indian systems is included for a clearer understanding.

# 2 Assessment Methods

Depending on the purpose and format, there are various ways of classifying assessment.

## *2.1 Formative and Summative*

Summative exams are qualifying high-stakes exams and do not provide for feedback and improvement. It has been proven that a programmatic assessment, which includes a well-designed longitudinal plan for "assessment for learning" (formative assessment) rather than "assessment of learning" (summative assessment) is effective in reaching desired outcomes. The progress of learners throughout the academic year is continuously monitored, and feedback is provided.

## *2.2 Format*

### 2.2.1 Written Tests

They are of two major categories: constructed-response tests and selected-response tests. For constructed-response tests, questions are presented, and the response is expected in writing (or typing) answers. Constructed-response formats include, for example, "Fill-in-the-blanks". Selected-response tests present a question or stimulus (referred to as a stem), followed by a number of option choices, e.g. multiple-choice (MC) questions.

### 2.2.2 Observation of Clinical Performance

This stage requires that students have an adequate knowledge base, the basic skills to perform fundamental tasks, and core attributes of commitment. Students at this stage are assessed such that they can answer the "What" questions about their patients. Assessment methods would therefore include case presentations and performance of clinical examinations (e.g. eliciting the Mental Status Examination).

This stage also requires the students to offer reasonable explanations for new problems and generate and defend a differential diagnosis. This step requires a greater knowledge base, increased confidence and skill in selecting and applying clinical facts to a specific patient. Students should be able to answer the "Why" questions about their patients. Assessment methods include viva voce, case discussions, and direct observation of procedural skills.

### 2.2.3 Performance Tests

A performance test is an examination designed to elicit performance on an actual or simulated real-life task. In contrast to observation of naturally occurring behaviour "in vivo", the task is contrived for the purpose of the examination and explicitly invites the examinee to demonstrate the behaviour to be assessed. Thus, a performance test is an "in vitro" assessment, at Miller's "shows how" level, involving all three domains, using methods such as Observation of Structured Clinical Examination (OSCE) and Observation of Structured Long Examination Record (OSLER). In vivo assessment methods include multisource feedback and mini-clinical evaluation exercise. These are often termed as work-based assessment.

### 2.2.4 Other Assessment Methods

This category includes miscellaneous types of assessments such as the formal oral exam, portfolios of student experiences, and case viva.

No assessment is ideal; all have their strengths and limitations (Table 13.1). An assessment tool is as good as the effort that is applied in training and utilization. It is therefore wise to choose according to context, stakes involved, feasibility, and acceptability. A well-planned programme would be the most appropriate way to plan.

## *2.3 Taxonomies of Learning and Their Assessment*

George Miller and Bloom have provided useful taxonomies, a classification system that organizes knowledge and skills into categories and subcategories. There are multiple assessment systems to gauge knowledge, skills, and attitudes at each level of these taxonomies.

I Miller proposed a framework for assessing clinical competence by dividing it into four hierarchical processes (Miller, 1990). At the lowest level of the pyramid is the assessment of knowledge (knows), followed by application of knowledge (knows how), performance (shows how), and action (does). This was later modified by Ten Cate et al. (2021) to include the dimension of "trusted" for coping with both familiar and unfamiliar situations in their practice and reflects the ability to adapt as per the context. The ability to trust is a hallmark of entrustable professional activities of assessment in a CBME curriculum.

**Table 13.1** Strengths and limitations of assessment methods

| Method | Domain assessed | Used currently | Drawbacks | Strengths |
|---|---|---|---|---|
| *Written* | | | | |
| MCQ | Knowledge, problem-solving | Summative and formative | Difficult to create<br>Not authentic | Quick, high reliability, technology can help |
| SAQ | Knowledge, problem-solving, clinical reasoning | Summative and formative | Training of raters critical | No guesswork |
| Structured essay | Synthesis, interpretation, and reasoning | Summative | Training of raters critical for reliability<br>Resource intensive | Can assess higher order cognitive domains |
| *Observation* | | | | |
| Oral | Knowledge, problem-solving, and clinical reasoning | Summative<br>Formative | Reliability is an issue, subjective with bias, resource-intensive | Feedback by an expert is valuable |
| Structured direct observation Mini-CEX/ DOPS | Clinical and communication skills | Formative | Selective observation<br>Not holistic | Feedback from expert is valuable |
| Global rating | Clinical and communication skills, teamwork | Formative | Subjective<br>Usually based on indirect observation | Improve use by having multiple experts rating |
| *Clinical simulations* | | | | |
| OSCE and standardized patients | Clinical communication and interpersonal skills | Summative<br>Formative | Not authentic, shortcuts penalized<br>Resources required | Reliable, consistent, observable |
| Technology-enabled simulation | Procedural skills | Formative | Not authentic, shortcuts penalized<br>Resources required | Reliable, consistent, realistic |
| *Multisource* | | | | |
| Peer | Professionalism, communication and interpersonal skills | Formative | Training of peers, confidentiality issues | Observes habits, authentic, credible |
| Patient | Ability to form rapport, communication skills | Formative | Global impression | Credible |
| Self | Knowledge, skills, and attitudes | Formative | Usually not accurate<br>Requires training | Encourages self-learning and reflection |
| Portfolios | Knowledge, skills, and attitudes<br>Competency of practice-based learning and system-based practice | Formative, occasionally summative | Time-consuming<br>Training required | Encourages self-learning and reflection<br>Technology can be incorporated and helps longitudinal tracking |

**Table 13.2** Levels and domains of learning and their assessment

| Level (domain-specific) | Level (Miller) | Level (Bloom) | Verbs Assessment tools | Type of assessment |
|---|---|---|---|---|
| Cognitive | Knows | Knowledge | Identify, define<br>Multiple-choice questions (MCQs) | Summative assessment |
| Cognitive | Knows | Comprehension | Describe, interpret, paraphrase, summarize -<br>Short answer questions, essays | Summative assessment |
| Cognitive + Affective | Knows how | Application | Practice, illustrate, problem-solving (case based)<br>Viva voce<br>Case presentation with feedback | Summative Formative |
| Cognitive + Affective | Knows how | Analysis | Differentiate, categorize, classify<br>Viva voce<br>Peer assessment, small group presentation | Summative Formative |
| Cognitive + Affective + Psychomotor | Shows how | Synthesis | Construct, organize, design<br>Multiple case studies, long case, OSCE, OSLER | Summative and Formative |
| Cognitive + Affective + Psychomotor | Does | Evaluation | Appraise, justify<br>Presentation DOPS<br>Mini-CEX, MSF<br>Debates | Summative Formative |

**Bloom's Taxonomy**

Bloom's Taxonomy is a hierarchical framework that organizes skills, helping teachers frame objectives and align assessments. It also describes the verbs that can be used to describe the desired objectives. The revised Bloom's Taxonomy (Anderson & Karthwohl, 2001) organizes learning objectives into six levels of cognitive complexity: Knowledge (lowest), Comprehension, Application, Analysis, Synthesis, and Evaluation (highest). Similarly, there is a hierarchy for affective and psychomotor skills. Table 13.2 illustrates the integration of these concepts.

## 3 Undergraduate Assessment

Compared to the global standards, the implementation of a competency-based assessment (CBA) framework with an all-encompassing model of teaching that was student- and skill-driven, with outcome-based assessment that furthered learning, was adopted early on in the Western world. In South Asia, however, implementation of such a CBA curriculum has been adopted relatively late, with implementation at different stages of CBA across countries in Asia. South Asian countries are now adapting to their local cultural context. Hence, in many ways, there are similarities across the countries with varying degrees of importance to psychiatry in the undergraduate curriculum (Table 13.3).

**Table 13.3** Curriculum and assessment of UG in South Asia (Arafat et al., 2021)

| Country | Training period | Curriculum and assessment details | Independent subject |
|---|---|---|---|
| Afghanistan | Two-week internship during the final year of training | | Not an independent subject |
| Bangladesh (Arafat, 2020, 2024) | 20 h: didactic lectures<br>3-weeks of clinical rotation in psychiatry<br>Years 4 & 5:<br>Ward placement in the third phase for clinical classes<br>Internship: as an elective for 5 days in some institutions. No mandatory placement in psychiatry | Psychiatry teaching starts late in medical course<br>-Receives less importance during internship (elective psychiatry posting) | Not an independent subject |
| Bhutan | Workplace-based assessment (WPBA):<br>The curriculum mandates that residents undergo WPBA sessions, with assessments like Mini-CEX, CbD, -DOPS 360-degree feedback.<br>Focus on core competencies:<br>to meet the needs of Bhutanese healthcare | The curriculum for the Bhutan Medicine Programme adopts an integrated approach for teaching-learning and assessments | Separate exam for graduation |
| Maldives | Recently introduced a 5-year programme with psychiatry in year 4 (32 credits) | | Not an independent subject |

(continued)

**Table 13.3** (continued)

| Country | Training period | Curriculum and assessment details | Independent subject |
|---|---|---|---|
| Nepal | 25–92 h didactic lectures<br>The clinical rotation for mental health is mostly 2 weeks to a maximum of 4 weeks<br>Internship posting: 2 weeks/1 week<br>Elective—2 weeks | Formative and summative assessment<br>competence assessed medical knowledge, patient care, professionalism, communication and interpersonal skills, practice-based<br>Assessment tools<br>Case presentation and assessment, seminars<br>MCQs, SAQs, modified essay questions,<br>OSCE, Viva, Mini-CEX<br>Exams<br>Included in the Internal Medicine paper, ranging from 3.75% to 31% of the total Internal Medicine marks<br>Practical exams:<br>Case presentation<br>Simulated clinical assessment | Not an independent subject |
| Pakistan | 4-week rotation during the 4th year of the MBBS programme, followed by an end-of-term examination and a written paper at the end of the year | | No separate examination for graduation |
| Sri Lanka | 40–75 h of lectures<br>8–12 weeks of clinical training<br>Clinical posting has two separate clerkships placed in the 4th and 5th year<br>Internship: Psychiatry posting isn't mandatory | Competencies assessed include diagnosing mental illnesses, core soft skills such as listening, empathy, effective communication and humanitarian values<br>Assessment tools<br>Case presentation using DOPS (formative assessment) written exams<br>Use of LMS for teaching and evaluation<br>The final qualifying examination in psychiatry<br>Given almost equal weightage as the other subjects.<br>It includes the following-<br>Essay and multiple-choice questions in theory exams<br>Practical exams in the form of objective structured clinical examinations and case viva | Evaluation as a separate subject<br>Integrates psychiatry with other medical disciplines, highlighting the importance of a holistic approach to patient care<br>Lacks depth in subspecialities |

## *3.1 Implementation in India*

In 2019, India moved towards a competency-based model. The new curriculum defined the roles of an Indian Medical Graduate (Box 13.1)

**Box 13.1 Roles of Indian Medical Graduate (IMG)**
An IMG ought to be a:

Clinician who understands and provides preventive, promotive, curative, palliative, and holistic care with compassion.
Leader and member of the healthcare team and system.
Communicator with patients, families, colleagues, and community.
Lifelong learner committed to continuous improvement of skills and knowledge.
Professional who is committed to excellence, is ethical, responsive, and accountable to patients, the profession, and community.
Critical Thinker who demonstrates problem-solving skills in professional practice.
Researcher who generates and interprets evidence to ensure effective patient care as well as contribute in the field of medical research and practice.

The curriculum and assessment changed from a knowledge-based curriculum to an outcome-based curriculum with specific competencies linked to the proficiencies required of the IMG (Box 13.2).

**Box 13.2 Psychiatry Goals for an IMG**
At the end of training, the learner should be able to

Promote mental health and mental hygiene.
Identify clinical features, make a diagnosis, and manage common psychiatric disorders across all ages.
Identify and manage psychotic disorders, mainly schizophrenia.
Identify and manage stress-related psychiatric disorders, institute preliminary treatment in disorders difficult to manage, and refer appropriately.
Identify alcohol/substance abuse disorders and refer them to appropriate centres
Assess the risk for suicide and refer appropriately.

For the first time, certifiable competencies related to diagnosing depression and suicide risk assessment were added to the curriculum. In 2024, based on Kern's six-step approach, there was a revision in the curriculum by the National Medical Council (NMC) (NMC Compendium, 2024; Sethi et al., 2024). The SWOT analysis of the CBME curriculum is outlined in Fig. 13.2.

The assessment can be categorized into the following:

### 3.1.1 Theory

The SAQs and MCQs would need to be scenario/case-based questions, which require not just rote, but application of analytical skills to be able to push the assessment higher up the Bloom's ladder.

### 3.1.2 Clinical Postings

The pedagogical tool used is DOAP (Demonstrate, Observe, Assist, and Perform) by the teachers, along with the use of role-plays, followed by formative assessment in the form of DOPS.

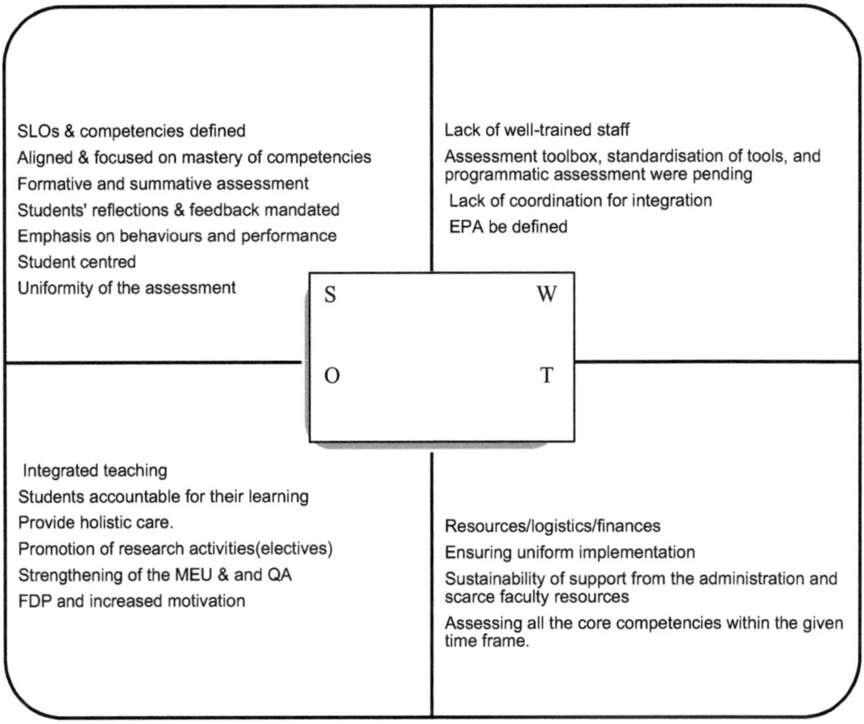


**Fig. 13.2** A SWOT analysis of CBME

The NMC has recommended outcome-based assessment metrics like OSCEs with objective checklists assessing the students across psychomotor, communication, affective, knowledge, and attitudinal domains. It prescribes formative assessment in that the feedback given to students is to be actualized for further learning.

**Self-Directed Learning**

Self-directed learning for a total duration of 10 h has been prescribed in phase 3, part 2. Topics can comprise those disorders which are seen relatively less often and those that would require the students to read in depth about, from the college library. Feedback is given by both the faculty and students.

### 3.1.3 Documentation

**Documentation in Logbooks as Reinforcers of Learning**

As opposed to earlier, the students now have a different logbook. The logbook had the competencies printed, against which the faculty had to document the number of attempts at the attainment of a specific competency as F (first), R (repeat), or Re (remedial). A decision of the faculty in terms of C (Completed), R (Repeat), and Re (Remedial) was also recorded so that remedial measures could be taken and recorded if required. A new column has been added to record the learner's reflection and feedback. Completion of certifiable competencies for that phase is to be recorded by the teacher in the logbooks.

A record of activities in the logbook is to be submitted as a prerequisite to be allowed to take their summative post-end exam. Assessment elements could include participation in grand rounds, seminars, case records, submission of assignments, reflection on learnings, and participation in patient education programmes. It is also imperative for the students to write down their reflections in their journals.

**Documentation in Journals**

Documentation of the cases that the students were assigned, psychological tests, drugs, and lab tests, e.g., Therapeutic Drug Monitoring tests, form a part of the formative assessment.

At the end of the posting, an exam, which consisted of OSCE and a viva, is conducted.

**Components of Internal Assessment (IA)**

Theory IA includes: SAQs, which are in the format of a case-based discussion.

Practical/Clinical IA includes practical/clinical tests, Objective Structured Clinical Examination (OSCE)/Objective Structured Practical Examination (OSPE), and Directly Observed Procedural Skills (DOPS).

Assessment of Logbook: The logbook records all activities like seminars, symposia, quizzes, and other academic activities. It is assessed regularly and submitted to the department. It constitutes 20% of the IA marks.

### 3.1.4 University Exams

Theory exams: As Psychiatry is not yet an independent subject and finds itself as a part of General Medicine and allied subjects, its weightage was 25% marks of General Medicine paper 2 (total out of 100 marks) in the final University exams. In theory examinations, the section B of paper 2 of medicine has been dedicated to the allied subjects, Psychiatry and Dermatology, with a weightage of 50% for each.

### 3.1.5 Electives

Electives provide interested students a chance to focus on a niche aspect in Psychiatry that is usually not covered during their routine lectures and postings.

They are divided into Block 1 and Block 2 electives. Block 1 (15 days) is non-clinical, in which the students can choose to do a preceptor-initiated research study. Assessment is based on the presentation of their research protocol, followed by feedback from the faculty. The student is observed for the implementation of ethical guidelines whilst conducting the research, and timely feedback is given when required to shape learning. Block 2 electives are "clinical" (for 15 days) wherein the students can benefit from a range of learning experiences including subspeciality OPDs and ward rounds, attend and participate in discussions, providing them with an immersive experience. Assessment is formative based on their reflections, completion of case presentations, and DOPS.

# 4 Postgraduate Assessment

The ultimate goal of postgraduate (PG) training is to make a doctor proficient in providing high-quality health care to patients in his speciality and advance the science of his speciality through research and training. The difference from UG training is that for postgraduates, students must ascend the Miller's pyramid from "knows" to ultimately "does" and be trusted. In South Asia, Afghanistan and the Maldives do not offer any postgraduate training. There are some variations in the other countries (Kallivayalil & Enara, 2021).

## *4.1 Assessment in India*

The postgraduate training is mainly monitored through the National Medical Council (NMC); there are a few centres of national importance that are run autonomously (Fig. 13.3).

Historically, PG teaching in psychiatry faces a myriad of challenges (Pal et al., 2024). This includes a lack of uniformity in training, insufficient training in

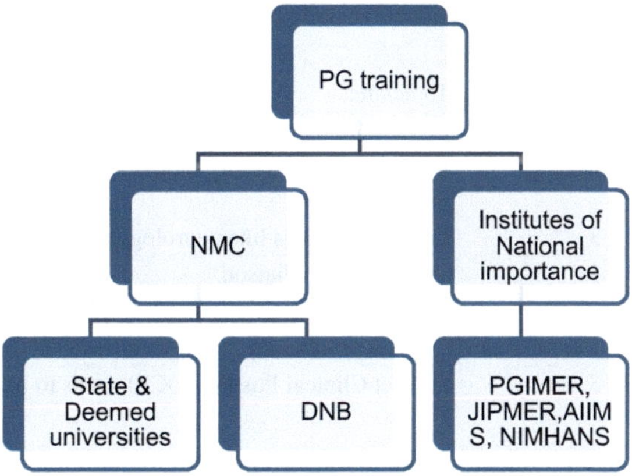


**Fig. 13.3** Organization of training in India. NMC, National Medical Council; DNB, Diplomate of National Board; PGIMER, Postgraduate Institute of Medical Education & Research; AIIMS, All India Institute of Medical Sciences, NIMHANS, National Institute of Mental Health & Neurosciences

psychotherapy, limited availability of training in novel modalities such as Repetitive Transcranial Magnetic Stimulation (rTMS) and Transcranial direct current stimulation(tDCS), a lack of robust assessment programmes, assessments mostly focusing on knowledge and less on skill, and finally, inadequate teacher training.

Attempts have been made in recent times to address some of these challenges. The Post-Graduate Medical Education Board (PGMEB) of the National Medical Council (NMC) of India, as part of the Competency-based Medical Education (CBME), has developed a curriculum to be followed by universities offering MD in Psychiatry (Medical Council in India, 2019). The National Board of Examinations in Medical Sciences (NBEMS), an autonomous body under the Ministry of Health and Family Welfare, Government of India, has developed a standardized assessment format for the Diplomate of National Board (DNB) examination for psychiatry. This assessment format aims to be more objective and aims to assess both knowledge and skills.

The new CBME curriculum document does a thorough job of defining competencies a student needs to learn by the end of the 36 months of postgraduate training in Psychiatry. These competencies are designed to ensure that students acquire knowledge (cognitive domain), skills (psychomotor domain), and an appropriate attitude (affective domain) by the end of the course. Based on these competencies, 19 SLOs (Specific learning objectives) are outlined.

The syllabus that needs to be taught has been meticulously outlined with 53 Must-know items and 7 May-know items. Specific competencies that the student must be able to demonstrate have been defined. The curriculum document elucidates the competencies students should be able to perform independently, under supervision, and with assistance from an expert. Along with core psychiatry, the curriculum gives importance to developing research, teaching, and leadership skills in students (Singh, 2022).

Each postgraduate trainee needs to go through a total of 36 months of psychiatry training in India, which is spread as depicted in Table 13.4.

Table 13.4 Breakdown of duration of psychiatry training in India

| Time (months) | Topic/area |
|---|---|
| 18 | In the ward and OPD |
| 9 | In various subspeciality clinics like forensic, child, de-addiction, community psychiatry |
| 3 | In allied sciences like neurology and internal medicine |
| 3 | In consultation liaison |
| 2 | Assigned as electives, can be decided by the institute |
| 1 | Clinical psychology |
| 3 | District Clinical Posting (DCP) needs to be factored into the schedule |

### 4.1.1 Summative Assessment

MD Psychiatry and the DNB Psychiatry summative exam has three parts: Thesis writing, theory examination, and practical examination, each of which will be discussed in detail below.

**Thesis Writing**

The thesis assesses concepts of research methodology. As soon as the PG trainee enters training, he is assigned a research guide who helps them select a topic within the first 6 months of their training and helps them conceptualize, plan, and execute the research. The completed thesis is to be submitted at least 6 months before the theory and practical examination and should be examined by at least three examiners (one internal and two external).

Strengths: For those who write their thesis sincerely and have active collaboration with their guide, writing the thesis can significantly help develop and enhance their skills and proficiency in research.

Weakness: The demanding nature of 3 years of training, along with a lack of research interest, makes it difficult for the trainee to devote time to thesis writing. Occasionally, the PG guides are not accessible because of their clinical, administrative, and personal commitments. These lead to impoverishing the quality of research and, in some cases, fabrication of data.

**Theory Examination**

MD course exams and DNB exams follow a similar format. It consists of 4 papers of 100 marks each. Paper 1 is basic sciences related to psychiatry. Paper 2 is clinical and organic psychiatry. Paper 3 is psychiatry subspecialties. Paper 4 questions regarding recent advances in psychiatry. Each paper is 100 marks and typically consists of 10-mark short answer questions (5 questions) and 25-mark long answer questions (2 questions).

Strengths: Excellent method to assess knowledge domain; questions can be framed as clinical case scenarios to gauge the "know-how" along with the "knows".

Weakness: Since these papers are only taken at the end of the trainee's 36-month course, they may struggle to write long and short answer questions. The evaluation of essay answers can be subjective and depend on the examiner.

**Practical Examination**

The practical examination for a trainee is taken on a single day after the theory examination.

It is conducted by four university-appointed examiners, of whom two are internal examiners and two are external examiners. Currently, the MD course candidates' practical examinations include four stations for assessment

(a) Presentation of a long case of psychiatry (100 marks)
(b) Neurology short case (50 marks)
(c) Short case—psychiatry (50 marks)
(d) Viva voce (100 marks).
(e) OSCE (80 marks)
(f) Thesis viva (20 marks)

The DNB psychiatry practical exam is of 300 marks in total. It contains 2 clinical cases for a total of 100 marks, ward rounds of 40 marks, Viva of 60 marks, and 20 OSCE stations of 100 marks.

Strengths: The format of the practical exam helps the examiners evaluate the "Know How" and "Show".

Limitations: Each student needs to be thoroughly evaluated in multiple separate stations, which is time and resource-intensive. Uniformity in scoring, bias of examiners are present, which OSCE aims to mitigate (Singh, 2022).

### 4.1.2 Formative Assessment

One simple way to understand formative assessment is that it gathers evidence of student learning and uses this evidence to guide student learning. It is a necessary part of self-directed adult learning where assessment monitors students' progress, helps identify their strengths and weaknesses, and encourages further learning.

According to the NMC guidelines, formative assessment should be continual and should assess medical knowledge, patient care, procedural & academic skills, interpersonal skills, professionalism, self-directed learning, and the ability to practice in the health system.

The NBE board, in its guidelines for competency-based training, has outlined a three-part scheme for formative assessment: part 1 is conducting a theory exam, part 2 is a feedback session on theory performance, and part 3 is a workplace-based clinical assessment.

The guidelines, however, lack a detailed framework for conducting formative assessments. Unlike summative assessments, there is no unified formative system across boards. This leads to significant variations in the techniques and approaches used. To counter this, the various subcommittees of the Indian Psychiatry Society (IPS) conduct digital mock exams for PG students.

**Internal Exams**

Some institutes hold formative exams (Theory and/or Practical) annually, whereas some hold them every 6 months.

**Academic Activities**
Feedback during academic activities is also a form of formative assessment. Institutes with PG programmes in India have various academic activities, including but not limited to case presentations, topic presentations, journal clubs, and academic discussions. These are typically presented by the PG students and are attended by faculty members. At the end of the activity, feedback is provided to the student presenting on the areas where they did well and areas where they could improve.

**Unstructured Work-Based Assessment**
A PG student as a part of his training needs to elicit and then present a detailed history, examination findings, their provisional diagnosis and the diagnostic formulation of the OPD/IPD patient to faculty of the institute; these faculty then independently assess the patient, give their diagnosis and collaborate on developing a management plan for the patient. This helps the student in two ways, one is that the faculty provides direct feedback to the student, and second, while observing the faculty eliciting history, the student gains insights into their errors in assessment (Kumar et al., 2024).

**Structured Work-Based Assessment**
Mini-CEX (Mini-Clinical Evaluation Exercise) and DOPS (Direct Observation of Procedural Skills) are workplace-based assessment tools used in medical training to evaluate trainees' clinical skills and performance in real-time clinical settings (Sethi et al., 2021). The scarcity of research makes it difficult to understand the practical applications of these tools in the country.

An Institute of National Importance in India assessed PG students on a 10 point scale every 6 months; the assessment was done in various domains such as clinical skills, history documentation, examination, routine notes, attitude, initiatives, interpersonal relationships with other residents, discipline, and punctuality; scores are collected from each faculty member of the team and at the end of the semester the students were shown a graphical representation of their scores in each domain helping each of them understand their strengths and weaknesses (Pal et al., 2024).

## 4.2 *Sri Lanka*

The Postgraduate Institute of Medicine from the University of Colombo has a board for study in Psychiatry (Kallivayalil & Enara, 2021). This board conducts a training programme and examination at the end of which an MD in Psychiatry is awarded to the students. The trainees are expected to develop competency in the following roles by the end of the training period: Medical expert, communicator, collaborator, health advocate, manager scholar, and professional (Board of study in Psychiatry, 2013).

The total training period is 5 years, which is divided into two parts:

(i) Stage 1 or Pre-MD training, which is a total of 36 months. At the end of the period, the trainee will have to pass the MD psychiatry summative examination.

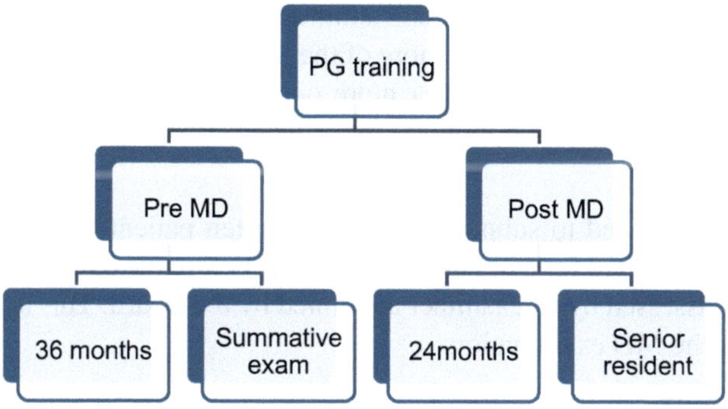


**Fig. 13.4** Organization of PG training in Sri Lanka

(ii) Stage 2 or Post-MD, which is a total of 24 months. In this stage, the trainee works as a senior registrar under the direct supervision of a consultant psychiatrist. The trainee has an option of doing 1 year of this training overseas. Trainees can also at this stage opt for superspecialization in Child and Adolescent Psychiatry or Forensic Psychiatry. However, if they choose to do so, their stage 2 training period would be 3 years instead (Fig. 13.4).

**MD Examination**

A trainee has to pass the MD Psychiatry exam at the end of phase 1 to move on to phase 2 of the programme. The total marks of the examination are 1000, of which 400 marks are for the theory component and 600 marks are for the clinical component. The pass mark is at 50% for the theory and clinical components separately.

The theory component consists of

(i) A multiple-choice question (MCQ): 200 marks
The MCQ paper consists of 60 questions to be answered in 2 h.
(ii) A structured essay question (SEQ) paper: 150 marks
The SEQ paper will consist of 10 questions to be answered in 3 h. Each question will be independently marked by two examiners.
(iii) An essay paper (one question on a given topic for 1 h): 50 marks

The clinical component consists of

(i) One long case: 300 marks
(ii) Two short cases: 200 marks
(iii) Viva voce examination on patient management problems: 100 marks

**Dissertation**

In stage two, the trainee needs to conduct a research project and submit a dissertation, which will be evaluated by two examiners appointed by the board.

**OSCE**

After the first 12 months of training in Stage I, trainees will be assessed on Objective Structured Clinical Examination (OSCE): The OSCE includes a minimum of four stations. Trainees are marked on a 5-point Likert scale for each OSCE station.

To pass, the candidate should obtain a minimum of 3 points on at least three stations and obtain an overall 50% or more of the total mark to be eligible to sit for the MD (Psychiatry) examination (10 or more out of 20). The OSCE examination is conducted approximately at 6-monthly intervals.

**Case Book**
The trainee is required to submit a case book of ten patient case notes. The case book is to be submitted for assessment 12 months before the date of the MD examination and is assessed by an examiner appointed by the Board. This is a prerequisite to appear for the MD examination.

**Progress Report**
In both phases 1 and 2, the consultant psychiatrist is to send a progress report of the trainee at the end of the trainee spending time in each subspeciality. The Consultant psychiatrist, if not satisfied with the progress, should send a report to the board, which will then take appropriate action.

**Challenges**
The country has lost many of its psychiatrists who do not return after their overseas training.

Lack of adequate funding is another issue (Hapangama et al., 2021).

## *4.3 Pakistan*

Postgraduate medical training in Pakistan is regulated by the College of Physicians and Surgeons of Pakistan (CPSP). The college offers Fellowship of the College of Physicians and Surgeons (FCPS) exams for assessment in psychiatry.

The FCPS exam has two parts (FCPS). Part 1 is like an entrance exam with eligibility criteria being MBBS or equivalent qualification, registered, and 1 year internship. After completing part 1, the trainee has to complete 4 years of training in psychiatry under a tutor in psychiatry. Tutors are psychiatrists with at least 5 years of experience in a medical college. Before being allowed to sit for the part 2 examination, the trainees must submit their logbook, dissertation, or two publications in a national journal, and proof of attendance at a workshop. The workshops could be in information technology, communication, and research methodology. The part 2 exam consists of two theory papers (MCQ in paper 1 and SAQ in paper 2). It also contains a clinical exam comprising one long case, two short cases, and a viva.

**Challenges**
Due to the unavailability of sufficient funding in medical colleges, there is a lack of structure and planning in training psychiatrists. The lack of training consultants makes it difficult to conduct subspeciality training in fields like child and adolescent psychiatry, forensic psychiatry (Naeem & Ayub, 2004).

## 4.4 Bangladesh

The Bangladesh College of Physicians and Surgeons (BCPS) is the governing organization regulating postgraduate medical education in Bangladesh. It offers a Fellowship (FCPS) and Membership (MCPS).

The Fellowship of the College of Physicians and Surgeons in Psychiatry (FCPS-Psych) is a 3.5–4 year course modelled on the UK-based systems. It comprises Part I, basic science, and Part II, clinical psychiatry. After completing Part I, candidates must complete 3 years of clinical training in psychiatry in a recognized institution and submit a dissertation before they become eligible for Part II. Trainees receive training in general adult psychiatry as well as subspecialities in psychiatry from qualified faculty members (Arafat, 2020; Siddiqui, 2016).

Various Universities in Bangladesh also offer an MD (Doctor of Medicine) in Psychiatry which is a 5 year course which is divided into two phases. It has a highly competitive entrance exam that can be given after internship (Arafat, 2024).

## 4.5 Nepal

Out of the 20 institutes in Nepal, only 12 offer postgraduate psychiatry training. The programmes in each of the institutes vary, and there is no centralized body guiding the process.

One such university—Tribhuvan University—has a 3-year programme for MD psychiatry training. They have set up eight different competencies that the trainee needs to achieve at the end of their programme (Rai et al., 2021).

## 4.6 Bhutan

In 2019, Bhutan started postgraduate training. Candidates are selected through a competitive selection examination, which includes MCQ and OSCE. There is a continuous assessment, a thesis, and a summative assessment. The summative is a combination of written and practical examinations (Objective Structured Clinical Examination (OSCE)/Objective Structured Practical Examination (OSPE)). For Postgraduate Residency Programmes, the pass mark shall be 50% each in all theory papers, OSCE/OSPE, thesis, and cases. The final cumulative is spread as follows (Khesar Gyalpo University of Medical Sciences of Bhutan, 2021).

Table 13.5 summarizes the differences between the assessment patterns in the South Asian countries.

**Table 13.5** Postgraduate assessment patterns in South Asia

| Country | Governing body | Duration of training | Theory assessment | Practical assessment | Thesis/ dissertation | Formative assessment | Challenges |
|---|---|---|---|---|---|---|---|
| Bangladesh | Bangladesh College of Physicians and Surgeons (BCPS) | 3.5–4 years | FCPS Part I (basic science) & Part II (clinical) | After completing part 1 & II | Mandatory post-Part I | Training under faculty supervision | Variable training standards; resource limitations |
| Bhutan | Khesar Gyalpo University of Medical Sciences of Bhutan (KGUMSB) | 4 years | Year-wise cumulative: Year I (15%), II (25%), III (25%), IV (35%) | OSCE/OSPE, viva, case-based exams | Mandatory; defended in Year III | Structured, ongoing internal assessments | System in early stages; limited infrastructure |
| India | National Medical Council (NMC); NBEMS | 3 years | 4 papers (MD & DNB)<br>Basic sciences, clinical, subspecialities, advances | MD: Long/short cases, viva, neurology case, OSCE<br>DNB: 2 cases, ward rounds, viva, OSCE | Mandatory; 3 examiners (1 internal, 2 external) | Mini-CEX, DOPS, internal exams, academic feedback; varies by institute | Inconsistencies in implementation; subjective grading; limited faculty training |
| Nepal | Individual universities (e.g. Tribhuvan University); no central body | 3 years | Varies by university | Varies by university | Mandatory before final exams | Depends on institutional policy; not standardized nationally | Decentralized structure; limited resources and specialization |
| Pakistan | College of Physicians and Surgeons Pakistan (CPSP) | 4 years | FCPS Part II: MCQ + SAQ | Long case, 2 short cases, viva | Mandatory; or 2 publications in national journals | Logbooks, required workshops (IT, research, communication) | Poor funding; lack of subspecialty training and structured curricula |
| Sri Lanka | Postgraduate Institute of Medicine, University of Colombo | 5 years (3 + 2) | MCQ (200), SEQ (150), Essay (50) | Long case (300), 2 short cases (200), viva (100), OSCE | Mandatory in Stage 2; 2 external examiners | OSCE at 12 months and 6-months intervals; periodic progress reports | Loss of psychiatrists overseas; funding shortages |

## 5 Recommendations

- Advocate for a separate subject status for psychiatry
- Encourage the implementation of competency-based psychiatry education
- Leverage technology
- Heed contextual and cultural factors
- Share best practices across the region
- Encourage research in innovative methods in psychiatry assessment
- Ensure Faculty Development

## 6 Conclusion

Psychiatric curriculum and assessment in South Asia are at an interesting stage of development. It is evolving from the colonial systems to include diverse cultural, socioeconomic, and healthcare realities. The region's enormous burden of mental illness, challenged with frugal resources and a high level of stigma, makes it imperative for context-sensitive and culturally competent assessment practices.

Despite challenges such as underfunded services, limited training opportunities, and a lack of standardized tools, there are hopeful developments. These include the gradual importance of psychiatry in undergraduate and postgraduate curricula, and research on contextually validated assessment instruments. Technology is also expanding the reach of assessments.

Going ahead, strengthening psychiatric assessment in South Asia will necessitate investment in mental health education and training, upscaling research on local epidemiology and tools, and finally, a policy commitment to improve training and faculty development. Eventually, the training and assessment should lead to better services in mental health. A regional approach that emphasizes collaboration, innovation, and cultural humility can help bridge existing gaps and promote equitable, effective psychiatric care across South Asia.

## References

American Educational Research Association, American Psychological Association, & National Council on Measurement in Education. (1999). *Standards for educational and psychological testing*. American Educational Research Association.

Anderson, L. W., & Karthwohl, D. R. (Eds.). (2001). *A taxonomy for learning, teaching, and assessing: A revision of Bloom's taxonomy of educational objectives*. Longman. ISBN 978-0-8013-1903-7.

Arafat, S. M. Y. (2020). The current status of psychiatric education in Bangladesh. *Asian Journal of Psychiatry, 52, 102108*. https://doi.org/10.1016/j.ajp.2020.102108

Arafat, S. M. Y. (2024). Psychiatric education and research system in Bangladesh. In S. M. Y. Arafat (Ed.), *Mental health in Bangladesh*. Springer. https://doi.org/10.1007/978-981-97-0610-5_12

Arafat, S. M. Y., Kar, S. K., Sharma, P., Marahatta, K., & Baminiwatta, A. K. A. B. (2021). A comparative analysis of psychiatry curriculum at undergraduate level of Bangladesh, India, Nepal, and Sri Lanka. *Indian journal of psychiatry, 63*(2), 184–188. https://doi.org/10.4103/psychiatry.IndianJPsychiatry_615_20

Board of Study in Psychiatry. (2013). *Prospectus—MD psychiatry and board certification in psychiatry.*

Hapangama, A., Kuruppuarachchi, K. A. L. A., & Hanwella, R. (2021). Country Initiatives psychiatric training in Sri Lanka and its relevance to South Asia. http://www.who.int/mental_health/policy/services/int.

Kallivayalil, R. A., & Enara, A. (2021). Education and training in psychiatry in South Asian countries. *Asia-Pacific. Psychiatry, 13(4)*. https://doi.org/10.1111/appy.12494

Kern, D., Thomas, P., Howard, D., & Bass, E. (1998). *Curriculum development for medical education: A six-step approach.* Johns Hopkins University Press.

Khesar Gyalpo University of Medical Sciences of Bhutan. (2021). *Academic regulations.*

Kumar, A., Singh, L. K., Somani, A., & Laxmi Nirisha, P. (2024). What we know, we see and do: Formative assessments practices of psychiatry: Postgraduate residency from a general hospital psychiatry unit in India. *Indian Journal of Psychological Medicine.* https://doi.org/10.1177/02537176241273711

Medical Council of India. (2019). *Assessment module for undergraduate medical education training program* (pp. 1–29).

Miller, G. E. (1990). The assessment of clinical skills/competence/performance. *Academic Medicine, 65*, 63–67. https://doi.org/10.1097/00001888-199009000-00045

Naeem, F., & Ayub, M. (2004). Psychiatric training in Pakistan. *Medical Education Online, 9(1), 4369.* https://doi.org/10.3402/meo.v9i.4369

NMC Compendium. (2024). *Competency based medical education curriculum (CBME) guidelines* (pp. 1–41).

Pal, A., Parmar, A., Nath, S., Chawla, N., Gupta, S., Vinay, H. R., & Kishor, M. (2024). Survey of felt needs among teachers of psychiatry in institutes of national importance (INI) to improve the quality of undergraduate and postgraduate training. *Indian Journal of Psychological Medicine.* https://doi.org/10.1177/02537176241273919

Rai, Y., Gurung, D., & Gautam, K. (2021). Insight and challenges: mental health services in Nepal. *BJPsych International, 18*(2), E5. https://doi.org/10.1192/bji.2020.58

Sethi, S., Srivastava, V., & Verma, P. (2021). Mini-clinical evaluation exercise as a tool for formative assessment of postgraduates in psychiatry. *International Journal of Applied and Basic Medical Research, 11*(1), 27–31. https://doi.org/10.4103/ijabmr.IJABMR_305_20

Sethi, S., Tekkalaki, B., Shah, N., Smitha, C. A., & Kumar, R. (2024). Undergraduate psychiatry CBME curriculum revision: The process and the way ahead. *Indian Journal of Psychiatry, 66*, 1066–1069. https://doi.org/10.4103/indianjpsychiatry.indianjpsychiatry_821_24

Siddiqui, M. T. H. (2016). Residency Program A new era in postgraduate medical education in Bangladesh. *Journal of Paediatric Surgeons of Bangladesh, 6*(1), 1–2. https://doi.org/10.3329/jpsb.v6i1.27738

Singh, O. (2022). Postgraduate psychiatry training in India—National Medical Council's competency-based PG curriculum. *Indian Journal of Psychiatry, 64*(4), 329–333. https://doi.org/10.4103/indianjpsychiatry.indianjpsychiatry_426_22

Ten Cate, O., Carraccio, C., Damodaran, A., Gofton, W., Hamstra, S. J., Hart, D. E., Richardson, D., Ross, S., Schultz, K., Warm, E. J., Whelan, A. J., & Schumacher, D. J. (2021). Entrustment Decision Making: Extending Miller's Pyramid. *Academic medicine: journal of the Association of American Medical Colleges, 96(2), 199–204.* https://doi.org/10.1097/ACM.0000000000003800

# Chapter 14
# Reflection and Feedback in Psychiatry Teaching

**Ajay Kumar, H. G. Kshamaa, and Vathsalya S. Gowda**

**Abstract** Education is the information we incorporate into our knowledge and the ability to continue learning by revisiting our skills. Reflection and feedback are critical components of medical education and allow evaluation of the core of teaching, suggesting possibilities for expanding and improving the knowledge acquired by the student. There is literature on reflective practice and feedback strategies in various medical specialities, but the literature has a dearth regarding psychiatry training. Hence, we attempt to gather information regarding the reflective practice and feedback mechanism in psychiatry training. It is indeed highly recommended when the mental health issues have crossed the critical level, and the suicide among medical residents and professionals.

**Keywords** Reflection · Feedback · Psychiatry training · Reflective practices · Medical education

## 1 Background

Education is the information we incorporate into our knowledge and the ability to continue learning by revisiting our skills. Reflection and feedback are critical components of medical education and allow evaluation of the core of teaching, suggesting possibilities for expanding and improving the knowledge acquired by the student. There is literature on reflective practice and feedback strategies in various medical specialities, but the literature has a dearth regarding psychiatry training. Hence, we attempt to gather information regarding the reflective practice and

A. Kumar (✉)
Department of Psychiatry, All India Institute of Medical Sciences, Raipur, Chhattisgarh, India

H. G. Kshamaa · V. S. Gowda
Department of Psychiatry, Kempegowda Institute of Medical Science, Bangalore, Karnataka, India



S. K. Kar et al. (eds.), *Teaching and Training in Psychiatry in South Asia*, South Asian Perspectives in Mental Health and Psychology,
https://doi.org/10.1007/978-981-95-1845-6_14

feedback mechanism in psychiatry training. Here, it is pertinent to understand the difference in the basic conceptual framework of reflection and feedback. Both reflective practice and feedback are crucial components in medical education and help residents develop self-regulated learning skills to enhance their competence and enable mentors to watch trainees' progress (Mamede & Schmidt, 2004; Mann et al., 2009; van den Berg et al., 2006; Winkel et al., 2017).

## 2 Reflection

A systematic literature review about reflection and reflective practice (Mann et al., 2009). Reflective practice is becoming more widely recognized as valuable for doctors' professional development. Case-based discussions are examples of reflective practice in psychiatric training that provide evidence of enhanced diagnostic accuracy in complex cases through reflection, offering us in general practice some helpful insights (Mamede & Schmidt, 2004; Mann et al., 2009).

### *2.1 Conceptual Framework of Reflection*

Mann and colleagues provide three different definitions or descriptions of reflection (Mann et al., 2009). These include describing reflection as:

(i) A critical thinking reflection
(ii) A purposeful form of reflection that is applied to a complex or unstructured issue
(iii) An approach to making sense of experience leading to new understanding

Reflection is principally about being able to think meaningfully, which promotes the integration of academic knowledge with implementation in clinical practice. There is also evidence that reflection relates to high standards of care being provided reliably. This is because thinking reflectively maintains enthusiasm and curiosity about professional practice, ensuring we use our experience to monitor, refresh, and update our learning. Reflective thinking is crucial for developing professional identity, an essential factor in general practice recruitment challenges. However, deeply analysing consultations and self-performance is demanding. It involves continuously questioning one's practice and learning from patient interactions. A study found that reflective levels decrease with more years in practice.

# 3 Feedback

Within health professional education, feedback has been described as 'Specific information about the comparison between a trainee's observed performance and a standard, given with the intent to improve the trainee's performance' (van den Berg et al., 2006). Feedback provides information on the learning process that matches pre-set objectives and complements traditional evaluation methods throughout the training course (Fornells et al., 2008; Ramaprasad, 1983). Feedback should be provided consistently throughout the learning period rather than only after evaluations. It can take various forms. The purpose of feedback is to convey information without making judgments (Ende, 1983).

Feedback can come from either the mentor or the resident. Traditionally, it has been educator-driven, focusing on mentor-to-resident content delivery. Medical education often follows a hierarchical model, with supervisors best positioned to give feedback. Learner-centred models, however, encourage residents to participate actively in the feedback process, promoting self-assessment and reflection to recognise strengths and weaknesses. Feedback can drive measurable improvements in clinical expertise, communication abilities, and patient satisfaction and enhance the quality of learning (Natesan et al., 2023). According to Ende, if there is no feedback in clinical medical education, errors will remain uncorrected, good performance will not be reinforced, and clinical competence will either be achieved empirically or not (Ende, 1983). This is true even though the acquisition of clinical skills arises directly from the clinical method. Although feedback plays a significant role in improving a resident's clinical skills and overall performance, it has been noted that not many residents receive timely feedback (Chur-Hansen & Mclean, 2006; De et al., 2004; Sender Liberman et al., 2005).

Mentors frequently believe they offer consistent feedback, but residents may not see it that way. This gap in perception regarding feedback between mentors and residents has been a longstanding problem (Gil et al., 1984). Additionally, even when residents receive feedback, they often consider it largely unstructured and lacking a systematic approach (Rubí González et al., 2019).

## 3.1 A Conceptual Framework for Feedback

By delivering constructive feedback, mentors can cultivate resident reflection, enabling them to assume responsibility for their learning through comprehensive planning and self-monitoring (Fig. 14.1). This results in improved learning outcomes (Maqsood et al., 2025).

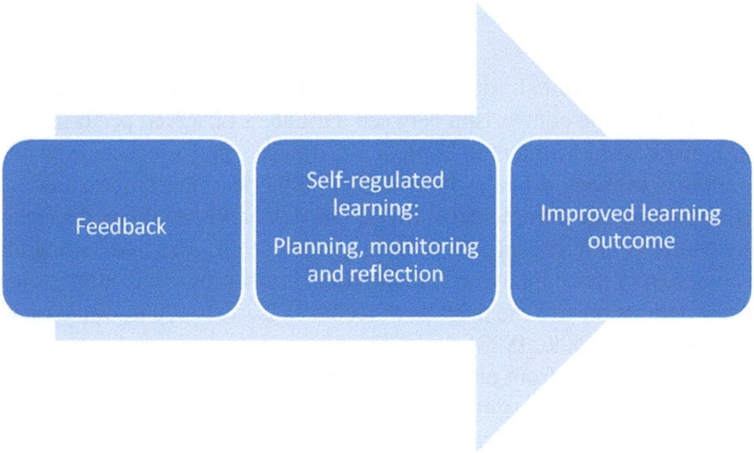


**Fig. 14.1** A conceptual framework of feedback

## *3.2 Types of Feedback*

It is essential to specify the feedback type. Feedback can convey appreciation, coaching, or evaluation (Lefroy et al., 2015).

(i) **Appreciation:** This feedback acknowledges and validates admirable actions, endeavours, and accomplishments. Its primary goals are to create a positive atmosphere, boost confidence, and reinforce desired behaviours. As a result, morale can be raised, and positive contributions can be made.

(ii) **Coaching:** Development and improvement are the main topics of coaching feedback. It points out areas where the resident can improve, makes recommendations, and assists them in learning new techniques or abilities. This kind of feedback frequently entails discussion and emphasising the next steps.

(iii) **Evaluation:** Evaluation feedback compares performance to predetermined benchmarks or requirements. It frequently entails rating and pinpointing areas that require significant improvement. It establishes the framework for a more formal assessment. Feedback can be given in the form of scores and percentages. This method helps in tracking residents' progress over time. However, individuals do not necessarily learn what they have done well and what they could improve. Conversely, conversational feedback involves the mentor highlighting the positive aspects and identifying the gaps in the resident's understanding, which can help them focus on areas. This enables individuals to plan strategically for forthcoming challenges. Once an individual comprehends the nature of their actions and the underlying rationale, they can cultivate a sense of control in managing their learning process (Bienstock et al., 2007).

### *3.3 Models for Giving Effective Feedback*

(i) **Pendleton's rules:** Pendleton's rules allow the mentor and the resident to comment on how well an activity was performed (Pendleton, 1984). The interview follows a format in which the resident and the mentor express what they think was done well, what aspects could be improved, and how these improvements might be achieved. The rules have been criticised for artificially separating the strong and weak aspects of performance and for spending too much time appraising the positive elements, leaving little opportunity for suggestions for change.

(ii) **The feedback sandwich:** It is beneficial at the start of a new mentor–resident relationship, allowing for the development and honing of specific skills and behaviours. The feedback sandwich allows criticism to be 'sandwiched' between two praise items. The mentor begins by commenting on a positive aspect of an activity and praising the resident for it. The 'meat' of the sandwich is the criticism, which should be constructive and include suggestions for improvement. The mentor then concludes the feedback with another positive remark regarding the resident's performance.

(iii) **Silverman's SET–GO (Calgary–Cambridge method):** Silverman's SET–GO involves detailed feedback. The residents review a video of themselves completing a task and discuss their thoughts and challenges with a mentor. Objectives are clarified, and strategies for achieving them are explored. This method is beneficial as it avoids relying on memory during feedback (Sommer et al., 2016).

(iv) **The six-step (problem-solving)** method effectively identifies a resident's performance issues. The mentor builds rapport, assigns a task with clear objectives, observes the execution, and then provides feedback. Flexibility in approach may be needed to ensure the resident understands and can act on the feedback (Ker, 2000).

(v) **The R2C2 (relationship, reaction, content, coaching) model:** The R2C2 feedback model, which stands for relationship, reaction, content, and coaching, aligns well with the Competency-Based Medical Education (CBME) framework by offering a systematic method for feedback and coaching of medical learners. It is grounded in robust theoretical principles, including person-centredness, informed self-assessment, and the science of behaviour change (Sargeant et al., 2015). The model encompasses four key phases: building relationships, examining reactions to feedback, understanding feedback content, and coaching aimed at enhancing performance. Key facilitators for successful implementation include the model's structure, self-efficacy, in-house educational expertise, learning culture, organisational readiness, and training support.

### 3.4 Feedback Tools

Feedback tools are available that briefly summarize various options, emphasizing their main features and offering relevant examples. The selection of a tool typically depends on the context, the kind of feedback needed, and the resources at hand. (Table 14.1).

### 3.5 Factors Influencing Feedback

Effective feedback helps residents improve their clinical and communication skills and enables self-reflection and self-assessment. However, several factors related to the mentor and the resident play a crucial role in the effectiveness of the feedback process.

(i) Factors related to the mentor
(ii) Factors related to the resident

### 3.6 Factors Related to the Mentor

Studies have shown that feedback is most positively received by a trustworthy mentor who has directly observed the residents during their clinical work (Table 14.2). Especially in psychiatry, residents accept the feedback positively when they are

**Table 14.1** Various feedback tools

| Feedback tools | Types | Description | Example |
|---|---|---|---|
| Physical tools | Feedback cards | Identify areas the learner wants feedback on | Debrief pads, Encounter cards |
| | Direct observation cards | Direct observation with written narrative feedback | Mini Cex |
| | Field note tool | Workplace assessment tool with the development of action plans | Field note tool |
| | Multisource feedback tool | Feedback from multiple assessors | Mini Pat, Tab |
| E tools | Web-based | Online survey platforms | Google forms, One-minute mentor-mentee feedback |
| | App-based | Feedback through apps, Accessible, low cost | RRC, SIMPL, M3APP |
| | Online social media platforms | Use of social media platforms to give feedback | Twitter, Instagram, Facebook |
| | Video recordings | Recordings of learners and feedback | OSCEs, OSTEs |

**Table 14.2** Qualities of effective feedback

| | |
|---|---|
| Related to feedback giver | • Providing clear, concise feedback based on observed skills<br>• A planed, timely feedback, keeping privacy/confidentiality<br>• Goal-references, with actionable inputs<br>• Being respectful and empathetic |
| Related to feedback receiver | • Having a learning attitude<br>• Being open to constructive criticism<br>• Willingness to overcome cognitive distortions |

followed by the mentor during clinical interviews and receive input regarding not just their skills but also observations on the personality factors that influence the interview (Rubí González et al., 2019).

Kumar, Nebhinani, et al. (2024) also pointed out organisational and work-culture-related hurdles, emphasising hierarchy flattening, facilitating unbiased feedback, and favouring a non-unit organisation with time-based clinical rotation conducive to learner-centred training and impartial feedback in a general hospital psychiatry Unit (GHPUs) (Kumar, Nebhinani, et al., 2024).

Other factors include the timing and specificity of the input, the environment where the feedback is given, and the mentors' communication and interpersonal skills (Bowen et al., 2017; Eva et al., 2012). The environment and tone in which the input is given seem to impact receptiveness—the residents better perceive feedback given one-to-one in a dyadic conversation. Residents get regular speaking opportunities, which empower them to identify their strengths and weaknesses, increasing the chance to apply the feedback for future improvement (Holmboe et al., 2004). Specific feedback with clear messaging, given respectfully and empathetically, helps residents self-reflect and develop their skills. Lack of confidence in mentors' skills or when the mentor is not modelling the feedback handed out leads to it being considered invalid. Providing feedback publicly in front of patients damages patient trust and can be perceived as demeaning by residents, hindering any positive impact (Bing-You et al., 1997).

The overwhelming majority of clinical mentors have received minimal or no formal instruction in providing feedback. Consequently, many are hesitant to deliver negative feedback, fearing potential detriment to their rapport with residents, a decline in their perceived popularity, or adverse effects on residents' self-esteem (Sender Liberman et al., 2005).

## 3.7 *Factors Related to the Resident*

The effectiveness of feedback is equally dependent on the receiver's perception and implementation. For any feedback to be effective, the resident must enter the conversation open-mindedly and with prior self-assessment. The resident's active involvement is essential to developing lifelong skills (Table 14.2).

Deci and Ryan developed Self-Determination Theory (SDT), which posits that fulfilling three crucial psychological needs—competence, autonomy, and relatedness nurtures and sustains intrinsic motivation in people (Deci & Ryan, 2008). A sense of competence drives individuals to participate in activities that allow them to showcase their skills. Autonomy signifies the ability to make choices and direct one's actions. Relatedness pertains to the aspiration to connect with others and gain acknowledgement as a valued member of a significant social group, such as family, friends, or colleagues. Any feedback that hinders these values acts as a barrier to receiving effective feedback.

Douglas Stone and Sheila Heen identified three common hindrances to effectively receiving feedback (Stone & Heen, 2015)

(i) **Truth trigger:** Feedback is rejected based on its content. The resident may believe the input is incorrect, biased, unhelpful, or vague. This can be overcome by allowing the resident to clarify their doubts, understand their perspective, and help them develop a willingness to learn.
(ii) **Relationship triggers:** Feedback can be rejected due to mistrust or lack of credibility in the feedback giver. Residents should separate the feedback from the person giving it and consider the situation objectively.
(iii) **Identity trigger:** Feedback that challenges a person's self-view can feel threatening, causing reactions based on their temperament and cognitive biases. Regardless of the feedback's accuracy or relevance, it may still affect their self-perception. To overcome these triggers, both givers and receivers should reflect on their responses to feedback. Cognitive behavioural therapy (CBT) techniques to identify and address cognitive distortions can help manage emotions and constructively process feedback. Giving feedback requires learning and adapting to the individual mentor, resident, and circumstances.

## *3.8 Feedback in Psychiatry*

A Pilot study conducted in the USA used Instant Feedback Cards during a 6-week psychiatry clerkship. The card aimed to help residents initiate feedback and help mentors standardise and structure that feedback (Bennett et al., 2006). They used feedback cards during mid-rotation and provided feedback without any tool at the end of the rotation. The card significantly increased the likelihood of residents receiving feedback (85%) compared to when no card was used (69%). This suggests the card acts as a prompt or structure that encourages supervisors to provide feedback.

Kumar, Singh, et al. (2024) developed a multilevel assessment model for psychiatry residents. The model uses progress graphs to show advancement in training areas like academic activities, clinical performance, work-based assessments, and mentor evaluations. At the end of the semester, mentors review scores visually and then discuss strengths, weaknesses, and challenges with the residents (Kumar,

Singh, et al., 2024). With technological advancement, cloud-based synchronous feedback is also possible using an eLogbook application, which has the advantage that student mentors are not physically present, as during the COVID-19 pandemic (Kumar et al., 2021).

### *3.9 Way Forward*

Reflection and Feedback are integral to the standard assessment process and evaluation and are incorporated into the actual script of evidence-based psychiatry training. Considering the profound inconsistency and non-uniformity in the practice of the art of reflection and feedback strategies in psychiatry training in India is one of the primary hurdles, not a lack of research in this context. It warrants a substantial boost to medical education-related programmes that should be conducted across the institutions, focusing on reducing unconscious biases and fostering an open environment for constructive criticism. Set clear goals and assignments, implement two-way feedback procedures, and offer professional development opportunities. Shift from performance-focused evaluation to learner-oriented feedback that encourages personal growth (Natesan et al., 2023; Ramani et al., 2019).

## 4 Conclusion

Reflective practice and feedback mechanisms should work together to help trainees and mentors achieve their goals. Reflection provides a qualitative, subjective account from the trainee, while feedback measures output quantitatively, compared with the resident's actual performance. Feedback identifies the gap between the desired standard and current performance, while reflection helps understand why the gap exists, the problems involved, and possible solutions. Reliable and unbiased feedback from multiple sources is essential, and a culture of feedback and reflection needs to be established in psychiatry training.

## References

Bennett, A. J., Goldenhar, L. M., & Stanford, K. (2006). Utilization of a formative evaluation card in a psychiatry clerkship. *Academic Psychiatry, 30*(4), 319–324. https://doi.org/10.1176/appi.ap.30.4.319

Bienstock, J. L., Katz, N. T., Cox, S. M., Hueppchen, N., Erickson, S., & Puscheck, E. E. (2007). To the point: medical education reviews—Providing feedback. *American Journal of Obstetrics and Gynecology, 196*(6), 508–513. https://doi.org/10.1016/j.ajog.2006.08.021

Bing-You, R. G., Paterson, J., & Levine, M. A. (1997). Feedback falling on deaf ears: residents' receptivity to feedback tempered by sender credibility. *Medical Teacher, 19*(1), 40–44. https://doi.org/10.3109/01421599709019346

Bowen, L., Marshall, M., & Murdoch-Eaton, D. (2017). Medical student perceptions of feedback and feedback behaviors within the context of the "educational alliance". *Academic Medicine, 92*(9), 1303–1312. https://doi.org/10.1097/ACM.0000000000001632

Chur-Hansen, A., & Mclean, S. (2006). On being a supervisor: The importance of feedback and how to give it. *Australasian Psychiatry, 14*(1), 67–71. https://doi.org/10.1080/j.1440-1665.2006.02248.x

De, S. K., Henke, P. K., Ailawadi, G., Dimick, J. B., & Colletti, L. M. (2004). Attending, house officer, and medical student perceptions about teaching in the third-year medical school general surgery clerkship. *Journal of the American College of Surgeons, 199*(6), 932–942. https://doi.org/10.1016/j.jamcollsurg.2004.08.025

Deci, E. L., & Ryan, R. M. (2008). Self-determination theory: A macrotheory of human motivation, development, and health. *Canadian Psychology/Psychologie Canadienne, 49*(3), 182–185. https://doi.org/10.1037/a0012801

Ende, J. (1983). Feedback in clinical medical education. *JAMA, 250*(6), 777–781.

Eva, K. W., Armson, H., Holmboe, E., Lockyer, J., Loney, E., Mann, K., & Sargeant, J. (2012). Factors influencing responsiveness to feedback: on the interplay between fear, confidence, and reasoning processes. *Advances in Health Sciences Education, 17*(1), 15–26. https://doi.org/10.1007/s10459-011-9290-7

Fornells, J. M., Julià, X., Arnau, J., & Martínez-Carretero, J. M. (2008). Feedback en educación médica. *Educación Médica, 11*(1). https://doi.org/10.4321/S1575-18132008000100003

Gil, D. H., Heins, M., & Jones, P. B. (1984). Perceptions of medical school faculty members and students on clinical clerkship feedback. *Academic Medicine, 59*(11), 856–864. https://doi.org/10.1097/00001888-198411000-00003

Holmboe, E. S., Yepes, M., Williams, F., & Huot, S. J. (2004). Feedback and the mini clinical evaluation exercise. *Journal of General Internal Medicine, 19*(5), 558–561. https://doi.org/10.1111/j.1525-1497.2004.30134.x

Ker, J. (2000). Teaching made easy: A manual for health professionals. *BMJ (Clinical Research Ed.), 320*(7250), 1677.

Kumar, A., Chandran, S., & M, K. (2021). Use of electronic logbook in psychiatry training and its relevance during COVID-19 pandemic in India. *Asian Journal of Psychiatry, 64*, 102763. https://doi.org/10.1016/j.ajp.2021.102763

Kumar, A., Nebhinani, N., Menon, V., Kishor, M., & Isaac, M. (2024). An overview of different clinical rotation styles and organizational strategies for postgraduate psychiatry training adopted in general hospital psychiatry units—A critical viewpoint from India. *Indian Journal of Psychological Medicine*. https://doi.org/10.1177/02537176241283372

Kumar, A., Singh, L. K., Somani, A., & Laxmi Nirisha, P. (2024). What we know, we see and do: Formative assessments practices of psychiatry: postgraduate residency from a general hospital psychiatry unit in India. *Indian Journal of Psychological Medicine, 46*(5), 466–470. https://doi.org/10.1177/02537176241273711

Lefroy, J., Watling, C., Teunissen, P. W., & Brand, P. (2015). Guidelines: the do's, don'ts and don't knows of feedback for clinical education. *Perspectives on Medical Education, 4*(6), 284–299. https://doi.org/10.1007/S40037-015-0231-7

Mamede, S., & Schmidt, H. G. (2004). The structure of reflective practice in medicine. *Medical Education, 38*(12), 1302–1308. https://doi.org/10.1111/j.1365-2929.2004.01917.x

Mann, K., Gordon, J., & MacLeod, A. (2009). Reflection and reflective practice in health professions education: a systematic review. *Advances in Health Sciences Education, 14*(4), 595–621. https://doi.org/10.1007/s10459-007-9090-2

Maqsood, Z., Sajjad, M., & Yasmin, R. (2025). Effect of feedback-integrated reflection, on deep learning of undergraduate medical students in a clinical setting. *BMC Medical Education, 25*(1), 66. https://doi.org/10.1186/s12909-025-06648-3

Natesan, S., Jordan, J., Sheng, A., Carmelli, G., Barbas, B., King, A., Gore, K., Estes, M., & Gottlieb, M. (2023). Feedback in medical education: An evidence-based guide to best practices from the Council of Residency Directors in Emergency Medicine. *Western Journal of Emergency Medicine, 24*(3). https://doi.org/10.5811/WESTJEM.56544

Pendleton, D. (1984). *The consultation: An approach to learning and teaching*. Oxford University Press.

Ramani, S., Könings, K. D., Ginsburg, S., & van der Vleuten, C. P. M. (2019). Twelve tips to promote a feedback culture with a growth mind-set: Swinging the feedback pendulum from recipes to relationships. *Medical Teacher, 41*(6), 625–631. https://doi.org/10.1080/0142159X.2018.1432850

Ramaprasad, A. (1983). On the definition of feedback. *Behavioral Science, 28*(1), 4–13. https://doi.org/10.1002/bs.3830280103

Rubí González, P. S., De la Barra Vivallos, L., Schaefer, H., & Vergara-Barra, P. (2019). The role of feedback in training psychiatrists. *The Journal of Mental Health Training, Education and Practice, 14*(4), 242–250. https://doi.org/10.1108/JMHTEP-02-2019-0009

Sargeant, J., Lockyer, J., Mann, K., Holmboe, E., Silver, I., Armson, H., Driessen, E., MacLeod, T., Yen, W., Ross, K., & Power, M. (2015). Facilitated reflective performance feedback. *Academic Medicine, 90*(12), 1698–1706. https://doi.org/10.1097/ACM.0000000000000809

Sender Liberman, A., Liberman, M., Steinert, Y., McLeod, P., & Meterissian, S. (2005). Surgery residents and attending surgeons have different perceptions of feedback. *Medical Teacher, 27*(5), 470–472. https://doi.org/10.1080/0142590500129183

Sommer, J., Lanier, C., Perron, N. J., Nendaz, M., Clavet, D., & Audétat, M.-C. (2016). A teaching skills assessment tool inspired by the Calgary–Cambridge model and the patient-centered approach. *Patient Education and Counseling, 99*(4), 600–609. https://doi.org/10.1016/j.pec.2015.11.024

Stone, D., & Heen, S. (2015). *Thanks for the feedback*. Penguin.

van den Berg, I., Admiraal, W., & Pilot, A. (2006). Peer assessment in university teaching: evaluating seven course designs. *Assessment & Evaluation in Higher Education, 31*(1), 19–36. https://doi.org/10.1080/02602930500262346

Winkel, A. F., Yingling, S., Jones, A.-A., & Nicholson, J. (2017). Reflection as a learning tool in graduate medical education: A systematic review. *Journal of Graduate Medical Education, 9*(4), 430–439. https://doi.org/10.4300/JGME-D-16-00500.1

# Chapter 15
# Developing Short Courses in Psychiatry

**Raj Kiran Donthu, Pooja Shatadal, Nitisha Verma, and Suhas Chandran**

**Abstract** Short courses in psychiatry serve as a powerful tool for mental health professionals to acquire relevant knowledge and skills efficiently. These courses are particularly valuable for busy healthcare practitioners seeking to enhance their expertise in specialized areas such as psychiatry research, teaching methodologies, or clinical topics (e.g., substance addiction, child and adolescent psychiatry).

This chapter presents a comprehensive framework for designing effective short courses in psychiatry. The process begins with establishing clear, audience-specific learning objectives, followed by structured curriculum development. Key considerations include identifying qualified resource persons, securing funding from potential agencies, and implementing strategic course promotion. This chapter also addresses common challenges encountered during course organization and provides practical solutions to overcome them.

To support organizers, a practical checklist is included to guide the systematic development of short courses. By offering this structured approach, this chapter aims to empower educators and institutions to create impactful training programs that meet the evolving demands of psychiatry education and mental health practice.

**Keywords** Short-term course · Correspondence course · Psychiatry · Academic training · Continuing medical education

---

R. K. Donthu
Department of Psychiatry, NRI Academy of Sciences, Guntur, Andhra Pradesh, India

P. Shatadal
Department of Psychiatry, Government Medical College Surat, Surat, Gujarat, India

N. Verma (✉)
Department of Psychiatry, ABVIMS and Dr. RML Hospital, New Delhi, India
e-mail: nitishaverma30@yahoo.com

S. Chandran
Department of Psychiatry, St. John's Medical College, Bengaluru, Karnataka, India



S. K. Kar et al. (eds.), *Teaching and Training in Psychiatry in South Asia*, South Asian Perspectives in Mental Health and Psychology,
https://doi.org/10.1007/978-981-95-1845-6_15

## 1 Introduction

A short course concentrates on a specific topic, such as a particular skill or area of knowledge. It offers immediate, practical skills within a certain field, enabling individuals to quickly gain new knowledge and skills that can be applied in the workplace (Online Jain University, n.d.). For example, a short course on "tobacco cessation" may focus on the burden of tobacco use, related legislation, evaluation, and intervention (NIMHANS E-Learning Hub, 2022). Similarly, a short course on research in psychiatry will cover topics related to research (Ameen, 2015). These courses will not include other psychiatry topics.

Short courses last from a few hours to several months, usually less than a year. They are offered by colleges, universities, or professional organizations, are cost-effective, and take less time to complete. Unlike traditional diploma or degree programs, these courses do not provide in-depth knowledge of the subject or any formal qualification upon completion. They typically offer a certificate of completion but do not grant a degree or license to practice as a psychiatrist.

Short courses can serve both professional and personal growth (Team, 2021). For instance, a short course on "stress management" or "anger management" may be used for personal development (NPTEL, n.d.). Psychiatrists may take short courses to update or refresh their knowledge and acquire new skills. These courses help them stay informed about the latest research, therapies, and technologies in psychiatry. Given the significant treatment gap for mental illness, these courses can also be used to train primary care providers, nurses, and other professionals to recognize and manage mental health issues effectively. Training more professionals to detect early signs of mental illness can aid in secondary prevention.

## 2 How to Organize a Short Course?

For effective course organization, the chairperson of the organizing committee should delegate responsibilities among team members so that accountability is ensured. Tasks can be systematically divided into five key domains:

(a) Faculty/Resource Person Management
(b) Course Curriculum Development
(c) Participant Administration
(d) Financial Management
(e) Venue Coordination

To ensure systematic course management, the organizational process is structured into three distinct phases: planning, implementation, and post-program. This triphasic approach provides organizers with a clear roadmap, ensuring all critical components of course management are addressed methodically at each stage of the process (Tables 15.1, 15.2, and 15.3).

**Table 15.1** Common challenges in organizing short courses in psychiatry and possible solutions

| Challenge | Description | Suggested solution |
|---|---|---|
| Participant engagement | Difficulty sustaining interest, especially in virtual settings | – Introduce mentorship programs for peer-to-peer interaction<br>– Use real-time polls and interactive breakout rooms<br>– Create post-course communities (e.g., WhatsApp/ Telegram groups) for continued discussion |
| Sustained engagement | Drop-off in participation post-course Lack of space for hands-on training in online-only courses contributes to drop-offs | – Schedule follow-up webinars or refresher workshops<br>– Share continuous learning materials via email/LMS<br>– Micro and macro credentialing: Offer certificates to incentivize repeat participation, especially for each module apart from the end course certification and awards<br>– Organizers must partner with institutions for shared resources and use open-access educational platforms for material distribution |
| Technological barriers | Technical issues (e.g., unstable Internet, platform glitches) and low participant tech literacy | – Provide pre-course tech orientation sessions or a dossier with tech-related FAQs or step-by-step tutorials, especially if the LMS is used<br>– Offer 24/7 technical support via chat<br>– Utilize user-friendly platforms (e.g., Google Classroom) |
| Varied skill levels | There are wide disparities in participants' prior knowledge (e.g., in the same course, a few participants could be PGs, a few could be junior faculty, and a few senior faculty) | – Conduct pre-course assessments to tailor content<br>– Provide beginner-friendly resources and advanced tracks<br>– Offer optional deep-dive materials for those who want advanced supplements<br>– A buddy system can be used to pair advanced participants with beginners for peer support during practical sessions |

(continued)

**Table 15.1** (continued)

| Challenge | Description | Suggested solution |
|---|---|---|
| Content relevance | Ensuring material aligns with participants' practical needs | – Use a pre-course Google Form survey to identify learning goals<br>– Include case studies from real-world psychiatry practice<br>– Train facilitators in cultural competency<br>– Delphi method: Conduct iterative expert consensus rounds post-course to refine content and objectives<br>– Advisory boards: Form panels of psychiatrists and educators to review outcomes annually |
| Time constraints | Participants are juggling clinical work/practice, family, and course commitments | – Offer flexible schedules (recorded sessions + live Q&A)<br>– Design modular content for self-paced learning |
| Sustainability | Difficulty maintaining course quality and participant engagement over multiple iterations | – Develop long-term funding strategies (e.g., grants, sponsorships)<br>– Create alumni networks for continued support<br>– Workload management of the course faculty by using rotational schedules and having workload caps is going to be key (max three sessions for a 3-month course, etc.) |

## *2.1 Planning (Pre-Program)*

This step is crucial and is described under various headings of practical relevance.

**The Organizing Team** (the advisors and implementing members): The course design team should comprise enthusiastic individuals from diverse backgrounds with complementary skill sets. A designated chairperson oversees task allocation and serves as a spokesperson, while a convener handles coordination. Team members require soft communication skills, financial acumen, subject matter expertise, and the ability to prepare for any in-person course elements. Experienced subject experts or event organizers can serve as advisors, offering guidance without micromanaging. Open communication between the team and advisors is essential.

**Aim and Objectives** When developing the course, the niche area of the subject needs to be articulated precisely. The aim and objectives of the said course should be clear. This clarity allows interested participants to evaluate the course objectives and ascertain its relevance to their needs. The organizing team must also determine the practicality of including all topics, as some may not be conducive to a brief course structure. Therefore, a concise promotional overview should be drafted early by the organizing team to engage potential attendees.

**Table 15.2** Checklist for organizing a short course in psychiatry

| Phase | Key steps | Details |
|---|---|---|
| Planning | Define course objectives<br>Define the target audience | – Outline goals (e.g., skill enhancement, certification)<br>– Identify participants (e.g., early career psychiatrists, PGs, mixed group, psychologists, etc.) |
| | Form an organizing team | – Assign roles and responsibilities (banners in charge, certificate developer, LMS in charge/Zoom in charge/food and accommodation, etc)<br>– Hold regular organizing committee meetings and document major action points and timelines |
| | Budget planning | – Cover venue, materials, speaker fees, prize money for awards, and contingencies |
| | Set timelines | – Create deadlines for planning, dissemination of course brochures, enrollment, and fee payment. |
| | Accreditation | – Apply in advance for any accreditation of the course, either to an organization or a medical council, as applicable |
| Curriculum design | Develop course content | – Include core topics (e.g., psychiatric disorders, research methodology, therapies) and practical components (case studies, assignments) |
| | Choose the core faculty, resource persons, and advisors for the course | – Send formal invitation letters using an email ID created uniquely for the course<br>– Decide on remuneration<br>– Delegate sessions |
| | Choose format and duration | – Online, offline, or hybrid<br>– Decide on schedule (e.g., weekend workshops) |
| Logistics | Select venue/platform | – If in-person, book the venue at least 3 months in advance or use reliable platforms (e.g., Zoom, Moodle) |
| | Arrange equipment | – Ensure projectors, mics, Internet access (in-person), or test virtual tools |
| | Set up registration | – Create user-friendly forms and payment methods |
| Promotion | Advertise course | – Create a dedicated course webpage with clear enrollment steps, FAQs, and downloadable brochures<br>– Use emails and partnerships with institutions/organizations (e.g., IPS, local psychiatry bodies, etc.)<br>– Ensure the affiliations of the resource persons are accurate |

(continued)

**Table 15.2** (continued)

| Phase | Key steps | Details |
|---|---|---|
| Execution | Conduct an orientation session | – Explain course objectives and schedule<br>– If there is an in-person component to the course, please ensure a dry run is done by the organizing team (refer to Table 15.3) |
| | Monitor sessions and engagement | – Use polls, breakout rooms, and Q&A sessions |
| Evaluation | Assess learning outcomes | – Pre/post-course quizzes or practical evaluations |
| | Collect feedback | – Distribute feedback forms to both participants and faculty |
| Follow-up | Issue certificates | – Provide completion certificates to eligible participants |
| | Share resources | – Email supplementary materials or session recordings |
| | Plan future iterations | – Document lessons learned for improvements<br>– Archive materials on LMS<br>– Update alumni database |

**Target Audience and the Number of Participants** This decision should be made beforehand and adhered to by the team. While occasional exceptions can be made for diverse participants (especially if it aligns with course objectives or if applications are low), short courses typically benefit from a limited number of attendees for easier logistical management. The participant count will also be influenced by the financial resources needed to organize the course, with online-only courses generally requiring less funding than in-person sessions.

**Time Frame and Schedule (Days & Dates)** The organizing team must determine the timeframe and session schedule before course preparation, incorporating insights from previous or similar course teams. It is advisable to consult potential speakers for topics and their availability before finalizing a tentative schedule. This schedule should be shared with applicants for review before they apply.

Maintaining a strict timeline is crucial to prevent participant disengagement. Any decision to add more topics should involve discussion with participants to ensure the course remains comprehensive and aligned with their interests. For online courses, consistency in the day of the week for classes is prudent, enhancing memorability and stakeholder arrangements. A fixed schedule promotes better participation, and polls can be used post-enrollment to determine preferred class days and times.

**Course Platform** Post-COVID-19, online learning platforms have gained widespread acceptance. Both online and offline platforms have their advantages and disadvantages. While online courses offer ease of conduct, reduced costs for organizers and participants, and flexible scheduling, they can suffer from a lack of participant

**Table 15.3** Dry run checklist for in-person course components

| Phase | Key steps | Details | Status (complete/in progress) | Person in charge of task |
|---|---|---|---|---|
| Venue setup & logistics | Confirm room layout matches planned activities<br>Test all equipment<br>Verify Internet stability | – Ensure layout aligns with group work/ lectures (small groups, tables, etc.)<br>– Check projectors, mics, and lighting (backup options)<br>– Ensure stable Internet for live demos | | |
| Materials & signage | Print/physical handouts/ worksheets ready<br>Check directional signage | – Organize handouts by session, name tags<br>– Place signs for bathrooms, exits, and key areas<br>– Create a list of house rules to be displayed outside the venue | | |
| Team briefing | Run through the roles and responsibilities with the team | – Define registration, tech support, and facilitator roles<br>– Cover medical/fire emergencies, evacuation routes | | |
| Emcee preparation | Review the emcee script and cues | – Verify script accuracy (agenda, speaker intros, key announcements)<br>– Train the emcee on transitions between sessions, Q&A handling, and timekeeping<br>– Simulate opening/ closing remarks, panel introductions, and emergency announcements | | |
| Schedule walkthrough | Simulate transitions<br>Confirm catering logistics | – Test timing between sessions<br>– Check break timings, food setup | | |
| Contingency planning | Identify backup plans<br>Share the vendor contact list | – Prepare for tech failures, no-shows, delays<br>– Provide AV/catering contacts to the team | | |

(continued)

Table 15.3 (continued)

| Phase | Key steps | Details | Status (complete/in progress) | Person in charge of task |
|---|---|---|---|---|
| Post-dry run debrief | Document issues<br>Update the run sheet | – Assign fixes for noted problems<br>– Adjust timing/ workflows for the final event | | |

and organizer cohesion, potentially leading to sparse attendance, decreased interest, and "ghost participation." Offline platforms, conversely, foster stronger cohesion and resemble traditional short courses completed in a few days, but they lack scheduling flexibility and cost-effectiveness. A hybrid model combines both, though physical attendees often remain more engaged than their online counterparts, who may feel less involved.

**Course Curriculum** The curriculum is "the heart and soul" of any course, demanding careful consideration and expert consultation before finalization. Organizers must align the curriculum with the course's stated aim and objectives. It is crucial to manage topic complexity, ensuring participants can understand and retain information, facilitated by adequate breaks. Certain topics or skills might be certifiable under the Competency-Based Medical Education (CBME) for undergraduates (e.g., suicide, depression) or involve basic training for primary healthcare physicians and educators in identifying common mental health disorders (like screening for depression, anxiety, and substance use among adolescents and college students). Furthermore, the course platform significantly impacts the curriculum; purely online formats may not support hands-on training, workshops, or direct patient/client interaction requiring instructor guidance.

**Course Material** There are two perspectives on distributing course materials. One advocates for providing materials such as presentation slides (acknowledged, de-copyrighted, preferably PDF) or speaker-prepared short notes. In online settings, recording sessions for participant access is feasible with prior speaker permission. If recordings are provided, however, it might reduce active participation and live attendance, as learners could defer viewing, potentially indefinitely. This could diminish enthusiasm for organizers, participants, and speakers. Conversely, withholding materials compels mandatory attendance and active engagement through questioning and note-taking. Yet, participants might then miss crucial details. An ideal compromise would be for speakers to provide topic summaries, offering essential points without negating the need for live class attendance, as summaries would not cover all the information.

**Assessments** Assessment is the key to participant learning. Formative assessments track progress, helping participants identify and improve weak areas. Summative assessments, as a final evaluation, gauge overall course benefit (Aboulsoud, 2011). The organizing team must decide on assessment types, frequency, and the grades required for certificates or prizes. Formative assessments can include pre-tests (to set expectations) and post-tests (for deeper understanding), with questions potentially being identical, favoring multiple choice questions (MCQs) or extended matching questions (EMQs). Resource persons are best suited to create questions based on content. To boost engagement, questions can sometimes be provided in advance for participants to prepare and discuss/present in class.

**Certificates and Prizes** Clear guidelines are essential regarding any certificates or prizes being offered by the organizing team. These guidelines, based on factors like scores on quizzes, active participation, or completion of assignments, should be transparent to all participants. Such transparency prevents future discrepancies, avoids participant discouragement, and boosts engagement in course activities. Although attendance can be easily tracked using software for online classes, manual screening is required for tracking active participation. Attendance and percentage scores may also be mentioned on certificates.

**Course Website** The team can develop a website using a content management system to enhance reach, publicity, and authenticity. This website can be expanded to include robust features such as a Learning Management System, tools for managing applications and payments, automated reminders, quiz posting capabilities, and a system for collecting feedback. Many of these features are available as extensions from service providers that support content management systems like *WordPress* or *Joomla*. Assigning website management to a knowledgeable team member is advisable. Furthermore, based on the specific needs of the course, budget constraints, and the level of team assistance, professional service providers may be engaged to construct the website. The option of having an Android application may be explored.

**Role and Benefits of Learning Management Systems** Learning Management Systems (LMS), such as Moodle or Canvas, serve as centralized digital platforms crucial for organizing, delivering, and overseeing short courses, especially in psychiatry. These platforms empower round-the-clock access to diverse course materials, including lecture recordings, handouts, and quizzes, making them ideal for professionals balancing work with studies. They significantly improve scalability, allowing organizers to manage large participant cohorts without physical venue limitations. Furthermore, LMS platforms facilitate personalized learning paths, ensuring modules are tailored to individual skill levels. Automated assessments provide immediate feedback, streamlining evaluation and reducing administrative effort, while integrated progress tracking enables early identification of disengaged learners for targeted support. Collaborative features like discussion forums enhance peer interaction, and digitized resources reduce operational costs by minimizing printing and venue expenses. Finally, it supports course sustainability through efficient content reuse and updates for future offerings, ultimately enhancing organizational flexibility, academic quality, and program continuity.

**Application Forms** In addition to the basic demographic information (name, contact details, postal address), participants may be asked to express their "statement of interest" or expectations from the course. This helps the team in selecting suitable applicants and also in refining the content of the course. Courses may have expected outcomes. For example, for a course on research methodology, the expected outcome could be publication of an original article in a reputable journal. Here, the "statement of interest" by a participant will give an idea of whether he/she can fit into the course. It may also act as a starting point for the participant to start working on a potential research idea. Sensitive issues like transgender candidates need to be respectfully addressed in the form.

Collecting application forms is simplified by free online services (e.g., Google Forms) or directly through the LMS platform via participant profiles. A comprehensive frequently asked questions (FAQs) section on the course website should handle queries, potentially managed by a designated team member. Prompt and official email responses are vital, using template messages for payment details. Payment information should follow the screening of applications if seats are limited or there are specific criteria for enrollment. Otherwise, it can be shared upfront with the application. An application form template (Brief Course in Psychiatric Research—BCPR) is provided in the appendix with due permission.

**Other Forms** It is essential to prepare feedback and assessment forms ahead of time, with the organizing team actively involved in formulating pertinent questions. While detailed participant feedback is invaluable for future course planning and necessary modifications, questions should be carefully designed to be brief and clear. This feedback provides a comprehensive understanding of the ongoing relevance of the course and areas for enhancement. Additionally, the organizing team can gather short testimonials from participants. Positive testimonials can be utilized in subsequent course brochures. They act as a significant incentive for future attendees.

**Payment Facility** If a professional society or institution sponsors the course, their existing payment mechanism can be utilized, with candidates asked to include a specific message for easy sorting. If no such system exists, the team should consider opening a dedicated bank account for the course and applying for a Tax Collection and Deduction Account Number (TAN). In India, UPI is the simplest payment method, and a QR code can be shared. Individual team members' bank accounts should be avoided due to potential income tax issues and inquiries from payment inflows. Additionally, the team must establish a clear refund policy, as there may be genuine reasons why a candidate could not attend the course. The amount to be refunded can be pre-decided, and also when the candidate will be given a full, partial, or no refund.

**Resource Person/Faculty** The effectiveness of a course largely depends on its resource persons or faculty. It has been observed that well-known speakers can significantly motivate interested participants to register and actively engage in course activities. Therefore, the organizing team should discuss and confirm speakers well in advance, securing their commitment before finalizing the course curriculum. Additionally, it is beneficial for faculty to represent diverse backgrounds to ensure a variety of perspectives. For example, in a course on research methodology, faculty could include non-psychiatrists, researchers from various institutes, or individuals from less privileged centers. Faculty can also assist in finalizing the curriculum. Before their sessions, faculty should be asked whether they consent to their class being recorded and shared with participants, and if any materials are needed for in-class group activities. The team should also finalize the honorarium, identify alternative speakers if the initial one is unavailable, and make arrangements for their stay and travel.

**Mentors** The team may also consider recruiting mentors to motivate participants in specific tasks and activities. A mentor is a person who gives advice and help to a less experienced person over time (Cambridge University Press, n.d.). They can bridge the gap between the faculty and participants. Each group of participants can be assigned a mentor, who can provide personalized help based on the activities designed in the course. Mentors can be selected based on various criteria that the team finds feasible, but they should be enthusiastic enough to guide the participants and actively engage in course activities.

**Venue and Hall (for Offline Course)** When selecting the venue, its accessibility, available accommodation options, and arrangements for snacks and meals must be considered. The team's budget should be the primary factor in choosing the location. Important details to check include the presence of a cafeteria or at least a coffee/tea vending machine, quality audio-visual equipment, suitable interior furniture such as round tables and chairs for group discussions , Wi-Fi connectivity (or mobile network coverage), accessible restrooms (especially for differently-abled or third-gender individuals), facilities for displaying course banners and directional signs, printers, lighting, ambiance, effective cooling and ventilation systems, and the availability of staff to manage hall arrangements.

**Stay and Travel Arrangements (for Offline Course)** Most cities would meet both requirements. It is always better for the organizing team to arrange accommodation for participants, as this saves them a lot of time and money. Additionally, participants staying together at a single location would help build their network, creating lasting memories. Care should be taken to make arrangements suitable for participants from different socio-demographic backgrounds. These details should ideally be provided to participants at the time of applying for the course, so that they can prepare accordingly. This also helps reduce unnecessary resource wastage by the organizing team. Another option is outsourcing to a local event management company, but the availability of funds should be considered before entering into an agreement.

**Advertising and Promoting** These play a crucial role in dispersing information and filling course seats. An effective course can reach its potential only when the right participants are present. There are various avenues to achieve this, like professional society platforms (WhatsApp, Google groups, website, etc.), word of mouth (especially when combined with personal experiences), official invitations to heads of departments, distribution of course brochures during conferences or CMEs, etc. A colorful brochure with all necessary details should be prepared and used both for advertising and as an official invitation to speakers or participants who wish to request official leave from their work. It can also feature three or four testimonials from previous participants (with prior permission) enhancing authenticity.

**Budget Planning** Budgeting is a vital task that requires a dedicated team member. While basic software like Microsoft Excel is sufficient, careful preparation of a budget is essential for two main reasons: its submission to potential funding agencies and its role in reporting the team's operational activities. When preparing the budget, several elements must be considered for both online and offline formats. These include honoraria for resource persons (which can be structured hourly or per session), allocations for certificates and prizes, fees for the LMS platform, and costs related to the course delivery platform (such as Zoom or Cisco Webex). For offline courses, additional budget is needed for participant accommodation and meals, stationery, travel and stay of resource persons, and rent of the venue. To demonstrate this process, a basic sample budget in Excel format has been prepared and shared as a supplementary material.

**Funding** A detailed budget must be prepared after gaining a clear understanding of all the above factors. The course can be funded by participant fees, especially when the expected demographic background of potential participants supports this. Charging participants often boosts their involvement and retention, though not always if the course is unique (skills not taught elsewhere) and participants recognize its potential. Funding can also come from the host institution or professional society, the Indian Council for Medical Research (ICMR), pharmaceutical company sponsorship, and other sources. Some host institutions and professional societies are willing to fund a part or all of the course. ICMR has a rolling application process inviting institutions and societies to apply for workshops under "Department of Health Research funded workshops" (Indian Council of Medical Research, n.d.). Applications, including all details and a detailed budget (up to 10 lakhs), must be submitted 3 months in advance and are limited to clinical training or translational research workshops. Sponsorship from pharmaceutical companies is less preferred, but possible if the team or professional society has favorable terms. However, this may impose restrictions or add conditions to certain aspects of the course or curriculum. For courses involving medical personnel, the team should review the guidelines issued by the National Medical Commission (NMC) regarding pharmaceutical company involvement (National Medical Commission, n.d.-b. Income Tax Department, Government of India. (n.d.).

**Psychological Support to the Team** This is often overlooked, and the team leader should ensure that support is accessible. During the organization process, various issues may arise where things do not go as planned, and scapegoating individual members should be avoided. Matters should always be openly discussed with members and resolved. This fosters trust and transparency, which is highly beneficial.

## 2.2 *Implementation (Program Per Se)*

It could be divided into the following subheadings:

**Platform for Communication** It can be a basic free messaging service like WhatsApp or an LMS (if the team has subscribed to it). Participants' ease of access to these services needs to be considered before finalizing. Most short courses can be easily managed through WhatsApp by creating a community, and, based on the course objectives, groups can be created within the community. An announcement group can be used to share schedules, reminders, post quizzes, etc. The community and each group should, in turn, be monitored by team members (by assigning admin status). This is not to invade participants' privacy, but to prevent unnecessary propaganda and keep them focused. Personalized messages can also be sent by creating a broadcast list of all participants/mentors/faculty to keep them updated.

**Schedule** The details of the course schedule and speakers should be shared with the participants once finalized. This can be distributed through multiple platforms such as messaging apps, emails, LMS, or a website. Reminders may also be sent periodically.

Online platforms have a mechanism to send reminder emails about the class 1 week, 1 day, and 1 h before the class. Even then, a few participants may not be well-versed in email. Hence, sending a reminder message to groups or communities is beneficial.

**Course Per Se** The preparatory phase of the course should establish a clear framework for participants, outlining expectations and objectives. The session may commence with introductions of faculty, advisors, mentors, and participants. If the course has been conducted previously, a brief history along with relevant photos or videos may be shared to foster engagement. Adherence to the schedule is essential for the success of the course. Materials for discussions or group activities should be distributed at the start of the session. To accommodate limited attention spans, scheduled breaks are recommended, during which activities such as stretching, peer introductions, sharing hobbies, or quick photo exercises can be incorporated to maintain engagement. Post-session or daily activities should include formative assessments, with answers reviewed to reinforce learning and encourage further participation. A comprehensive summative assessment should be scheduled at the conclusion of the course, with prior notification. For online courses, participants should be instructed on maintaining decorum, including keeping videos on, muting microphones when not speaking, and adhering to video etiquette such as facing the camera, being aware of surroundings, blurring backgrounds, and avoiding eating during sessions. Throughout the course, the team should monitor participation and record relevant details to facilitate recognition of participants or groups based on predefined criteria.

**Mentors** Mentors can serve as initial points of contact for various issues that participants may be reluctant to discuss with faculty members. They can share their experiences and challenges and guide the participants to facilitate successful completion of the course. Additionally, they can be integrated into participant groups to oversee discussions and, when necessary, stimulate further engagement to ensure continuous progress.

**Discussion Groups During the Class** During scheduled class sessions, participants can be systematically divided into groups to facilitate collaborative tasks. These activities promote active engagement, foster consensus building, and help mitigate monotony. In online settings, platforms such as Zoom offer features to assign participants to breakout rooms, with a designated host overseeing the discussions. Offline classes can utilize separate round tables to enable small group discussions on assigned tasks, enhancing interaction and participation.

**Valedictory** The key considerations include the outcomes of summative assessments, the distribution of awards and certificates, the collection of feedback and testimonials (both written and video formats), the dissemination of information regarding support and supervision (if planned), recognition of resource persons and mentors, and a formal vote of thanks.

## *2.3 Post-Program*

Before concluding the course, especially if it is intended for future continuation, several considerations should be addressed.

**Availability of Course Materials** Course materials may include presentation slides (preferably in PDF format), resources prepared by faculty, video recordings of sessions (for online classes), and materials distributed during group discussions. If an LMS platform is available, sharing these materials becomes more efficient, with access restricted to authorized participants. The timing for hosting materials on the LMS should be predetermined and communicated to participants in advance.

**Preparation of Invoices and Reports** This is a detailed process that demands careful attention and accuracy. It is essential to maintain proper backups of payment receipts for all relevant stakeholders. Additionally, participants should be provided with the necessary payment documentation to meet their requirements.

**Support and Supervision** In some courses, faculty and mentors need to be accessible to participants for ongoing support when they face challenges. Specifically, in psychotherapy-related courses, participants might require supervision from qualified experts. It is recommended to establish clear arrangements regarding supervision responsibilities before the course begins.

## 3 A Few Short Courses

Below is an overview of short courses available in Psychiatry within the South Asia Region:

1. **Certificate Course in Child & Adolescent Psychiatry for General Psychiatrists:** An initiative of the Indian Association of Child and Adolescent Mental Health (IACAM), this certificate short course is of 1-year duration and has run successfully for four batches. The course content is directed toward increasing the knowledge and skills of MD Psychiatry doctors in diagnosing and treating child and adolescent psychiatry patients (Indian Association for Child and Adolescent Mental Health, n.d.).
2. **Indian Teachers of Psychiatry-Scholarship for Teachers toward Enrichment in Psychiatry Teaching Skills (IToP-STEPS):** This is a 20-h-long short course specifically targeted toward psychiatry teachers and educators to increase their skills and gain further knowledge in areas of psychiatric medical education. Four scholars are selected annually and awarded Rs 10,000/- on successful course completion. A chance to engage with leading psychiatric educators and mentors is an added advantage (Indian Teachers of Psychiatry, n.d.).
3. **National Programme on Technology Enhanced Learning (NPTEL) Swayam:** This is an online portal, an initiative of the Ministry of Education and Human Resource Development. It hosts multiple short courses digitally and aims to bridge the education gap by providing free access to quality education. Examples of courses relevant to psychiatry are Basics of Mental Health and Clinical Psychiatry. Many courses are also available on psychology, e.g. Positive Psychology and Abnormal Psychology. It also hosts many courses related to research methodology, such as the Basic Course in Biomedical Research(BCBR), which has been made mandatory by NMC for postgraduate students, as well as faculty, and the Short Course on Statistical Package for the Social Sciences(Ministry of Education, Government of India, n.d.).
4. **Brief Course in Psychiatric Research (BCPR):** Run under the aegis of IPS-South Zone, this 6-month course offers training in research methodology

specifically for psychiatrists. It has both online and in-person sessions (Ameen, 2015).

5. **NIMHANS Digital Academy (NDA):** It runs approximately 27 certificate courses on topics like counseling, psychotherapy, and mental health from beginner to advanced levels.
6. **NIMHANS Virtual Knowledge Network(VKN):** It is also an online e-learning platform that offers short-term certificate courses on deaddiction topics. It is run by the Center for Deaddiction, NIMHANS. For example, a few courses are Primer on Tobacco Cessation, Primer on Motivational Interviewing, Primer on Relapse Prevention Substance Use Disorders, etc. (NIMHANS Virtual Knowledge Network, n.d.).
7. **Basic Course in Medical Education (BCME):** Run by NMC nodal centers, it is a 3-day short course teaching the basics of Competency-Based Medical Education (CBME) and principles of Medical Education (National Medical Commission, n.d.-b).
8. **Curriculum Implementation Support Program (CISP I, II, III):** Similarly run by NMC nodal centers, it is a 2-day course that focuses on developing a yearly curriculum and timetable for each phase of MBBS under CBME (National Medical Commission, n.d.-a, n.d.-b).
9. **Advanced Course in Medical Education (ACME):** This is a 6-month course run at various NMC nodal centers focusing on advanced skills in medical education (National Medical Commission, n.d.-a, n.d.-b).
10. **National Teacher Training Center (NTTC) JIPMER:** A 15-day in-person training program conducted by JIPMER to train faculty of all disciplines, including psychiatry (Jawaharlal Institute of Postgraduate Medical Education & Research | Government of India, n.d.).
11. **Indira Gandhi National Open University (IGNOU):** It offers courses like the Postgraduate Diploma Course in Mental Health and the Postgraduate Diploma Course in Counseling and Family Therapy for professionals with a background in psychiatry, psychology, social work, and nursing. Duration of the courses is a minimum of 12 months, maximum 36 months, and the fees are Rs. 9000 for Indian Nationals (Indira Gandhi National Open University, n.d.-a, n.d.-b).
12. **Certificate courses in conferences:** Sometimes, conferences also provide short-term courses on specific topics. For example, the 19th Indian Association of Biological Psychiatry annual conference hosted a 3-h certificate course in sexual medicine covering seven modules (Indian Association of Biological Psychiatry, n.d.).

Short courses in niche areas, such as sleep disorders, psychoanalysis, Women's Mental Health, etc., are run occasionally.

Infrastructure deficits, shortage of skilled instructors, financial constraints, regulatory hurdles, and perceived lack of usefulness of these courses by the audience, as they do not provide certification similar to professional courses, are some challenges faced in developing short courses in Psychiatry in South Asian countries. The way forward is to focus on identifying felt learning needs of the targeted mental health professionals, digital-based infrastructure, collating financial and human resources across the country and the region to benefit all, open communication amongst the organizing team, maintaining motivation, and a positive working environment.

## 4 Summary

This chapter offers a comprehensive framework for designing effective short courses in psychiatry, aimed at enhancing healthcare professionals' knowledge and skills.

Key insights include:

1. Short courses are intended to deliver immediate, practical skills applicable in clinical settings
2. A well-defined framework is essential for developing courses tailored to the specific needs of the target audience
3. Engaging qualified faculty members is vital for course success, providing diverse perspectives within the curriculum
4. Identifying potential funding sources, such as professional societies or grants, can mitigate financial constraints
5. Implementing formative and summative assessments is crucial for evaluating participant learning and increasing engagement
6. Organizing short courses promotes collaboration and networking among participants, supporting professional development
7. Supporting and valuing team members throughout fosters a positive working environment
8. Open communication and mutual support are key to overcoming challenges and maintaining motivation
9. Addressing common organizational challenges effectively ensures smooth delivery of the course

**Acknowledgement** The authors thank Dr. Shahul Ameen and Dr. RaviTeja Innamuri for their valuable inputs to improve the content.

## References

Aboulsoud, S. H. (2011). Formative versus summative assessment. *Education for Health, 24*(2), 651. https://doi.org/10.4103/1357-6283.101431

Ameen, D. S. (2015, January 22). *Brief course in psychiatric research—Home*. https://www.bcpr.in/.

Cambridge University Press. (n.d.). Mentor | English meaning. In *Cambridge dictionary*. Retrieved January 24, 2025, from https://dictionary.cambridge.org/dictionary/english/mentor.

Jawaharlal Institute of Postgraduate Medical Education & Research. (n.d.). General info [Department of Medical Education]. Government of India. Retrieved July 7, 2025, from https://jipmer.edu.in/department/medical-education/general-info

Income Tax Department, Government of India. (n.d.). *Frequently asked questions on TAN*. Retrieved January 18, 2025, from https://incometaxindia.gov.in/Pages/faqs.aspx?k=FAQs+on+TAN&c=7.

Indian Association for Child and Adolescent Mental Health. (n.d.). *IACAM academy—An initiative of the Indian Association for Child and Adolescent Mental Health*. Retrieved February 12, 2025, from https://iacamacademy.com/.

Indian Association of Biological Psychiatry. (n.d.). *Midyear conference*. Retrieved May 1, 2025, from https://iabp.org.in/midyearconference.php.

Indian Council of Medical Research. (n.d.). *Workshop funding support programme*. Retrieved January 16, 2025, from https://www.icmr.gov.in/workshop-funding-support-programme.

Indian Teachers of Psychiatry. (n.d.). *STEPS & MUST—Indian Teachers of Psychiatry*. Retrieved February 12, 2025, from https://indianteachersofpsychiatry.com/scolarship/.

Indira Gandhi National Open University. (n.d.-a). *Post graduate diploma in mental health*. Retrieved April 30, 2025, from https://www.ignou.ac.in/schools/programme/PGDMH.

Indira Gandhi National Open University. (n.d.-b). *Post graduate diploma in counselling and family therapy*. Retrieved April 30, 2025, from https://www.ignou.ac.in/schools/programme/PGDCFT.

Ministry of Education, Government of India. (n.d.). *Swayam*. Retrieved February 12, 2025, from https://swayam.gov.in/explorer.

National Medical Commission. (n.d.). *Registered medical practitioner (professional conduct) regulations, 2023 - reg*. Retrieved January 16, 2025, from https://www.nmc.org.in/rules-regulations/national-medical-commission-registered-medical-practitioner-professional-conduct-regulations-2023-reg/.

NIMHANS E-Learning Hub. (2022, December 20). *Primer on tobacco cessation*. https://nimhanselearning.org/courses/primer-on-tobacco-cessation/.

NIMHANS Virtual Knowledge Network. (n.d.). *Empowering providers, transforming lives*. Retrieved February 12, 2025, from https://vknnimhans.in/.

NPTEL. (n.d.). *Stress management—Announcements*. Retrieved February 12, 2025, from https://onlinecourses.nptel.ac.in/noc24_hs163/announcements?force=true.

Online Jain University. (n.d.). *Short-term course vs full-time degree: Which is better for upskilling?* Retrieved February 12, 2025, from https://onlinejain.com/blogs/short-term-course-vs-full-time-degree-which-better-upskilling.

Team, E. (2021, October 31). *What is an online short course?* UK Study Online. https://www.ukstudyonline.com/what-is-an-online-short-course/.

# Chapter 16
# Newer Teaching-Learning Methods in Psychiatry Teaching

**Varchasvi Mudgal, Priyash Jain, and Varun Mehta**

**Abstract** The evolution of teaching methodologies has significantly transformed the landscape of education, particularly in medical and psychiatric training. Traditional pedagogical approaches, while foundational, often fail to fully engage students or cater to diverse learning styles. Newer teaching methods, such as problem-based learning (PBL), flipped classrooms, simulation-based education, and artificial intelligence-based digital tools, have emerged as effective alternatives. These approaches foster critical thinking, active participation, and improved retention of knowledge.

Despite their advantages, newer teaching methods present challenges such as resource constraints, faculty adaptation, and student acceptance. A balanced integration of these methodologies with traditional formats is essential to optimize learning outcomes. As medical education continues to evolve, a hybrid approach that combines evidence-based pedagogical strategies with emerging technologies appears to be the most effective way forward. Further research and institutional support are necessary to refine these methods and assess their long-term impact on professional competency.

**Keywords** Medical education · Teaching-learning · Self-directed learning · Problem-based learning · Technology-enabled learning · Innovative methods of teaching

V. Mudgal (✉)
Department of Psychiatry, MGM Medical College, Indore, Madhya Pradesh, India

P. Jain
AIIMS Bhopal, Bhopal, Madhya Pradesh, India

V. Mehta
CIP Ranchi, Ranchi, Jharkhand, India



S. K. Kar et al. (eds.), *Teaching and Training in Psychiatry in South Asia*, South Asian Perspectives in Mental Health and Psychology,
https://doi.org/10.1007/978-981-95-1845-6_16

## 1 Introduction

Over the years, several deficiencies have been found in medical education including psychiatry, which has contributed to misalignment in the content (what people learn), pedagogy (how people learn), and culture (why people learn). The need for a change in approach led to the shift in the process from knowledge-oriented learning having focus on the number of hours spent sitting in lecture halls or behind computer screens to skill-based learning based on what medical students can do, know, and value known as outcome-based medical education (OBME) (Davis et al., 2009). "Competency-based medical education (CBME) is one such OBME, that intends to address this misalignment by creating a medical student who can practice medicine at a defined level of proficiency, in accord with the societal expectations, to meet local needs" (McGaghie et al., 1978). This ambitious aim for medical education is achieved by developing a curriculum framework against these competencies. The new curriculum also provided an opportunity for departure from the traditional mode of teaching, i.e., teachers and what they teach, to a student-centred approach, in which the emphasis is on students and what they learn. This also required a fundamental change in the role of the teacher from that of a didactic educator to that of a facilitator of learning. The focus is now on bedside clinics, small group discussion, and demonstration-observe-assist-perform sessions apart from traditional lectures. Teaching methods are methods that deliver content or facilitate the learning process to acquire new knowledge or skills, with the intention of changed behaviour in practice, or as actionable educational practices to facilitate learning and development (Matinho et al., 2022; Ramani et al., 2019). For a meaningful practice change, teaching methods should adopt the principles of adult learning and utilize learning activities such as feedback, reflection, or team-based activities. This chapter discusses some of these new Teaching-Learning (TL) methods based on the principles of adult learning in Psychiatry Medical Education (PsyME).

## 2 Competency-Based Medical Education in Psychiatry

The past few years have witnessed CBME being adopted by different low- and middle-income countries across South Asia. The National Medical Commission (NMC), responsible for medical education, practice, and expertise in India, introduced CBME for all the undergraduate medical colleges in the country from August 2019. Out of the 412 topics for learning and 2949 outcomes to be mastered, Psychiatry received its due importance with competencies related to mental health and illness being divided into 19 topics and 117 outcomes (Jacob, 2019). In addition, there are 45 competencies across nine subjects where Psychiatry is either vertically or horizontally integrated, specifically with General Medicine, Geriatrics, Paediatrics, and Community Health (Jacob, 2019). For each topic, the competencies, domains of learning (knowledge, skill, attitude, and communication), and expected level of achievement (Knows, Knows How, Shows How, and Performs) have also been identified along with the TL and the assessment method. The duration of psychiatry training has increased to at least 40 h of teaching and around 4 weeks of clinical rotations for medical students.

The affective (communication and professional skills) and psychomotor (physical skills) domains of CBME take priority for psychiatry teaching (Kishor et al., 2016). For instance, in a session on depression, the emphasis can be on building rapport with patients and effectively eliciting mood, which primarily falls within the affective domain. Here, psychiatry educators and students must engage actively. In contrast, the cognitive domain (knowledge-based learning) is well-covered in standard textbooks, allowing teachers to provide guidance while students engage in self-learning. For example, understanding the diagnostic criteria for depression is a cognitive task. When addressing the psychomotor domain, direct demonstration by the teacher becomes essential. In the case of alcohol dependence syndrome, for example, students must learn how to recognize and demonstrate alcohol withdrawal tremors, a crucial clinical skill. A clear understanding of these domains facilitates competency acquisition within the available time, allowing for a greater focus on fostering self-directed learning among medical students. There are various methods of teaching—traditional and newer methods. A brief comparison can be seen in Table 16.1.

# 3 Effective and Innovative Teaching Methods

## *3.1 Self-Directed Learning*

Malcolm Knowles, the champion of theory of andragogy, defined self-directed learning (SDL) as "*…a process in which individuals take the initiative, with or without the help of others, in diagnosing their own learning needs, formulating goals, identifying human and material resources for learning, choosing and implementing*

**Table 16.1** Comparison of traditional and newer teaching methods in Psychiatry

| Feature | Traditional learning | Newer learning methods |
|---|---|---|
| Learning approach | Teacher-centred | Student-centred |
| Teaching methods | Lectures, textbooks | CBL, PBL, TBL, flipped classrooms |
| Role of Faculty | Instructor/lecturer | Facilitator/guide |
| Student engagement | Passive | Active and participatory |
| Assessment style | Exams, rote memorization | Competency-based, interactive evaluation |
| Use of technology | Minimal | High (VR, AR, AI, interactive platforms) |

*appropriate learning strategies, and evaluating learning outcomes*" (van der Walt, 2019). In simpler words, it can be put as a gradual transition from teacher-led education to student-led education. It is an outcome that empowers students to pursue the information regarding the skills that they want to become proficient in.

In traditional learning, an instructor provides the learning objectives, learning materials and resources, assessments, and feedback. However, in SDL, the underpinned principle is that the student takes complete responsibility of learning by identifying their learning needs, setting learning objectives, gleaning resources, planning assessments that allow feedback. The Self-Directed Learning (SDL) approach represents a significant transformation for educators, shifting their role from merely delivering information to actively facilitating learning. In this model, educators act as motivators, designers of learning experiences, and often co-learners alongside students, developing both instructional skills (such as facilitation) and expanding their own knowledge beyond their areas of expertise. SDL fosters learner autonomy and mastery while bringing a greater sense of purpose to education. When effectively implemented, SDL enhances students' motivation, strengthens their sense of control, and boosts their confidence and self-belief (Knowles, 1975).

SDL must be differentiated from self-regulated learning and self-paced learning. Self-paced learning is when students are given a learning objective, resources, and a deadline by which to complete their reading, allowing them to follow their own pace. For example, giving a deadline to study a particular set of topics by a certain date.

Self-regulated learning is a narrower construct than SDL, in a way that SDL takes place outside of the traditional classroom, while self-regulated learning occurs in an environment controlled by an instructor and the task is imposed by the instructor. Self-regulated learning enables learners to regulate their impulses and prioritize their well-being. This process involves adjusting emotional, cognitive, and behavioural responses throughout the learning experience to achieve desired outcomes. Another key distinction between self-regulated learning and self-directed learning is that the former originates from cognitive psychology, whereas the latter is rooted in adult education (Saks & Leijen, 2014).

Self-directed learning can be developed with the help of a scaffolding process. Initially, self-paced learning activities are introduced via didactic lectures early on, enabling students to become more self-regulated. Gradually, learning is moved from the classroom to experiential settings. Several educational components can help students achieve this goal, like—flipped classrooms, learning contracts, and minimal guidance instructions (Robinson & Persky, 2020).

In a flipped classroom approach, students learn some foundational material on their own prior to the class based on the resources provided by a teacher. Then, with the help of the instructor, the learned content is applied, expanded upon to reinforce and deepen the learning. When the students learn the material by themselves, it helps them build confidence and develop self-paced learning as well as self-regulated learning, which serves as the foundation for self-directedness. The flipped classroom approach can be further used to direct students to explore even more by encouraging them to make plans on how to explore the topic further (DeLozier & Rhodes, 2017).

Learning contracts can be used by the instructors to develop SDL. It involves making an agreement between an instructor and a student, which specifies that particular work will be completed by a student in a given period of time. The contract consists of specific steps similar to SDL that the student has to go through in order to learn a particular topic. Such learning contracts induce a sense of responsibility coupled with a sense of autonomy, empowering students further.

The last method is a minimally guided instructional approach. This approach is based on the premise that people learn best in a minimally guided environment. Problem-based learning (PBL) involves use of this approach. Problem-Based Learning (PBL) as an educational approach in medicine was first introduced at McMaster University in Canada in 1969. This approach moved away from traditional lecture-based teaching, shifting the focus to student-centred learning. In its original form, PBL begins with a real-world problem or scenario, prompting students to develop hypotheses and identify learning needs to better understand the issue and achieve specific learning objectives. Because of the minimal guidance provided, this type of instruction encourages self-directed learning (Robinson & Persky, 2020). Problem-based learning is based on the premise that learning is enhanced if the student is able to attach new pieces of information to the existing foundation (Trullàs et al., 2022).

PBL is typically conducted in small groups of around 8–10 students, guided by a tutor. During group sessions, students analyse a given problem or scenario, define key concepts, brainstorm potential solutions, and establish important learning goals. They then independently research these topics and reconvene in subsequent sessions to share and discuss their findings (Trullàs et al., 2022).

## *3.2 Case-Based Learning*

Traditionally, students in healthcare usually received didactic lectures in the initial years, followed by a transition to internships. But policymakers have realized the importance of introducing clinical exposure early in the education and have been moving towards vertical integration of basic sciences with clinical sciences in what is also called as "spiral curriculum". With this motive, using clinical cases to facilitate learning has been termed case-based learning (Thistlethwaite et al., 2012).

Case-based learning has been defined as "learning and teaching approach that aims to prepare students for clinical practice, through the use of authentic clinical cases. These cases link theory to practice, through the application of knowledge to the cases, and encourage the use of inquiry-based learning methods" (Thistlethwaite et al., 2012).

Successful implementation of CBL requires at least:

1. A clinical case
2. Some kind of inquiry on the part of the learner, which is all of the information to be learned is not presented at first
3. Enough information presented so that there is not too much time spent learning basics and
4. A faculty member teaching and guiding the discussion, ensuring that learning objectives are met

CBL is often contrasted with PBL. Both fall into the category of inquiry-based learning; however, the difference is in the approach towards the objectives in both. While in CBL the objective is pre-defined, PBL encourages students to come up with their own objectives and explore the problems. The role of the instructor in CBL is to provide a structure to the discussion, while there is minimal intrusion from the instructor in PBL. PBL facilitates self-directed learning where students are the drivers, while in CBL, it is the instructor who drives the discussion (Thistlethwaite et al., 2012).

CBL encourages students to develop high-order thinking skills and the use of reasoning, helping them develop decision-making skills. An important part of the process is the opportunity provided to the students to reflect on the problem, allowing them to apply previously acquired knowledge. It also requires creativity and reduces focus from the traditional didactic lectures. Case-based learning also led to an improvement in student motivation and engagement.

### *3.3 Team-Based Learning*

Team-based learning (TBL) is defined as "*an active learning and small group instructional strategy that provides students with opportunities to apply conceptual knowledge through a sequence of activities that includes individual work, team work, and immediate feedback*" (Parmelee et al., 2012).

Team-Based Learning (TBL) is an active learning strategy designed for small group instruction, allowing students to apply conceptual knowledge through structured activities. It can be implemented in both large classes (over 100 students) and smaller ones (fewer than 25 students), with multiple teams of 5–7 students working within the same classroom.

TBL is defined by three essential components (Table 16.1):

- Independent Pre-Class Preparation
- Readiness Assurance Process
- Application of Knowledge in Teams

This method is highly student-centred but guided by faculty expertise. It incorporates grading, peer evaluation, and immediate feedback to ensure individual and team accountability (Parmelee et al., 2012).

Sometimes introduced as an alternative to problem-based learning (PBL), in comparison to PBL, TBL maintains the advantages of small group teaching and learning, but importantly, without the need for large numbers of tutors (Parmelee et al., 2012).

There are various advantages to the TBL, as it helps students to develop professional attributes, keeps them motivated to reflect on their own strengths and weaknesses as members of a team, teaches them the value of working and collaborating in teams, and provides an opportunity for structured learning (Parmelee et al., 2012).

## *3.4 Role of Technology in Psychiatry Education*

Rise of technology has enabled newer avenues for imparting education. Technology-enabled learning (TEL), augmented reality, virtual reality, artificial intelligence, interactive learning platforms are some of the cutting-edge advancements in medical education. Technology has been serving as a conduit for learning on the foundation of existing learning methods like CBL and PBL. Challenges faced during the COVID-19 pandemic further facilitated the transition towards technology-enabled learning.

### 3.4.1 Technology-Enabled Learning

While the COVID-19 pandemic may have facilitated the transition of learning towards TEL, the use of TEL has not been new. Online or TEL-based small group learning was introduced to leverage both asynchronous and synchronous collaboration, providing students with continuous engagement opportunities. This approach minimizes the constraints of face-to-face interactions, addressing challenges such as limited availability of expert faculty, scheduling physical learning spaces, and ensuring greater flexibility for students. Institutes across the world have attempted using various platforms like WeChat and Zoom (Donkin et al., 2023).

### 3.4.2 Virtual Reality and Augmented Reality

Augmented Reality is a type of mixed reality in which the real-world experience is modified/enhanced using specialized tools. This is usually achieved with the help of specialized headsets like devices or even glasses. Caudell first introduced the term "augmented reality" (AR) in 1990 while working for Boeings Computer Services when he guided workers using head-mounted display devices to guide the wiring work of aircraft equipment (Barsom et al., 2016).

Virtual Reality, on the other hand, refers to a digital environment in which the user interacts as if the interaction is happening in the real world. AR differs from VR in terms of the focus of interaction, as in AR it lies within the real world (AR) instead of the digital environment (VR) (Barsom et al., 2016).

Within healthcare, augmented reality applications are being designed to supplement medical education, as a navigation tool in surgery, and even as a therapeutic tool in the treatment of phobia (Bretón-López et al., 2010). Significant strides have been taken in the field of medical education with the use of apps like HoloHuman that provide a virtual cadaver which can be interacted with using of HoloLens headset (Dhar et al., 2021). In psychiatry education, in 2021, Libera et al. introduced a method of assessing paranoia using 360° immersive videos to elicit emotions like fear, distress, and curiosity (Della Libera et al., 2021).

American Psychiatric Association (APA) Council on Medical Education and Lifelong Learning report on Training Psychiatrists for Integrated Behavioral Health Care advocated for the development of resource materials to simulate experiences, aiding psychiatry trainees in learning psychiatric-medical clinical care (Summers, 2015). In light of this, Pedersen et al. in their review proposed the development of a phenomenologically driven approach to the design of AR/VR scenarios to aid in psychiatry education (Pedersen & Musaeus, 2023).

However, there are certain challenges that need to be addressed before pushing for the use of these newer learning aids. One of the major concerns is regarding the availability of technological infrastructure. Another constraint would be training of the students as well as the instructors regarding the use of these technological aids. Another hurdle faced for the adoption of these technological aids is cost of designing these equipment and the programs (Dhar et al., 2021).

Augmented Reality (AR) and Virtual Reality (VR) present medical educators with a unique opportunity to design an immersive and interactive curriculum, allowing students to not only acquire knowledge but also experience the learning process firsthand. The shift away from traditional classroom teaching, accelerated by the COVID-19 pandemic, has driven widespread adoption of digital education tools. This transition has underscored the crucial role of technologies like AR in maintaining uninterrupted student learning. Effective integration and sustained use of digital learning tools hold the potential to significantly transform medical education.

### 3.4.3 Web-Based and Mobile-Based Applications in Psychiatry Education

The rapid advancements in web-based and mobile technologies over the past decade have significantly transformed how individuals engage with digital platforms. Smartphones equipped with app capabilities represent a new era of technology, offering extensive computing power and constant Internet access, enabling users to interact with a wide range of applications (Zhang et al., 2015).

Mobile applications, or apps, are specialized software programs designed for computers, tablets, and smartphones to perform specific functions. In the field of medical education, these applications have become indispensable tools for both healthcare professionals (HCPs) and students, enhancing their training and clinical practice. Medical education, in particular, benefits from the accessibility and flexibility of mobile and web-based applications, which support learning in diverse settings. These applications aid in critical functions such as clinical documentation, time and health record management, professional networking, decision support, and continuing medical education. Their interactive and multimedia features—including images, videos, text, and podcasts—make them engaging and effective tools for learning, ultimately contributing to the enhancement of psychiatric training and patient care (Chandran et al., 2022).

Globally, there have been numerous efforts towards the integration of mobile phone technologies in medical education across various specialities, including paediatrics, ophthalmology, nephrology, plastic surgery, orthopaedics, pharmacology, and urology. For instance, a neonatal intubation app has been developed to improve intubation skills in paediatrics, while in plastic surgery, 16 apps have been identified as valuable educational tools for surgeons (Zhang et al., 2015).

Given this widespread adoption, it is important to assess the extent to which psychiatry has incorporated web-based and mobile applications for educational purposes. A literature review indicates that while psychiatry has explored digital learning tools, their use remains relatively limited compared to other medical fields. Notable advancements include the application of virtual reality for role-play simulations in child and adolescent psychiatry, the use of telemedicine for peer-to-peer learning between medical students in different countries, the integration of simulation for performance evaluation in psychiatry, and the development of virtual patients as training tools for clinical interviewing skills. However, there is still a gap which underscores the need for further exploration into how digital tools can enhance psychiatric training and practice (Zhang et al., 2015). More models need to be explored integrating SDL, PBL, TBL with mobile and web-based applications in order to empower students in their learning.

Mobile and web-based applications offer numerous advantages over traditional methods as they can be considered as an effective adjunct tool in medical education by considering the low expense, high versatility, reduced dependency on regional or site boundaries.

### 3.4.4 AI-Powered Chatbots in Psychiatry Training and Education

AI-powered chatbots have emerged as a transformative element in the evolution of psychiatry training, offering a dynamic supplement to traditional educational methods. These systems are designed to streamline complex psychiatric information into concise, accessible summaries, ensuring that students can quickly assimilate critical concepts and stay informed about emerging developments in the field. By reducing the cognitive load associated with deciphering intricate clinical data, chatbots facilitate a deeper understanding of theoretical principles, thereby enhancing overall learning efficiency (Ghorashi et al., 2023).

Moreover, these advanced tools simulate real-world patient interactions, providing trainees with the opportunity to engage in realistic clinical scenarios in a controlled environment. Through simulated dialogues and case-based learning, learners can practice diagnostic assessments and therapeutic communication without the immediate pressures of real patient care. This interactive practice not only helps in honing clinical decision-making skills but also builds confidence by allowing for repeated trial and error in a safe setting. Immediate and personalized feedback from the chatbot further enables learners to identify strengths and address areas needing improvement, bridging the gap between classroom theory and practical application (Ghorashi et al., 2023).

The adaptability of AI-powered chatbots makes them a particularly valuable resource in modern psychiatric education. They offer on-demand access to curated information, enabling self-directed learning that can be tailored to the individual needs of each trainee. Whether used as a supplementary study tool or an integral part of simulation training, chatbots help create a more engaging and flexible educational experience. This not only supports the continuous professional development of trainees but also ensures that emerging psychiatrists are well-equipped to meet the challenges of clinical practice with both updated knowledge and refined interpersonal skills (Ghorashi et al., 2023).

### 3.4.5 Simulation-Based Training in Psychiatry

Simulation-based training represents a critical educational strategy in psychiatry, effectively bridging the gap between theoretical instruction and clinical practice. By employing controlled, realistic scenarios, simulation modalities allow trainees to develop and refine essential clinical competencies in a safe environment.

The use of standardized patients (SPs) is a well-established method in psychiatric education. SPs are trained individuals who reliably reproduce clinical scenarios, enabling students to practice diagnostic interviewing, formulate treatment plans, and develop effective communication strategies. This method provides consistent exposure to a range of psychiatric conditions, fostering skill acquisition through repeated, realistic interactions and enabling immediate, structured feedback.

Role-playing exercises further enhance learning by allowing trainees to assume both the clinician and patient roles within a simulated clinical encounter. This dual perspective not only cultivates empathy and a deeper understanding of patient experiences but also encourages critical reflection on clinical decision-making processes. Such exercises promote adaptability and improve interpersonal communication skills, which are vital in managing complex psychiatric cases.

Virtual reality (VR) simulations represent a novel and increasingly popular approach to psychiatric training. VR creates immersive, high-fidelity environments in which learners can engage in realistic, interactive clinical scenarios. This technology is particularly valuable for simulating high-stakes or rare psychiatric events, allowing trainees to practice crisis management and rapid decision-making in a controlled, risk-free setting. The immersive nature of VR also supports the development of technical and non-technical skills in a manner that closely mirrors real-life clinical situations.

Collectively, these simulation-based training modalities contribute significantly to the development of clinical competence in psychiatry. Research indicates that simulation enhances self-confidence, improves diagnostic accuracy, and fosters effective therapeutic communication. Furthermore, by providing a structured setting for reflective practice, simulation training encourages continual learning and adaptation, which are essential for effective clinical practice in the ever-evolving field of mental health care.

In conclusion, the integration of standardized patients, role-playing exercises, and VR simulations into psychiatric education provides a robust framework for experiential learning. These methods collectively enhance clinical readiness, promote the development of critical thinking, and ultimately contribute to the delivery of high-quality psychiatric care. The comprehensive review by Piot et al. (2021) underscores the value of simulation-based training as a cornerstone of modern psychiatric education (Piot et al., 2021).

A variety of teaching and learning methods can be implemented according to the learner's requirements, the instructor's proficiency, the group size, and the availability of resources. A comparison of various teaching-learning methods is provided in Table 16.2.

## 4 Addressing Challenges in Psychiatry Teaching in South Asia

Innovative teaching methods in psychiatry offer a pathway to transform mental health education in South Asia; however, the region faces unique challenges that complicate the transition from traditional didactic methods to more dynamic, learner-centred approaches. In India, where there are only about 0.75 psychiatrists per 100,000 population, far below the desirable threshold of 3 per 100,000 thus, the urgency for reform is compounded by both systemic constraints and cultural factors (Garg et al., 2019). Furthermore, the mental health treatment gap remains wide, with national surveys reporting gaps as high as 70–92% for various disorders (Murthy, 2017). Psychiatry education in South Asia faces several unique challenges, shaped by cultural, systemic, and resource-related factors. Despite growing awareness of mental health issues, psychiatric training often remains underdeveloped due to a lack of standardized curricula, inadequate faculty training, and stigma surrounding mental illness. These challenges not only affect the quality of psychiatric training but also contribute to a shortage of skilled professionals in the region. Addressing these barriers requires a multifaceted approach, including curriculum reforms, faculty development, and greater integration of psychiatry into general medical training.

**Table 16.2** Highlighting the core aspects of various teaching methods

| Method | Description and strategy | Instructor vs. learner role | Key pros & cons |
|---|---|---|---|
| Self-directed learning (SDL) | Learners independently diagnose needs, set goals, gather resources, and evaluate outcomes; often scaffolded from self-paced to experiential activities | **Instructor:** Facilitator and co-learner **Learner:** Drives all stages of learning | **Pros:** Enhances autonomy and confidence **Cons:** Demands high self-motivation |
| Case-based learning (CBL) | Uses authentic clinical cases with pre-defined objectives to link theory with practice | **Instructor:** Structures and guides discussion **Learner:** Applies prior knowledge to analyse cases | **Pros:** Strengthens critical thinking **Cons:** Less learner-driven exploration |
| Team-based learning (TBL) | Involves pre-class preparation, individual/team assessments, and group application exercises with immediate feedback | **Instructor:** Designs activities and offers feedback **Learner:** Prepares individually and collaborates in teams | **Pros:** Fosters collaboration and accountability **Cons:** Requires strong team coordination |
| Technology-based learning | Leverages digital tools like AI, VR, Chatbots, etc., for both synchronous and asynchronous learning, increasing flexibility | **Instructor:** Guides virtual interactions **Learner:** Engages with online resources independently | **Pros:** Flexible and accessible **Cons:** Relies on technology and digital skills. Risk of false information |
| Simulation-based training | Employs controlled, realistic scenarios (standardized patients, role-play, VR) to practice clinical skills | **Instructor:** Designs and oversees simulations **Learner:** Participates actively and reflects on performance | **Pros:** Improves diagnostic and communication skills **Cons:** Resource-intensive |

## *4.1 Faculty Preparedness and Attitudinal Barriers*

One significant challenge in the South Asian context is the readiness of faculty to adopt and implement new pedagogical methods. Many educators in India and its neighbouring countries were trained under traditional, teacher-centred models and may be less familiar with student-led methodologies such as self-directed learning, problem-based learning (PBL), and team-based learning (TBL) (Kishor et al., 2016). This gap necessitates comprehensive faculty development programmes that not only impart technical skills—such as using digital platforms, simulation software, and virtual reality (VR)—but also promote a paradigm shift towards interactive, student-centred learning. Targeted training initiatives must focus on both the acquisition of these new skills and on overcoming the entrenched attitudes that have historically characterized psychiatric education in the region.

## *4.2 Resource and Infrastructure Constraints*

In many parts of South Asia, and India in particular, infrastructural and financial limitations pose formidable barriers to innovation. Integrating technology-enhanced learning modalities, including simulation-based exercises and VR/AR applications, requires significant investment in hardware, software, and robust Internet connectivity (Barsom et al., 2016). Many institutions—especially in rural and semi-urban areas—lack high-speed Internet or modern teaching facilities, leading to an uneven distribution of educational opportunities. Addressing this digital divide will require not only institutional commitment but also partnerships with government bodies and the private sector to upgrade technological infrastructure and secure necessary funding.

## *4.3 Societal Stigma and Cultural Nuances*

Psychiatry in South Asia is burdened by persistent societal stigma, influencing both the perception of the discipline and the willingness of students to engage deeply with it. In India, for example, mental health is often shrouded in cultural taboos and misconceptions that can diminish interest in psychiatric careers (Kallivayalil, 2012). This stigma extends into academic settings, where psychiatry is sometimes relegated to a minor component of the undergraduate curriculum. Overcoming these challenges demands curricular reforms that emphasize the scientific underpinnings of psychiatry while integrating patient narratives and community-based learning to humanize mental illness. By exposing students early to authentic clinical scenarios and culturally relevant case studies, educators can help dispel myths, foster empathy, and ultimately attract a more committed cohort of future mental health professionals (Kishor et al., 2016).

## *4.4 Rapidly Evolving Mental Health Science*

The dynamic nature of psychiatric research and clinical practice means that curricula must be continuously updated to reflect the latest evidence and techniques. In South Asia—where mental health resources are already stretched thin—ensuring that teaching materials remain current is an ongoing challenge. Institutions must establish agile systems for curriculum review and revision that incorporate emerging research findings and best practices from both regional and international sources

(Gupta & Menon, 2022; Kishor et al., 2016). This approach will help ensure that graduates are not only clinically competent but also well-versed in the latest diagnostic and therapeutic strategies relevant to the South Asian context.

### *4.5 Integration into the Undergraduate Curriculum*

In India, psychiatry is often subsumed under general medicine within the undergraduate MBBS curriculum, leading to a diluted focus on the subject. This limited exposure contributes to a reduced interest in psychiatry among medical students and reinforces the societal stigma associated with mental health. A reformed curriculum that elevates psychiatry to a core subject is essential. Such a curriculum should include a mix of traditional lectures, interactive case-based learning, and hands-on clinical experiences (Gupta & Menon, 2022). By integrating psychiatric education more fully into the undergraduate training programme, institutions can better prepare future physicians to address the significant mental health challenges faced in the region.

## 5 Future Directions in Psychiatry Education

The future of psychiatry education in South Asia, and particularly in India, holds promise through the adoption of cutting-edge pedagogical approaches and technology-driven innovations. Emerging trends suggest that the region's educational paradigm will evolve to meet both the unique challenges and vast opportunities presented by modern mental health care.

### *5.1 Advanced Digital Technologies and Telepsychiatry*

One of the most promising avenues for the future is the integration of advanced digital technologies into psychiatric education. With the expansion of telemedicine and digital health solutions in India, digital platforms can be leveraged not only for patient care but also for training purposes (Barsom et al., 2016; Chakrabarti, 2015). Telepsychiatry, in particular, has been highlighted as a cost-effective strategy for providing mental health care in resource-limited settings, making it an essential component of future psychiatric training in South Asia. Augmented reality (AR) and virtual reality (VR) tools can simulate clinical environments that mimic real-world scenarios, allowing students to practice diagnosing and managing complex psychiatric conditions in a controlled, risk-free setting (Pedersen & Musaeus, 2023). For instance, VR has been explored in psychiatric education by creating immersive experiences that allow learners to understand patient perspectives. A research by

Della Libera et al. (2021) demonstrated the use of 360° immersive videos to assess paranoia, highlighting the potential of VR in training clinicians to recognize and empathize with psychiatric symptoms (Della Libera et al., 2021). Moreover, digital technologies can facilitate remote learning, a significant advantage in regions marked by geographical and infrastructural disparities. With robust digital platforms, students from remote areas can access high-quality educational content, participate in virtual case discussions, and receive real-time feedback, thus reducing regional inequities in education.

## 5.2 *Personalized and Adaptive Learning Platforms*

The future of psychiatry education in South Asia is likely to be shaped by personalized learning platforms that harness the power of big data and artificial intelligence (AI). These adaptive systems can tailor educational content to meet the individual needs of each student, ensuring that learning is efficient and targeted. For example, AI-driven platforms can analyse a student's performance on diagnostic assessments, identify areas of weakness, and provide customized learning modules to address those gaps (Sharma et al., 2017). Such individualized approaches not only enhance the learning experience but also ensure that educational outcomes are closely aligned with the specific needs of a diverse student body across the region.

## 5.3 *Interprofessional and Collaborative Education*

Psychiatry is inherently multidisciplinary, intersecting with fields such as neurology, psychology, social work, and pharmacology. Future educational frameworks in India and across South Asia should promote interprofessional education (IPE) to encourage collaboration among various healthcare disciplines. Joint learning activities—such as interprofessional simulation exercises, case conferences, and team-based projects—can help students develop a holistic understanding of patient care (Parmelee et al., 2012). This collaborative approach mirrors the realities of modern clinical practice and helps dismantle traditional silos in healthcare education, fostering a culture of teamwork and shared responsibility.

## 5.4 Emphasis on Outcome-Based and Evidence-Driven Education

With the rapid evolution of psychiatric knowledge, there is an increasing need to ground teaching methods in evidence-based practices. Future curricula in South Asia should be structured around clearly defined competencies that align with the latest clinical guidelines and research findings. Problem-based learning (PBL) and self-directed learning (SDL) have been shown to improve clinical reasoning, critical thinking, and long-term retention in medical education (Trullàs et al., 2022). Outcome measures—such as Objective Structured Clinical Examinations (OSCEs), peer reviews, and digital assessments—can offer detailed insights into student performance, ensuring that educational interventions are both effective and adaptable to changing clinical needs. In the context of India, where the mental health burden is high and resources are limited, an outcome-based approach is crucial for translating training into improved clinical practice and better patient outcomes.

## 5.5 Sustainable Faculty Development and Institutional Support

For transformative change in psychiatry education to be sustainable, ongoing support for faculty is essential. In South Asia, and particularly in India, long-term investments in faculty development are vital. Institutions must establish continuous professional development programmes that not only introduce innovative teaching methods but also build supportive communities among educators (Kishor et al., 2016). Faculty must be trained in modern pedagogical approaches such as team-based learning (TBL), problem-based learning (PBL), and self-directed learning (SDL) to enhance student engagement and clinical reasoning (Gupta & Menon, 2022; Parmelee et al., 2012). Furthermore, interprofessional collaboration must be a core focus of faculty training, ensuring that psychiatrists, psychologists, and other healthcare professionals can work effectively as a team. Additionally, partnerships with international academic institutions, technology developers, and government agencies can provide the necessary resources and expertise for long-term curricular innovation.

## 5.6 Cultural Adaptation and Contextual Relevance

Psychiatric education in South Asia must be culturally sensitive and adapted to regional socio-economic realities. Cultural competence training should be integrated into curricula to help students understand the role of sociocultural determinants and traditional healing practices in mental health. The South Asian context—with its unique social, cultural, and economic landscape—requires that psychiatric education be tailored to address local realities. Stigma remains a significant barrier, often leading to delayed help-seeking. Incorporating community-based learning and mental health literacy programmes can equip students with skills to engage patients effectively and combat stigma. Additionally, telepsychiatry and digital platforms can enhance accessibility in rural and underserved areas, ensuring broader mental health coverage. By fostering community engagement and leveraging technology, psychiatric education can become more inclusive and contextually relevant, improving mental health outcomes across the region (Chakrabarti, 2015; Rukadikar et al., 2022).

## 6 Conclusion

Psychiatry education in South Asia is at a critical juncture, with innovative teaching methods offering promise amid persistent challenges. India faces a severe psychiatrist shortage and a wide mental health treatment gap, exacerbated by resource constraints, societal stigma, and outdated educational models. Psychiatry education is undergoing a transformative shift from traditional, teacher-centred models to innovative, learner-centric approaches. This chapter has highlighted the importance of competency-based education and the integration of methods such as self-directed, case-based, and team-based learning, which foster critical thinking, clinical reasoning, and active engagement. A multifaceted strategy is needed, beginning with faculty development and a shift towards student-centred learning. Investments in digital infrastructure and curriculum reforms—including the integration of psychiatry as a core subject are essential. Emerging technologies like AR/VR, use of AI, chatbots, simulation-based learning, adaptive learning, and telepsychiatry can enhance training accessibility and effectiveness. However, progress must be culturally grounded, incorporating relevant case studies, reducing stigma, and fostering interdisciplinary collaboration to produce competent, empathetic psychiatrists suited to the region's unique mental health challenges.

Despite significant challenges such as resource constraints, cultural stigmas, and the need for robust faculty development, these innovative strategies are paving the way for a more dynamic and effective educational framework in psychiatry. Looking ahead, future directions will likely emphasize strengthening digital infrastructure, promoting continuous faculty training, and fostering interprofessional collaboration. In conclusion, the evolution of psychiatry education in South Asia is more than an academic pursuit—it is a critical investment in the future of mental health care. By addressing the present challenges and strategically planning, we can bridge the gap between the current state of mental health care and the evolving needs of our communities. This educational revolution will not only elevate the standard of psychiatric practice but also contribute to reducing the pervasive stigma surrounding mental illness, ultimately leading to more compassionate and effective mental health services. The transformation of psychiatric education is an ongoing process—one that calls for collaboration among educators, policymakers, and stakeholders across the region. With sustained commitment, strategic partnerships, and a clear vision for the future, a robust, adaptive, and inclusive educational framework could be created that meets the evolving needs of South Asia.

## References


Barsom, E. Z., Graafland, M., & Schijven, M. P. (2016). Systematic review on the effectiveness of augmented reality applications in medical training. *Surgical Endoscopy, 30*(10), 4174–4183. https://doi.org/10.1007/s00464-016-4800-6

Bretón-López, J., Quero, S., Botella, C., García-Palacios, A., Baños, R. M., & Alcañiz, M. (2010). An augmented reality system validation for the treatment of cockroach phobia. *Cyberpsychology, Behavior, and Social Networking, 13*(6), 705–710. https://doi.org/10.1089/cyber.2009.0170

Chakrabarti, S. (2015). Usefulness of telepsychiatry: A critical evaluation of videoconferencing-based approaches. *World Journal of Psychiatry, 5*(3), 286–304. https://doi.org/10.5498/wjp.v5.i3.286

Chandran, V. P., Balakrishnan, A., Rashid, M., Pai Kulyadi, G., Khan, S., Devi, E. S., Nair, S., & Thunga, G. (2022). Mobile applications in medical education: A systematic review and meta-analysis. *PLoS One, 17*(3), e0265927. https://doi.org/10.1371/journal.pone.0265927

Davis, M. H., Amin, Z., Grande, J. P., O'Neill, A. E., Pawlina, W., & TR, V. (2009). Case studies in outcome-based education. *Medical Teacher, 29*(7), 10 1080 01421590701691429.

Della Libera, C., Quertemont, E., Laloyaux, J., Thonon, B., & Larøi, F. (2021). Using 360 immersive videos to assess paranoia in a non-clinical population. *Cognitive Neuropsychiatry, 26*(5), 357–375.

DeLozier, S. J., & Rhodes, M. G. (2017). Flipped classrooms: A review of key ideas and recommendations for practice. *Educational Psychology Review, 29*(1), 141–151. https://doi.org/10.1007/s10648-015-9356-9

Dhar, P., Rocks, T., Samarasinghe, R. M., Stephenson, G., & Smith, C. (2021). Augmented reality in medical education: Students' experiences and learning outcomes. *Medical Education Online, 26*(1), 1953953. https://doi.org/10.1080/10872981.2021.1953953

Donkin, R., Yule, H., & Fyfe, T. (2023). Online case-based learning in medical education: A scoping review. *BMC Medical Education, 23*, 564. https://doi.org/10.1186/s12909-023-04520-w

Garg, K., Kumar, C. N., & Chandra, P. S. (2019). Number of psychiatrists in India: Baby steps forward, but a long way to go. *Indian Journal of Psychiatry, 61*(1), 104–105. https://doi.org/10.4103/psychiatry.IndianJPsychiatry_7_18

Ghorashi, N., Ismail, A., Ghosh, P., Sidawy, A., & Javan, R. (2023). AI-powered chatbots in medical education: Potential applications and implications. *Cureus, 15*(8), e43271. https://doi.org/10.7759/cureus.43271

Gupta, S., & Menon, V. (2022). Psychiatry training for medical students: A global perspective and implications for India's competency-based medical education curriculum. *Indian Journal of Psychiatry, 64*(3), 240–251. https://doi.org/10.4103/indianjpsychiatry.indianjpsychiatry_187_22

Jacob, K. S. (2019). Medical council of India's new competency-based curriculum for medical graduates: A critical appraisal. *Indian. Journal of Psychological Medicine, 41*(3), 203–209.

Kallivayalil, R. A. (2012). The importance of psychiatry in undergraduate medical education in India. *Indian Journal of Psychiatry, 54*(3), 208–216. https://doi.org/10.4103/0019-5545.102336

Kishor, M., Isaac, M., Ashok, M. V., Pandit, L. V., & Sathyanarayana Rao, T. S. (2016). Undergraduate psychiatry training in India; past, present, and future looking for solutions within constraints!!. *Indian Journal of Psychiatry, 58*(2), 119–120. https://doi.org/10.4103/0019-5545.183794

Knowles, M. S. (1975). *Self-directed learning: A guide for learners and teachers*. Adult Education.

Matinho, D., Pietrandrea, M., Echeverria, C., Helderman, R., Masters, M., Regan, D., Shu, S., Moreno, R., & McHugh, D. (2022). A systematic review of integrated learning definitions, frameworks, and practices in recent health professions education literature. *Education Sciences, 12*(3), article 3. https://doi.org/10.3390/educsci12030165

McGaghie, W. C., Miller, G. E., Sajid, A. W., & Telder, T. V. (1978). *Competency-based curriculum development in medical education: An introduction* (Issue http://apps.who.int/iris/bitstream/10665/39703/1/WHO_PHP_68.pdf). World Health Organization.

Murthy, R. S. (2017). National mental health survey of India 2015–2016. *Indian Journal of Psychiatry, 59*(1), 21–26. https://doi.org/10.4103/psychiatry.IndianJPsychiatry_102_17

Parmelee, D., Michaelsen, L. K., Cook, S., & Hudes, P. D. (2012). Team-based learning: A practical guide: AMEE Guide No. 65. *Medical Teacher, 34*(5), e275–e287. https://doi.org/10.3109/0142159X.2012.651179

Pedersen, K., & Musaeus, P. (2023). A phenomenological approach to virtual reality in psychiatry education. *Frontiers in Virtual Reality, 4*. https://doi.org/10.3389/frvir.2023.1259263

Piot, M.-A., Attoe, C., Billon, G., Cross, S., Rethans, J.-J., & Falissard, B. (2021). Simulation training in psychiatry for medical education: A review. *Frontiers in Psychiatry, 12*, 658967. https://doi.org/10.3389/fpsyt.2021.658967

Ramani, S., McMahon, G. T., & Armstrong, E. G. (2019). Continuing professional development to foster behaviour change: From principles to practice in health professions education. *Medical Teacher, 41*(9), 1045–1052. https://doi.org/10.1080/0142159X.2019.1615608

Robinson, J. D., & Persky, A. M. (2020). Developing self-directed learners. *American Journal of Pharmaceutical Education, 84*(3), 847512. https://doi.org/10.5688/ajpe847512

Rukadikar, C., Mali, S., Bajpai, R., Rukadikar, A., & Singh, A. K. (2022). A review on cultural competency in medical education. *Journal of Family Medicine and Primary Care, 11*(8), 4319–4329. https://doi.org/10.4103/jfmpc.jfmpc_2503_21

Saks, K., & Leijen, Ä. (2014). Distinguishing self-directed and self-regulated learning and measuring them in the E-learning context. *Procedia—Social and Behavioral Sciences, 112*, 190–198. https://doi.org/10.1016/j.sbspro.2014.01.1155

Sharma, N., Doherty, I., & Dong, C. (2017). Adaptive learning in medical education: The final piece of technology enhanced learning? *The Ulster Medical Journal, 86*(3), 198–200.

Summers, R. F. (2015). Integrated behavioral health care and psychiatric training. *Academic Psychiatry, 39*(4), 425–429. https://doi.org/10.1007/s40596-015-0326-9

Thistlethwaite, J. E., Davies, D., Ekeocha, S., Kidd, J. M., MacDougall, C., Matthews, P., Purkis, J., & Clay, D. (2012). The effectiveness of case-based learning in health professional education. A BEME systematic review: BEME Guide No. 23. *Medical Teacher, 34*(6), e421–e444. https://doi.org/10.3109/0142159X.2012.680939

Trullàs, J. C., Blay, C., Sarri, E., & Pujol, R. (2022). Effectiveness of problem-based learning methodology in undergraduate medical education: A scoping review. *BMC Medical Education, 22*, 104. https://doi.org/10.1186/s12909-022-03154-8

van der Walt, J. L. (2019). The term "self-directed learning"—Back to knowles, or another way to forge ahead? *Journal of Research on Christian Education, 28*(1), 1–20. https://doi.org/10.1080/10656219.2019.1593265

Zhang, M. W., Cheok, C. C., & Ho, R. C. (2015). Global outreach of a locally-developed mobile phone app for undergraduate psychiatry education. *JMIR Medical Education, 1*(1), e3. https://doi.org/10.2196/mededu.4179

# Chapter 17
# Online Teaching-Learning in Psychiatry: Opportunities, Challenges, and Best Practices

**Gopal Das M. Chikkerahally**

**Abstract** Online Psychiatric education dates back as early as invention of communication technology and gained momentum after the multimedia and Internet-enabled videoconferencing. It has been considered as a complement to existing methods but the real impetus derived from COVID-19 pandemic has propelled the innovation as well as adoption of online learning. This chapter attempts to briefly discuss the concept, relevance, and evolution of online education particularly in the context of psychiatry and briefly introduce online teaching-learning modalities, frameworks, and models across the globe with South Asian and Indian perspectives. The aim of this chapter is to review and discuss opportunities and challenges in online psychiatric education, best practices and future directions with brief recommendations to educators and institutes who would take up online education in psychiatry in days to come.

**Keywords** Medical education · Distance education · Online learning · Psychiatry · Mental health · Active learning

## 1 Introduction

Intellect and Learning are the two important abilities that put humans at the pinnacle of creation. Learning has always been at one of the top most priorities after the basic physiological needs. The evolution of teaching-learning practices is like a flowing river that has grown with scientific progress, adopting the best possible applications

G. D. M. Chikkerahally (✉)
Department of Psychiatry, Dr. Chandramma Dayananda Sagar Institute of Medical Education & Research Institute (CDSIMER), Dayananda Sagar University (DSU), Bengaluru, Karnataka, India



S. K. Kar et al. (eds.), *Teaching and Training in Psychiatry in South Asia*, South Asian Perspectives in Mental Health and Psychology,
https://doi.org/10.1007/978-981-95-1845-6_17

of inventions. Health being the overarching need, the health practices as well as medicine need knowledge and skill transfer down the generations, where medical education has been one of the most important aspects all the time. The best practices of teaching-learning have been reflected in medical education and it also applies to technology-facilitated teaching and learning. Virtual learning is as much the part of traditional learning where learners and teachers may not be in the same place when knowledge transfer and skills acquisition happen at different times. This requires the use of learning material and mode of delivery to be facilitated by the use of means other than direct in-person instruction. Technology through the electronic form has enormously enabled virtual learning and facilitated learning called by different names such as distance learning, virtual learning, e-learning, online learning, and so on. These terms are used interchangeably but there exist differences between them. Let us know the difference between the two terms which are often used nowadays, the e-learning and online learning.

## *1.1 Concept and Evolution of E-Learning and Online Learning*

Learning has been traditionally happening with tutors and pupils being together in a place. It has long been equated to chalk, blackboard, and lectures. But, the unquenchable thirst for learning has always attempted to break these barriers and a concept of distance learning probably originated long before the inventions of communication technologies. It dates as far back as the postal system existed. Learning primarily requires the communication between learners and the teachers and then the learning material. They traditionally engaged visual and auditory senses of learners but not limited to it. The printing and mailing have been perhaps the oldest form of virtual learning that could have happened.

Then came the inventions of recording the visual and auditory materials in the form of photo-videography and audio recording that opened up Pandora's box. As the fields developed, the materials expanded and the exchange of materials too, in the context of learning. The first real impetus for distance learning started after the inventions of communication technology, first in the form of wireless and then wired transmissions. Then came the era of computers, which opened up the possibilities of data recording, storage, and dissemination, yet confined to the local machines. The analogue signals shifted to digital as the machines evolved. This gave rise to the new concept of e-learning, where the electronic material is used to replace the traditional print material that is needed for learning. It is the Internet that revolutionized e-learning and led to an era of online learning, expanded the area enormously so as to connect multiple individuals in the process of learning, yet being at their places. This really broke the geographical barriers, and the learning took the true global stage. The technology is a restless and tireless area that keeps outdating itself in the next minute. The COVID-19 pandemic posed an unprecedented challenge to mankind, and education obviously took a severe hit. The need for learning ruffled the feathers and took off to the skies which gave an enormous impetus to the relatively sluggish progress of online learning in the pre-pandemic times. Even the core traditionalists had to gear up to adapt to the inevitable need to try online modes. The 'why-not' and 'what else but this!' experience bought in many revelations that online teaching-learning is not as ineffective as earlier thought. Of course, who does not like the idea of sitting at their places and being able to access material and interact with teachers who are elsewhere. Though, it may not really match the true human interaction of traditional learning, the integration of technology certainly adds up to enhance the learning experience, and overcomes the barriers. The momentum derived led to innovations in the virtual learning. The advent of virtual and augmented realities (VR and AR), the Artificial Intelligence (AI), and newer computing systems (Graphic Processing Units—GPUs, Quantum computing) gave the thrust to already existing technologies leading to newer learning experiences in mixed reality-based teaching-learning environments and gamification-based teaching-learning (TL) and assessments.

The so far discussed evolution can be thus categorized into five eras as follows:

1. The pre-digital era of distance learning (before 1980)
2. The e-learning era (1980–2000)
3. The Internet era of blended learning (2000–2019)
4. The pandemic driven thrust for online learning (2020–2022)
5. The post-pandemic era of hybrid learning (2022 onward)

## *1.2 Relevance in Contemporary Medical Education*

Though the learning mind remains the same, the need, method, and learning environment keep evolving hand in hand with the generational trends and lifestyle. A century ago, the world was fascinated by the introduction of telephones but now the world is unable to function without them. The predominant generation currently in medical education is Late gen Zs (1996–2009) and upcoming are gen alpha (born 2010–2024) who are digital natives, i.e. they are born with technology in their cradles! They are exposed to screens more than the meaningful human interactions, and probably more comfortable handling a gadget than a human. In a generation who is so natural with the available technology, would normally incline to use the same in accessing information and expect their senses to be engaged in a manner which is known to them, even while learning. Whether it is a boon or bane is left to the debate but what we cannot deny is that there is a generational shift in teaching-learning methods. Senior professors who would be heading institutions would not have seen such a technology during their undergraduate training, that is now considered as a basic minimum (e.g., like slide presentations) which s/he uses now in their own teaching sessions. The amount of medical knowledge and new skills to be acquired have amassed to such an extent that no trainee would be stopping the medical education at the basic undergraduate level anymore. Whichever field they choose, the rapidity with which things are evolving needs a constant updating of skills and knowledge whereas the available time then and now remains the same which is 24 h a day and 365 days a year! A trainee or an aspiring learner has to accommodate so much of new knowledge and skills traversing the challenges of place and time yet come out successful. It requires engaging multiple senses in learning, accommodating parallel learning, inputs from several sources, easy access to information and moreover an easily accessible learning environment at their disposal to enable these. Online learning can provide all these requirements and hence the medical education is embracing more elements of e-learning and online learning. Depending upon the outcomes, there are two contexts where medical education can be understood. There are traditionally two contexts, formative and summative. The latter refers to the completion of basic training to reasonably good standards of professionalism and can be called as high-stake learning. The other is continuous updating and upgrading of skills and knowledge which can be formative and low-stake learning. While the high stake remains more or less traditional, yet with elements of online learning and technology in it, but it is the low-stake learning which has bloomed post-pandemic era that has provided an unprecedented opportunity for the learners to choose and take up different courses and certifications through online learning.

## *1.3 Evolution of Online Education in Psychiatry and Impetus Derived from COVID 19 Situation*

The trajectory of evolution of online learning in psychiatry can be closely traced along with other fields as described above. Starting from the computer-assisted training with recorded interviews, it moved into the era of live videoconferencing using available technology that was used to teach, assess, and evaluate. It has been in the brackets of novel and experimental section even in high-resource settings while low-resource areas had not considered it. A scoping review on Online-Based and Technology-Assisted Psychiatric Education for Trainees (Kassim et al., 2025) describes the initiatives, trends, and work done in this area pre and post pandemic. Before the pandemic, the studies were predominantly from west, the USA and Canada, used methods like videoconference-based learning, use of online modules or e-learning platforms, development of software or applications, adoption of virtual patient approaches, and use of social media as a learning tool. As the Internet accessibility improved with greater coverage, speeds, and stability, there occurred increased efforts to conduct online modules to complement traditional methods. Efforts to move structured assessments like OSCEs into online mode for practice and actual exams as an experiment. Various tools like Case-Based Learning (CBL), Problem-Based Learning (PBL), Simulation-Based Education (SBE), and Virtual Patients (VP) are tried as experimentation.

The true impetus was derived when the world locked down with severe social restrictions, and the training had no other means than to adopt the virtual means of interactions and teaching. The need drove the innovations and there was a spike in the studies describing various methodologies and how to use existing resources to suit the needs.

### *1.4 Contexts of Online Learning in Psychiatry*

Psychiatry being a branch of medicine which deals with keen behavioural observation, communication and analysis, and comparatively lesser demonstrable psychomotor skills unlike surgical branches, is perhaps more suited for online learning contexts than those branches. Nevertheless, online learning trends, in general, are increasing in medical education as a whole, and not just Psychiatry. We can understand online learning in Psychiatry under the following contexts:

- Basic science or pre-clinical training as a foundation for neuro-behavioural sciences and Psychology. These fall under predominantly cognitive domains, and a flexible self-paced asynchronous online models may serve the purpose well as the learners are preparing for other aspects as well
- Clinical skills training which are meant to develop interviewing skills, therapeutic communication, and formulation of diagnosis. Virtual patient interaction, simulations, and live feedbacks can serve the purpose well, providing safe as well as repeatable practice environment for the learners
- Telepsychiatry training
- Psychotherapy training
- Continued Medical Education (CME)/Continued Professional Development (CPD)
- Skills and capacity building
- Promoting mental health advocacy and literacy

## 2 Online Teaching-Learning Modalities

When we see the term 'online' the typical picture we get is a 'videoconferencing' session just like the picture of classroom with an ongoing lecture when we hear traditional learning. But there are mixed elements of technology, may it be a streaming video or a guest speaker in a conventional class or face-face (F2F) elements in an online class, famously called as HyFlex learning (Beatty, 2019) which stands for Hybrid-Flexible course design.

Depending upon the learning process and the timing of learner interactions, there can be four types of online learning broadly (NMC, 2020)

I. Synchronous learning—Where learning interaction happens at a same time and learners are at different places of their convenience.
II. Asynchronous learning—It is also called as self-paced learning where learning interactions happen at different times for each learner, and learners may be at different places of their convenience.
III. Conventional or face-to-face learning—Where learning interactions happen at same time, and learners are in the same place regardless of their convenience.
IV. Blended learning—It can be a mixture of any of the above in different proportions.

## *2.1 Online Teaching-Learning Frameworks*

Online teaching-learning frameworks are a set of standards which provide structure for designing and delivering online course effectively. These guide teachers to effectively engage and employ active learning strategies and creating an overall supportive learning environment. Association for Medical Education in Europe (AMEE) Guide 161 Online Learning in Health Professions Education. Part 1: Teaching and Learning in Online Environments (MacNeill et al., 2024) discusses on online teaching frameworks and theories, models in detail, which is a must read for all the faculty who would like to know more about online learning.

The guide describes three important frameworks, namely, PICRAT matrix, the community of inquiry, and connectivism theory.

PICRAT matrix looks at two main questions: How students interact with technology, and how teachers use technology in their pedagogy. The elements of PICRAT form a matrix, where rows are formed by PIC—Passive, Interactive, Creative elements which describe how students interact with technology and coloumns are formed by RAT—Replacement, Amplification, Transformation elements which examine how technology impacts teacher pedagogy. This is generally for beginner online educators and is commonly used in schools.

The Community of Inquiry (CoI) model is one of the most widely used and studied online learning models and is well-suited for intermediate online educators. Three interconnecting presences: social presence (SP), cognitive presence (CP), and teaching presence (TP), create overlapping domains from which to start conversations around considerations in designing and researching online learning.

Connectivism is a more advanced theory, which prompts educators to consider how technology may assist in changing education systems from those that merely allow transmission of information from teacher to learner, to systems and networks that transform learning through connections.

Another important takeaway from the above guide worth mentioning here is the multimodal learning. One of the major benefits of online learning is the ability to provide multimodal methods to meet diverse learning objectives and learner needs. Of particular interest is the Hybrid model also called as Hyflex model originally used by Dr. Brian Beatty (2019). It is based on four principles: Student Choice/

Learner Control, Equivalent Learning, Reusability, and Accessibility (Beatty 2019). Learners have the ability to choose which path and pace best suits their needs, leading to increased appreciation for the flexibility of their learning and feeling supported by their teachers.

## *2.2 Strategies of Online Teaching-Learning*

- **Clear communication:** Set expectations, provide feedback, and encourage discussion.
- **Interactive content:** Use of multimedia, gamification, and simulations to engage students.
- **Collaborative tools:** Utilize discussion boards, group projects, and live sessions.
- **Continuous assessment:** Monitor progress, provide feedback, and adjust instruction.
- **Technical support:** Ensure reliable infrastructure and offer technical assistance.

## *2.3 Essentials for Online Teaching-Learning*

This section would just contain brief mention of tools and methods in order to avoid the risk of expansion as the header itself is worth a book or at least a chapter.

### 2.3.1 E-Learning Infrastructure (Fig. 17.1)

- **Delivery** of e-learning—Learning Management System (LMS)
- **Organizing** e-learning and outcomes—Course management system (CMS)
- **Resource** management, funding & accreditation
- Programme **evaluation** system

### 2.3.2 Online Teaching-Learning Methodologies

- Simulations and case-based learning
- Telepsychiatry-based teaching-learning models
- Use of newer tech like VR, AR, and MR in online learning
- AI in online teaching-learning

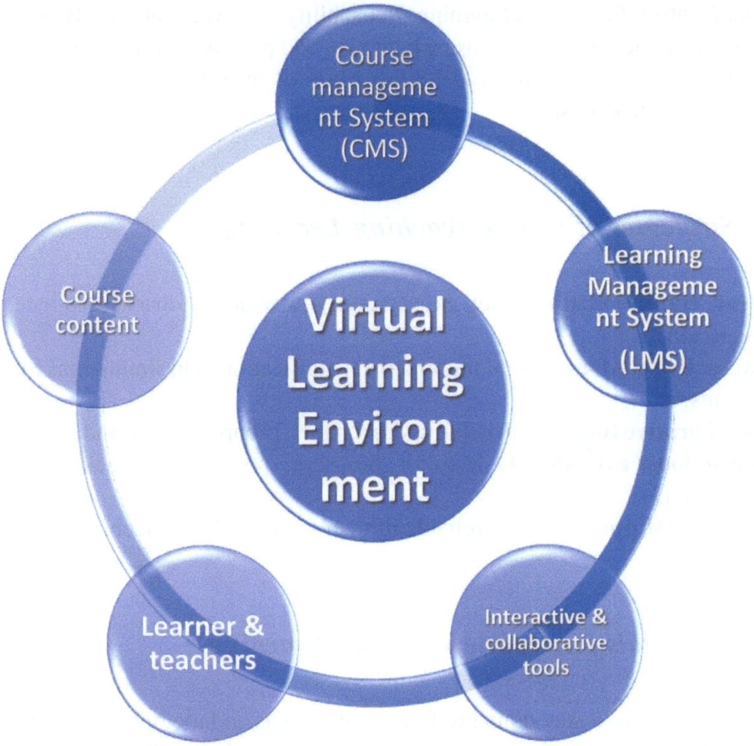


**Fig. 17.1** Online learning infrastructure

## 3 Online Teaching-Learning Models Across the Globe, South Asia, and India

Online teaching-learning modalities in Psychiatry have undergone significant transformation over the past decade. This section provides a comparison of the models used globally, in South Asia, and in India. It explores technological integration, pedagogical innovations, and challenges specific to each region. The review highlights how different countries have adapted to changing educational demands, especially post-COVID-19, and offers recommendations for future improvements in psychiatric education.

Psychiatric education is a vital component of medical training, requiring a strong foundation in both theoretical knowledge and interpersonal skills. The rise of online learning, particularly catalysed by the COVID-19 pandemic, has redefined the way psychiatry is taught and learned.

## 3.1 *Global Models of Online Psychiatry Education*

**Blended and Hybrid Learning** In North America and Europe, psychiatry education typically employs a blended learning model combining asynchronous video lectures, live discussions, and clinical case simulations. Learning Management Systems (LMS) such as Canvas, Blackboard, and Moodle support content delivery.

**Simulated Patients and OSCEs** Virtual Objective Structured Clinical Examinations (OSCEs) and simulated patient interactions are standard practices. Students engage in case-based learning using digital platforms that mimic real psychiatric consultations.

**Telepsychiatry Training** Telepsychiatry is integrated into both undergraduate and postgraduate training, preparing students for remote clinical practice in diverse settings.

**Massive Open Online Courses (MOOCs) and International Access** Universities like Harvard, Yale, and King's College offer open-access psychiatric modules through MOOCs, expanding access to quality psychiatric education globally.

## 3.2 *South Asian Perspective*

Before COVID, many studies were from the West and high-resource countries. Asia, being the largest and most populous continent, due to the predominance of developing economies, wide disparities in education, basic resources, geopolitical instabilities, and many other factors have affected the training and innovations. China, South Korea, and Japan have been leading in technological innovations and parallelly, on innovations in educational technologies (edutech). Singapore, Malaysia, and Indonesia have been innovating and refining their medical education practices. When it comes to South Asia, it was COVID situation that gave momentum to innovate in online methodologies. An analytical study on opportunities and challenges of E-learning in South Asia (Mittal, 2021) discusses the South Asian perspective, challenges and opportunities in e-learning, and emerging markets. India, being the prominent economy in South Asia, is one of the few nations to have highly penetrated infrastructure in Information Communication Technology (ICT). It has the largest skilled workforce in the Information Technology (IT) sector and the highest Internet users. The nation having worked in the steps of technological development and has embraced ICT for educational purposes, is now leading in online education in the region. It is one of the emerging markets for edutech industry. Though there is a considerable improvement in ICT infrastructure and development of edutech industry, the collaboration, funding, and, most importantly, the technical expertise particularly in health profession academia, adoption of online education and e-learning methods are not matching. However, most of the countries having realized the opportunities that online and blended models can deliver, are slowly adopting the same. Mental health training is now being increasingly regarded as a necessity, where online learning can be a game changer.

**Emerging Adoption of Online Learning** Countries like Pakistan, Bangladesh, Nepal, and Sri Lanka have adopted online platforms such as Zoom, Moodle, and Google Classroom for delivering psychiatry education. A study on designing and implementing an innovative digitally driven primary care psychiatry programme in India (Manjunatha et al., 2018) describes an adopted psychiatric curriculum designed in 'Clinical Schedules for Primary Care Psychiatry' (CSP), which is an integral part of the primary care psychiatry programme. The CSP and Tele-psychiatric 'On-Consultation Training' (Tele-OCT) are two path-breaking innovations having inbuilt higher clinical translation value when extended country wide.

**Digital Psychiatry Training** Limited but growing trend of incorporation of tele-psychiatry training, particularly in private institutions and urban medical colleges is noted. Non-governmental organizations also play a role in facilitating online mental health education. A web-based International Survey to evaluate the level of training, knowledge, experience, and perception regarding the topic of digital psychiatry (Orsolini et al., 2021) discusses a perspective from Asia Pacific region on training and education in digital Psychiatry and reports an overall lack of theoretical and/or practical training on new digital tools and digital health interventions, and implementing psychiatry training programmes may significantly improve the level of knowledge and use of digital tools in mental healthcare.

**Competency-Based Medical Education (CBME)** India adopted the CBME framework in 2019 (NMC, 2019), integrating psychiatry into undergraduate curricula. Online learning became essential during the pandemic, supported by recorded lectures, assessments, and interactive modules. NMC has published a comprehensive guiding document on online teaching (NMC, 2020) which prescribes the TL methods and assessments that may be used by institutes in India.

**National Platforms and Initiatives** Institutions like NIMHANS in India lead online psychiatry training through the Digital Academy and Virtual Knowledge Network initiatives. Platforms such as SWAYAM and NPTEL provide MOOCs covering mental health topics and cater to wide and diverse learner groups.

**ECHO Model for Professional Training** The ECHO (Extension for Community Healthcare Outcomes) model (Arora et al., 2017; ECHO, 2008) is used extensively in postgraduate and continuing medical education, enabling case-based virtual mentorship. This model, though resembles telemedicine, is defined more in terms of tele-mentoring where participating care provider as participants become part of a knowledge-sharing platform for building capacity and sharing best practices through case-based learning.

**Telepsychiatry and Virtual Clinics** Medical colleges increasingly include telepsychiatry modules, where students observe or participate in supervised virtual consultations (Basavarajappa et al., 2022). An article on designing and implementing an innovative digitally driven primary care psychiatry programme in India (Manjunatha et al., 2018) discusses about the telepsychiatry implementation, advantages, and disadvantages. This will be discussed in detail in further sections.

**Mental Health Literacy and Student Well-Being** Workshops, online counselling, and peer-led initiatives are being employed to enhance mental health awareness and resilience among medical students.

Psychiatry education has become integral to contemporary medical training. While high-income countries lead with advanced simulations and structured telepsychiatry curricula, South Asia and India have made significant strides by leveraging scalable, context-sensitive models. Moving forward, enhancing infrastructure, faculty development, and regional collaborations will be key to sustaining and advancing psychiatric education globally.

## *3.3 Author's Experience in an Indian Model of Indian Teachers of Psychiatry (IToP) Online Programmes for Teachers of Psychiatry and Its Evolution*

With due respect to educators and researchers whose works are cited in this chapter, I must admit that my interest in the area is relatively recent. . Online education has long been an area where the curiosity and experimentation constantly prevailed. My involvement with this area was rather serendipitous that started when I was selected as one of the first four candidates into this novel programme called as Scholarship for Teachers towards Enrichment of Psychiatry Teaching Skills (STEPS) (Kishor et al., 2023). While all other training programmes and initiatives focused heavily on research or patient care related skills, practically none focussed on teaching skills per se. This came as a game changer in the difficult scenario in India where Undergraduate (UG) training in Psychiatry is neglected from decades (Kallivayalil & Enara, 2020) and lack of teachers who can motivate and kindle interest in UGs. The pandemic hit the world in an unprecedented manner and its impact does not need an explanation. It is interesting to note that, the programme's online and blended mode of teaching and learning was thought and planned well before anyone imagined a situation like COVID. However, onset of the programme was delayed because of the pandemic and aligned with the global surge of online methodologies. Prior to this, it was only an intellectual awareness of having heard of online methodologies and their pros and cons. When we actually go through the interaction ourselves, the experiential learning provides us with emotional insights. The module consisted of 20 sessions of two hours spread over 20–25 weeks with assignments and presentations and thus involving both synchronous and asynchronous engagement. It involved mentors from across the globe, yet managing their enthusiastic participation in live meetings, despite the time zone differences. The best part was the synchronous element where the presentation, assessment, and feedback happened in real-time, with senior mentors who role modelled as ideal teachers and true ambassadors of teachers of Psychiatry. The in-person arm of the programme consisting of 1-week contact sessions could not happen in first edition of the programme. This initiative has successfully completed 4 years and is up to starting the fifth on a bigger stage. Trainees who successfully completed the programme are taken into peer mentoring roles and retained in the programme to adapt to newer roles. It has evolved continuously integrating blended elements increasingly and in an effective manner, managing to bring in learners from different parts of the vast country like India and institutes which has wide disparity of resources. This programme is an example on how a determined team committed to a specific goal can achieve the outcome despite having low resources and nominal funding, utilizing existing open-source tools in a very difficult situation, and in a system where outcome is not rewarded or readily recognized. Many research conclusions in low-resource settings have echoed similar finding thatwhen recognition, funding, and learning infrastructure are provided, the committed and focussed groups can make difference in teaching and learning.

## 4 Opportunities in Online Teaching-Learning in Psychiatry

Mental health in the twenty-first century is being increasingly perceived as a need, especially by younger generation who are vocal on various new world issues like global warming, life style, and work–life balance. Addressing mental health is being increasingly perceived as a necessary rather than the optional skill by the younger generation of doctors who would aspire to be globally relevant and competent. This has opened up opportunities for training needs and opportunities not just in formal speciality training in Psychiatry but relevant mental health skills for doctors from other specialties, primary care physicians and in general, any health professional. Increased access to information and rising social trend towards mental health care has made the potential learners even from underprivileged, remote areas, conflicted zones, etc., to reach out for the training. Online methods offer accessibility and flexibility by overcoming geographical barriers, high cost of immigration, and other issues in conventional training. Asynchronous and self-paced models also offer safe space and flexibility for the students to adjust to time zone differences, work shift balances yet continuing to serve their primary responsibilities.

## 4.1 Accessibility and Flexibility

Online modes of learning have a global reach, accommodating learners from diverse demographic backgrounds and regions. Cultural and language barriers can also be addressed as the learning material can be translated or subtitles be added to engage the learners from diverse backgrounds. Advent of AI-driven models exploiting large language models and natural language processing has made the online models much more engaging and helpful overcoming language barriers. A review on challenges and solutions when developing online interactive psychiatric education (Warren et al., 2020) discusses accessibility and flexibility as one of the benefits of online education by the virtue of ability to share ideas and complete activities without time and environmental restrictions of a classroom/lecture, improved rural and remote access, and flexibility for those with family, work, and other commitments.

## 4.2 Self-Paced and Asynchronous Learning Options

As described above, the self-paced asynchronous options are particularly helpful for busy professionals who would like to update their knowledge, students in the main stream academic or practice but would like to learn parallel skills, collaborate with other peers and mentors worldwide, for micro-credentialing and skill stacking (described in sections ahead). In an article on Asynchronous Technologies in Mental Health Care and Education, Lagera et al. (2023) discuss on asynchronous technologies in psychiatric education. It describes the use of asynchronous modes in training of psychotherapy through digital recordings, use of social media as a valuable e-tool and its effective utilization. Another article, Media-Related Education in Psychiatry Residency Programs (Morris et al., 2018) suggests three core domains to incorporate into basic media-related education: (1) effects of media coverage around mental health on public attitudes towards these topics, (2) clinical scenarios related to media that may arise during the practice of psychiatry, and (3) education for psychiatry residents around media participation. For medical student training in psychiatry during COVID times, asynchronous modalities were used effectively to make up shortcomings of synchronous online education. These included watching pre-recorded lectures prior to attending synchronous sessions and also as an alternative when Internet connection and data were severely limited.

The asynchronous model may be roughly compared to a model where students study regularly after the active classroom learning activity, only with better structure and guidance. when such asynchronous methods are effectively blended in the curricula, they can significantly benefit the learning outcomes.

## *4.3 Global Collaboration, Networking and Overcoming Geographical Barriers*

Online learning has created a stage not only for learners to connect across the globe but various international conferences and organizations with experts from different regions to collaborate and create course and programmes for online learning. In the simplest form, invited lectures and international guest lectures, seminars involving learners from universities across the regions can participate, which can be scaled up to faculty and student exchange in a virtual setup.

### 4.3.1 Online and Blended Mentoring and Exchange Programmes

A virtual international exchange programme for early career psychiatrists (Naskar et al., 2022) describes the experiences of online academic mentoring to trainees and early career Psychiatrists especially from the regions where they lack access to resource and opportunities, like Low & Middle Income (LMIC) countries. World Psychiatric Association (WPA) Exchange programme for early career Psychiatrists is one such initiative that is worth mentioning here (Pinto da Costa et al., 2023).

Training the trainers initiatives—WPA initiatives during the pandemic like train the trainer initiative (Baessler et al., 2021) has created opportunities not just for learners but for the teachers and mentors to collaborate network and put in their expertise in capacity building programmes which happened online in 2020.

Training Initiative for Psychiatry Post-graduate Students (TIPPS) (Suhas et al., 2022)—a Unique Early Career Psychiatry Training Initiative in India—is a peer mentored online platform started in 2015 and led by early to mid-career psychiatrists who have completed their training from India's different medical universities.

Brief Course in Psychiatric (Ameen, 2015)—An online mentoring and capacity building programme is the flagship programme of the Research Capacity Building Committee of the Indian Psychiatric Society South Zonal Branch. It is a 4-month course with online and offline components covering research planning, conduct, and publication. Faculty includes experts in psychiatry and related fields like statistics and library science.

IACAM certification course in Child and Adolescent Psychiatry (IACAM Academy, 2025)—This platform focuses on educating and mentoring psychiatrists across India, with a focus on child and adolescent psychiatry. The platform features mentors with expertise in various areas of psychiatry, including child mental health and addiction psychiatry.

Indian Teachers of Psychiatry (IToP) forum along with MINDS united for Humanity trust funded by Infosys foundation has initiated two courses in capacity building and mentoring teachers of Psychiatry in psychiatric education methodologies and research, namely, IToP-STEPS (Scholarship for Teachers towards Enrichment of Psychiatry Teaching Skills) (Kar et al., 2022; Kishor et al., 2023) and

ITOP MUST Enrich grant and scholarship programme (Indian Teachers of Psychiatry (IToP), 2024; Verma et al., 2024)

Virtual Conferences and Webinars

These are held as much or perhaps more regularly than in-person events in major Psychiatric organizations across the globe and particularly helped to continue the learning and socialize in virtual space during the pandemic. Though the main stream conferences have reverted back to in-person mode, what remains a new norm in post-pandemic conference is that online element or the blended approach which is helping for those who are unable to make it due to various causes. There is an increasing trend in webinars and online continued professional development activities that keep interested learners active by wide offerings of topics and courses to choose.

Massive Open Online Courses (MOOCs)

Massive Open Online Courses (MOOCs) are the most important and popular online learning mode offered by various universities and organizations. They give a space for educators and technical team to interact and design courses and learning materials and collaborate with many platforms which offer MOOCs to host and deliver their courses. Some of the notable platforms are Coursera, edX, Canvas academy, Udacity (US), FutureLearn (UK), EPA e-learning platform (European Psychiatric Association), SWAYAM-NPTEL (India), and many others with millions of registered students and thousands of courses available. The list is exhaustive and hence not given.

## *4.4 Evolution of Edutech Industry*

The edutech industry refers to the broad field of educational technology, encompassing various tools, platforms, and approaches that utilize technology to enhance learning and teaching. It started from VCRs and CD-ROMs for recordings as computer-assisted learning. The first of the companies to start solutions for education is Blackboard LMS, in 1997 (Anthology Inc., 2025) and participation of industry, universities in efforts to enhance learning experiences led to many initiatives like MIT OpenCourseWare in 2001 (Massachusetts Institute of Technology, 2025). The suit was followed by many leading universities and investors resulting in development of Learning Management Systems (LMS) and digital transition in many universities between 2000 and 2010. The emergence of MOOCs during 2011–2015 led to global access of online learning. Various edutech companies and platforms like Coursera, edX, Udacity, FutureLearn, etc., partnered with leading global universities giving access to education across the world, led to development of mobile apps, various software and social media integration which revolutionized the perspective of learning and learning ecosystem. Initially USA, Canada, UK, and Australia had considerable boom of edutech start-ups but the countries like China, India, Korea, Japan, and the Middle East soon caught up, particularly driven by the pandemic. A review article (Ravichandran et al., 2024) discusses edutech evolution with Indian perspective. It reports that projections outlined by the India Brand Equity Foundation (IBEF) suggest remarkable growth potential for the Indian edutech industry, with figures expected to climb from $700–800 million in 2021 to $30 billion by 2031. The second largest market for e-learning is now held by India, surpassing the United States as stated by KPMG International (2025) with projections from IBEF showing a growth to $30 billion in the edutech sector by 2031. The future of edutech is propelled by adaptive learning, learning analytics, integration of AI, simulations, VR and XR (virtual and extended reality), and other futuristic technologies. A time has come that no education programme can be delivered without some technology in the process, and utilization of edutech in one or the other way has become the new norm, with more integration in the days to come.

# 5 Assessments in Online Teaching Learning

It is well said that assessments drive the learning. Without knowing the benchmarks of what needs to be learnt, a learner's competence cannot be assessed and the gap remains unaddressed. One needs to be clear of what domain is being assessed, select the method of assessment based on it and the validity and feasibility of the method is important in determining how reliable assessment is. The stakes of outcome is also an important factor. Feedbacks are part of the well performed assessments and are the part of any learning programmes. Assessments pose a challenge in online learning as the learner may not be physically present with assessor, and sometimes temporally disconnected as well. Hence, it is more important to plan the assessments in online or blended methods carefully.

## *5.1 Contexts and Methods*

Most common and important contexts of assessments are formative and summative with low and high stakes, respectively. While the former is used for monitoring learning, providing feedback, and identifying gaps, the latter is used for certifying competence and evaluating course outcomes. Common methods to assess cognitive domain are quizzes employing multiple choice questions (MCQs) and essay based short and long answers. Higher cognitive domains like synthesis, analysis, critical thinking, reasoning, and problem-solving may be targeted by clinical and problem-based questions. Skills are tested by various methods like direct observation, demonstration, OSCE (Objective Structured Clinical Examination), OSLER (Objective Structured Long Case Record), MiniCex, and other workplace-based assessments. Affective domains are also tested using clinical interviews, roleplays, reflective writing apart from above methods. While these are relatively convenient in face-to-face settings, teaching in online mode poses numerous challenges.

### *5.2 Challenges in Assessments in Online Teaching and Learning*

Technical Challenges—Instability in Internet connection, bandwidth issues, hardware incompatibility, server and platform slowing down or crashes, technical glitches, bugs that are not identified, media compatibility, data loss or corruption, malwares or cyber-attacks, etc.

Maintaining Integrity - Impersonation, unethical collaboration, difficulty in monitoring during assessments, ineffective proctoring, use of unauthorized access to materials and resources, AI and other tools are few of the common challenges faced in assessments. The AMEE Guide 146 on ethical teaching in medical education (Masters et al., 2022) discusses the delicate issues of ensuring fairness and balancing the proctoring to maintain ethical privacy and consent issues arising in this context.

Equity and Accessibility—Students from low-resource settings, diverse ethnic-religious-linguistic groups, and differently abled students may undergo incomplete or unfair assessments if not previously planned on how to accommodate them.

Validity, Reliability, and Standardization—Psychiatric education often involves subjective and behavioural competencies, which are harder to measure objectively online.

Clinical and Affective Skills—Real-time and reliable assessment of empathy, nonverbal communication, and psychomotor skills may not be easy to assess in online only mode and may lead to deficient or ineffective feedback. An article describing the experience of the virtual Clinical Assessment of Skills and Competence (Chu & Sathanandan, 2023) discusses the lack of empathy involved in virtual assessment environments may lead to questionable reliability.

Faculty Training and Skills in online assessment methodologies, grading systems, and technical competence are very important and requires faculty development programmes which are resource intense and challenging.

Ethical, Security, and Privacy concerns—Data storage, security, and privacy maintenance are difficult to achieve and often come at a premium price. Unauthorized access (to answer keys, responses, and evaluation systems) with malicious intent leads to leaks and tampering which are far easier done in online than physical mode of assessments.

### 5.2.1 Validity of Credentialing and Regulatory System

Selecting the universities and courses has always been a matter of pride, and, on the other hand, done after thorough thought and enquiry. This is because of the academic culture, outcomes, and real-world performance by the professionals educated in the university. When it comes to online education, the reputation often carries forward. But online learning is altogether a different ballgame and it may not guarantee the same without a valid system that credits the learning. It should maintain certain standard and ensure the knowledge and skills to be translated into clinical care or other relevant output in the real world. Hence, credentialing is a vital process where universities and organizations conducting online or blended learning courses award badges or certificates of completion, diplomas or degrees based on various criteria to learners who meet specific benchmarks and competency-based criteria. This needs rigorous assessment standards, verification processes for assessments, and accreditation of the university or institute providing the credentials. Some of the important terms those need to be understood in credentialing are

- Construct validity—True reflection of competencies needed in real-world performance.
- Reliability—Ability of the assessments to produce similar pattern of results across the various groups.
- Recognition—It is the course recognized by an accrediting body and valid across the globe.

Accreditation and licentiate bodies are those which regulate medical education standards and norms in that particular region or country. To cite a few prominent agencies, ACGME, Liaison Committee on Medical Education (LCME) & American Osteopathic Association, Commission on Osteopathic College Accreditation (AOA COCA) in USA, Royal College of Physicians and Surgeons in Canada, GMC in United Kingdom National Medical Council (NMC) and National Assessment and Accreditation Council (NAAC) in India, Japan Accreditation Council for Medical Education (JACME), Australian Medical Council (AMC) for Australia & New Zealand, Independent Agency for Accreditation and Rating (IAAR) for Russia and many Eastern European countries, World Federation for Medical Education (WFME) provides recognition for accrediting agencies, ensuring global standards.

## 5.3 *Tools for Online Assessment*

Many online tools which may be integrated into LMS platforms are now available to address these challenges and are discussed in further sections. These platforms have proctoring facilities and various levels of proctoring can be predetermined, from open book variant to highly restricted access to other material and technology-enabled monitoring like microphone or webcam monitoring. Interactive online quizzes, online synchronous discussions, interviews with real, simulated, or standardized patients and with AI technology-based virtual patients diverse modes of online assessments are now possible. VR and XR technology have the potential to enable a virtual assessment environment which are designed to simulate the real assessments when assessors and learners are embodied in virtual environments. The sophistication, however, requires considerable resource, including financial requirement and technical expertise along with academic planning. A course is said to deliver best outcomes only when the assessment is feasible, reliable, ethical, and equitable. Let us discuss a few nuances on assessments in online education.

## *5.4 Evaluating the Online Teaching-Learning Programmes*

### 5.4.1 Data-Driven Learning and Assessment

Online learning generates a lot of data, not just in learning related content but also from the participation and behaviour of students and teachers. This data is collected carefully and analysis can be done using various techniques. Machine learning algorithms and AI are being seamlessly integrated in this process to identify patterns and trends, which provide deeper insights into many aspects that can be measured in various metrics related to learning. This helps in defining a personalized learning path, catering to learner-specific needs, adaptive assessments based on the level of performance, with targeted and personalized feedback leading to enhanced learning. It also helps in resource optimization and efficient use rather than generalized resource allocation like 'one-size-fits-all'. Some of the learning analytics are listed in the next subsection.

### 5.4.2 Learning Analytics for Performance Tracking

Traditional learning had direct observation and supervision while online modalities pose challenges in tracking the learning process and evaluate what is learnt by the students. Learning analytics is a process where data related to learning is collected from various sources and metrics which are then analysed to understand and improve learning and performance. It includes various metrics and key performance indicators like completion rates, time spent on course or its content, engagement metrics, drop off rates, user satisfaction, assessment scores & pass rates, return on investment (ROI), net promoter scores, etc. These metrics help in evaluating how a course is performing in terms of its effectiveness and impact. Some of the course evaluation metrics are Learning Effectiveness (LE), Return on Learning (ROL), Time to Proficiency (TTP), Knowledge Retention Rate (KRR), and Application Rate (AR). These metrics evaluate higher levels of Kirkpatrick's model of programme evaluation (Kirkpatrick, 2007). Due to the risks of expansion, these indices are not elaborated on in this section. Most of the LMS, whether designed for universities or open source, commercially available free and subscription-based platforms like Moodle,

Canvas, etc., has an inbuilt analytic system which automatically derives these metrics and publishes in the learners' and course dashboards.

### 5.4.3 Adaptive Learning Systems

Adaptive learning is an approach that personalizes learning experiences by adapting to individual student needs. A review on Adaptive Learning in Medical Education by Sharma et al. (2017) describes adaptive learning, at the most basic level, as a process that provides an individualized learning experience with technologies designed to determine a learner's strengths and weaknesses. Once an individual's strengths are recognized, the computer-based technology can modify the learning material to ensure that there is greater focus on an individual's limitations. A Forbes article (Zimmer, 2014) describes the evolution of adaptive learning technology reports a considerable increase in pass rates and much more decrease in withdrawal rates from courses with incorporation of adaptive learning systems in their courses. A review on Adaptive Learning Systems in Medical Education (Prabhakar, 2024) discusses the application of AI-powered adaptive learning in medical education. The AI-Driven Data Analytics in Adaptive Learning consists of

- Data Collection & Analysis—Use of higher-level NLP algorithms
- Personalized Learning Paths
- Predictive Analytics for Early Intervention
- Automated Feedback & Adaptive Assessments—Adaptive testing and real-time re-evaluation based on individual performances

Benefits of adaptive learning are Student-Centred, Personalized Learning, Augmented Instructed Decision-Making with Real-Time Data, Augmented Competency-Based Learning & Testing, On-Demand Learning & Continuing Medical Education, Greater Engagement & Motivation.

The future trends as described in above article are Virtual Reality (VR) and Augmented Reality (AR) in Medical Training, AI-Powered Chatbots & Virtual Tutors, Blockchain Credentialing in Medical Education involving career tracking, automated verification of licences and credits, cross-institutional sharing of the same to enhance global validity and mobility for students and professionals, Predictive Analytics for Personalized Learning, and Robotics & AI Integration in Medical Training.

## 6 Challenges in Online Psychiatric Education

While much of the discussion thus far has focused on the benefits of online education, types, and opportunities, it is equally important to understand the significant challenges in technical, pedagogical, and systemic aspects, starting from designing to delivering and certifying. An Australian review by Warren et al. (2020) describes the challenges in three areas, namely, challenges in the content of online courses, format, and conveying the art of Psychiatry in an online format. The content discusses about various materials, engaging the learner and preventing overburdening with information. The format discusses the ease of accessing the material, resources available to learners, cost and infrastructure needed to host and deliver this material. Conveying refers to suiting the online content to match the richness of physical interaction between learners, patients, and teachers. Adding on to these, challenges in online psychiatry education can be discussed in the following areas.

## *6.1 Enabling and Accessibility*

### 6.1.1 Accessibility and Equitable Distribution:

As psychiatric education is increasingly moving into digital and online platforms, questions of **access** and equity have emerged as key areas of concern. While online formats can extend the reach, they also carry the concerns of worsening of already existing disparities particularly in low- and middle-income countries (LMICs), rural and remote settings, marginalized communities and conflicted zones. There is a great digital divide that exists, which makes it challenging to provide uniform education to those who need it most. A review article discussing digital psychiatry in low-and-middle-income countries (Chakrabarti, 2024) states that the greatest paradox of digital psychiatry is that those with the greatest need and those most likely to benefit from such services are least likely to have access to them. Many barriers, such as service costs, underdeveloped infrastructure, lack of trained professionals, and significant disparities in access to digital services, impede the progress of digital psychiatry in LMICs. While this is mainly described in the context of digital mental health as a whole, psychiatric education is not very far from this reality. A survey on training and education in digital psychiatry: A perspective from Asia-Pacific region by Orsolini et al. (2021) describes more or less similar findings in South Asian countries, which are predominantly LMICs. Urban and rural divide, differences in metropolitan and lower-tier cities are also prominent in such countries which further pose challenges for the implementation of training within the region. Online courses offered by reputed organizations such as the Royal College of Psychiatrists, UK, and Harvard University online programmes, to name a few, that are developed in high-income countries (HIC) may be difficult to afford for the people from LMICs. Even if they afford it, these high-quality courses may not be designed for the low resource, language and cultural challenges. Other resources like databases and premium journal access, simulation tools may not be affordable in LMICs where the resource grants are very less, unequally distributed, and policy making may not be keen on developing these resources.

### 6.1.2 Challenges in Online TL Infrastructure

Online learning entails far more than merely providing a screen, stable Internet connection for the learner or uploading learning materials and scheduling sessions. It requires a digital ecosystem to create a virtual learning environment which consists of appropriate specifications of hardware, legitimate and licenced software, simulation tools, a responsive IT support team, and data security. Live streaming, live sessions, and e-simulation require substantial bandwidth and a consistent Internet service provider. This comes at a premium cost to subscribe and maintain. Apart from this, learning management software, online simulation tools are expensive to procure and maintain. It also requires internal training before it can be effectively used by instructors. Bandwidth choking, loss of quality, disruption in live participation, and difficulty in accessing larger files of course content can act as challenges, especially where a digital divide exists.

### 6.1.3 Organizational Support and Funding

Planning online curricula and delivering courses requires considerable teamwork with diverse expertise, a well-established e-learning infrastructure and collaboration. This requires organization policies, investment and budget allocation, sustainable funding and leadership with commitment and vision. Many universities, standalone medical schools especially in LMICs lack dedicated budget for sustaining online learning. Even if they have, they seem to be fragmented, outsourced, or under-funded and sustenance becomes difficult. The need and enthusiasm in a situation like COVID did make it obligatory on many universities to take up online teaching-learning but once the situation eased and conventional learning resumed, most of them reverted back and cut down on funding to divert and prioritize to other essential needs despite being aware of the shifting trend and benefits of online models. The commitment and prioritization have not been the same as the COVID 19 situation. This may mean lesser faculty development and capacity building, lesser incentives to learners and instructors to pursue online TL, lesser support from technical team and infrastructure, fatigue and burnout of existing faculty, less focus into quality improvement and programme evaluation thereby leading to numerous challenges in this area.

### 6.1.4 Technical Competence and Online Instructional Skills

Another important challenge is the technical or digital competence of the stakeholders, specifically the teaching faculty. In resource-limited settings, the absence of adequate infrastructure to support the development, delivery, and evaluation of online courses can pose significant barriers. Additionally, faculty members who lack prior exposure or formal training in online pedagogical methods may face difficulties in adopting and implementing contemporary online curricula and instructional models. Some of the important competences that a teacher or facilitator must possess are skills in working with LMS platforms and online collaboration tools. Creating and managing digital content, planning online assessments, and providing feedback at the other end are equally important. This requires considerable exposure, availability, and some basic training in using this technology. A qualitative study on instructors' experience and acceptance of online mental health training in its thematic analysis (Chalmers et al., 2024) reported that drawbacks faced by instructors are distractions, fatigue, and sub-optimal interpersonal and emotional connections. Instructors perceived the course to be effective in meeting learning outcomes; however, providing more opportunities to practice skills and apply course content was strongly suggested as a valuable and necessary addition. Instructors grappled with how to best use online technology for skill instruction and to meet learning objectives, and whether their online instruction style aligned with their face-to-face pedagogical style.

## *6.2 Learner-Related Challenges*

### 6.2.1 Engagement and Interactivity Issues

Learner engagement, motivation, and interaction play a very important role in participating in the learning process, assimilating and internalizing the learnt material. A review on measuring student engagement in technology-mediated learning (Henrie et al., 2015) describes three domains of engagement, namely, cognitive, behavioural, and emotional engagement. A research article on the concept of School engagement by Fredricks et al. (2004) states that behavioural engagement includes the observable behaviours necessary to academic success, such as attendance, participation, and homework completion. Emotional engagement includes both feelings learners have about their learning experience, such as interest, frustration, or boredom, and their social connection with others at school. Cognitive engagement is the focused effort learners give to effectively understand what is being taught, including self-regulation and metacognitive behaviours. Cognitive engagement and behavioural engagement centre on actions by the learner. Cognitive engagement differs from behavioural engagement because it focuses on the less observable effort expended in the mind. Online learning has both synchronous and asynchronous and blended sessions. Information or cognitive overload can happen in online sessions due to a large amount of information that may need to be processed. If coupled by attentional lapses or fatigue that frequently results when focusing on screens may in turn lead to reduced or poor engagement in the learning. Physical isolation from other peers limits peer interactions in online learning, which may affect emotional support and interpersonal connection.

### 6.2.2 Screen Fatigue and Mental Well-Being of Learners

Online learning often requires extended screen time and sustained attention, which may lead to many issues often termed as 'zoom fatigue'. A study on medical students in Thailand (Charoenporn et al., 2024) describes that Zoom fatigue is linked to the excessive use of nonverbal communication in video conferencing. In comparison to regular meetings, videoconferencing requires heightened concentration and attention. Various factors contribute to Zoom fatigue, including eye strain from prolonged close-range staring, increased cognitive load processing information in video calls, self-consciousness from constant self-reflection during calls, and restricted body movements in online sessions. Additionally, external factors beyond one's control, such as Internet disruptions, the pressure to respond to speaker questions, and environmental conditions, can exacerbate it. Therefore, the condition of Zoom fatigue may impact individuals' overall well-being. The study also describes a significant correlation found in the students with depression. This study has used Zoom Exhaustion & Fatigue (Fauville et al., 2021) developed by Stanford university, which is a specific assessment tool to measure video-related fatigue. A study on theorizing spatial dynamics in Zoom fatigue (Nadler, 2020) described the 'third skin concept' which is a 'flattened' totality that comprises person, background, and technology and participants are not engaged as human actors. This transformation results in exerting substantial cognitive efforts to maintain the interaction that can result in exhaustion. A study at Brazil, on medical students using hybrid and problem-based learning (PBL) methods over traditional teaching (de Oliveira Kubrusly Sobral et al., 2022) reported a higher Zoom fatigue in the former group with overall 48% prevalence, with higher frequency of wanting to be alone after a video conference session. However, the article also takes a reference of Kaplan's Attention Restoration Theory (Kaplan & Kaplan, 1989) and states that is not just the videoconferencing that leads to fatigue but the compatibility and motivation described as perception of belongingness in the learners' group and soft fascination which are associated with lower degree (Basu et al., 2019). Another study in Iran (Mosalanejad et al., 2024) describes about 'Zoom dysmorphia', a phenomenon where users felt discomfort regarding their appearance. Virtual learning, especially online and synchronous learning involves prolonged interactions involving videoconferencing platforms which poses a constant presence of one's own face which can serve as a 'mirror' promoting the awareness of self and prompting a feeling of 'being seen constantly' by everyone and critical evaluation by others. Several studies (Chen & Zhou, 2023; Gasteratos et al., 2021; Huang & Pricer, 2024; Wegge, 2006) have described this concept on Zoom dysmorphia along with challenges and consequences it poses in online learning. The above Iranian study (Mosalanejad et al., 2024) aimed to explore how students' self-efficacy and dysmorphic concern influence Zoom dysmorphia and found that self-efficacy had a reducing effect on Zoom dysmorphia, while dysmorphic concern had a positive correlation and an increasing effect on Zoom dysmorphia. A Canadian study (Desai et al., 2024) assessed educator burnout and has used a validated scale called the Maslach Burnout Inventory-Educators Survey (MBI-ES) (Mind Garden, Inc, 2025). The study reported a high degree of emotional exhaustion, depersonalization, and a moderate degree of personal accomplishment in surgeon educators. Among the learners, it is the lack of connection to learners that resulted in burnout while the largest mitigating factor was decreased travel time.

### 6.2.3 Maintaining Learner Participation and Reducing Passive Learning in Virtual Settings

Distractions in Informal Environments Other Than Traditional Settings

The inherent nature of online learning is the accessibility at the place of the learner that brings in the informal nature of home-based working. It is susceptible to distractions, which are otherwise eliminated in formal settings of traditional teaching by the supervision of a facilitator. Many factors like differences in seating or workspace, ambient conditions, noise and intrusion of informal interactions, out of the context of learning environment, etc., play a role. Another important aspect is the digital distraction inherent to online learning. The presence of gadgets and screens or even a single computer may potentially enable the learner to engage into different parallel tasks or processes. This may result in fall out of attention towards other out-of-context material, like gaming, streaming media, and social media. Each learner has a different ability at different times and also temperamental factors influence the ability to focus and prevent getting distracted in such unsupervised settings. However, various levels of formality and accountability may be brought in synchronous sessions by enabling video feed and mandating the focus alike the traditional settings, yet it may be difficult to monitor as it is easier to cut off from the feed citing technical glitch or connectivity where such things are beyond the control of both facilitator and learner. A review on what distracts the students from online learning (Wang, 2022) describes distraction as diverting attention from primary task to secondary task or paying partial attention to task-irrelevant information with negative effects on task performance. The review describes three main types of distraction, namely, multitasking, mind-wandering, and using digital devices and also proposed two new types of distraction, namely, unexpected interruption and consistent interference. It is hence imperative for the stakeholders to be aware of distractions and minimize the obstruction in learning. It requires higher levels of self-regulation and reaching the 'state of flow' (Csikszentmihalyi, 1990). A Romanian study on college students (Aivaz & Teodorescu, 2022) reported that the students were twice likely distracted by multitasking during online classes, more lenient and less bothered in using digital devices than in face-to-face classes and also the instructors in online classes are less likely to have a policy on use of digital devices for off-task purposes. An Indian survey on medical students (Grover et al., 2021) also reported that students often indulge in different activities while attending online classes; surfing Internet and chatting on instant messenger platforms being the most common and a small proportion of students does this very frequently.

### Lack of Structured Routine and Physical Inactivity

The home comfort and not needing to get ready to reach the classroom physically may be the most convenient aspect of online learning. Though it results in considerable time saving but the same can result in disruptions of routine. However, it is highly variable on how the learners use this extra availability of time which is saved in reaching to conventional settings but generally expected that they fill in some other tasks. The qualitative study on lived experiences of medical students of online learning (Rajesh et al., 2024) reported the online classes during pandemic resulted in considerable overeating of junk and lack of physical activity and weight gain, reported mostly by male students of upper socio-economic classes. But this was contrasted by female students to have been beneficial effect. A study on female medical students in Saudi Arabia (Almeheyawi et al., 2024) reported that online learning has negatively affected physical activity in a 'dose dependent manner', i.e., more online hours, worse the physical activity and most of the students perceived that online learning has affected their overall physical activity. Another study on Taiwanese university students (Chu & Li, 2022) reported a drastic reduction of physical activity during online learning period and it is particularly evident in vigorous physical activity among male students than their female peers.

All these studies however were done mostly during COVID-19 situation where there were social restrictions along with online classes and hence it may have affected the physical activity and promoted sedentary lifestyle. Hence, it cannot be generalized to online or blended learning in post-COVID era. Nevertheless, online learning may promote physical inactivity and appropriate measures, both at personal and institutional levels may be designed to address this issue.

### Low Motivation and Accountability

The very characteristic of online learning, i.e., accessibility at one's convenience also has a flip side of making the person isolated leading to a lack of real-time interaction and collaborative work, lack of the feeling of peer and facilitator presence and supervision during the active learning process. Also, the online methodologies require innovation and high knowledge-skills in assessors which may lead to reduced priorities on assessment and feedback compared to delivery of the learning content. This leads to a shift towards self-directed learning and require more self-regulation than in conventional learning. Also, students have reported being frequently disconnected, either deliberately or unintentionally during learning and assessments using online methods owing to technical or other reasons. Students were noted to access online content during less rigorous online assessments, such as MCQs and other simpler methods thereby rising issues of accountability. This may lead to lower motivation and accountability towards attending classes or assessments.

Limited Opportunities for Active Participation

Online learning isolates a learner physically and it may be difficult to engage in various interaction that happen in conventional learning as in a small group methodology where various types of interaction happen, namely, student–student, student–content, and student–teacher interactions that facilitate learning. An editorial in American Journal of Distance Education (Moore, 1989), described three such interactions which are vital to any learning process and need to replicate in online learning as well, to be more effective. It emphasizes real-time interaction between learners and teachers and not only with content. It also mentions about how this opportunity is frequently misused by instructor presentations and how teleconferencing bridges this gap. One needs to note that this editorial has been written in the pre-COVID and pre-Internet era but yet, the recommendations are still relevant. A mixed method study done in India on student perceptions towards online learning (Barche et al., 2022) showed similar findings that students engaged better with live lectures and interactions than recorded videos and regarded as superior by students largely due to the opportunity to directly communicate with the instructor and peers and receive quick feedback.

Technical Issues

Regardless of the need for citing literature, technical issues form one of the most common and serious challenges that any online learning programme can face. Almost all the articles discussing about online learning in medical education have invariably commented on the technical issues each emphasizing about various aspects. Overall, from the learner's perspective, these can be classified as challenges in accessibility and digital divide, Internet connectivity & bandwidth related issues, and availability of appropriate gadgets required for online learning. Most of the studies report these issues from LMIC countries while HIC discussed about online learning platforms and online teaching-learning skills of teachers rather than students.

### 6.2.4 Challenges in Assessing Clinical Empathy and Communication Skills

Psychiatric education requires considerably high emotional understanding, empathy, communication, and reflective skills. It is typically done in face-to-face interactions with either real patients or standardized patients and interaction with mentors and peers serve as continuous informal feedbacks which facilitate learning. Online education has limited opportunities to observe subtle changes in nonverbal behaviour, and feeling of presence which may pose a difficulty in empathizing, rapport, and interviewing. It may also be difficult to assess the skills that are imparted through online modes because of above reasons. A study on virtual Clinical

Assessment of Skills and Competence (CASC) (Chu & Sathanandan, 2023) discusses about the impact and challenges of a digitized final examination which is a high-stake assessment. The trainee experience mentions about the lack of peer interaction and the 'exam environment', sharing of experiences, reassurances, and the sense of camaraderie may be missing in virtual formats. Apart from technical concerns, the sense of disconnect between stations and lack of framework to mentally reset is mentioned.

## *6.3 Ethical and Privacy Concerns*

Ethical considerations in medical education are by no means unfamiliar to the medical educators. The emergence of the main stream online education brings its own set of special concerns. The COVID 19 situation resulted in urgent adaptation of online methodologies, with almost no conventional teaching-learning being possible then, gave rise to the actual realization of many possible ethical concerns which were mostly read than seriously given a thought. The AMEE guide No. 146 (Masters et al., 2022) discusses in detail the ethical teaching in online medical education. This article outlines the following six broad ethical principles applicable to online medical education:

1. Transparency, disclosure, and informed consent: Ensuring that there is full disclosure about the course layout and requirements, gathering, storage, sharing of data, and ensuring that consent when required is truly informed.
2. Equality, equity, diversity, and accessibility: Ensuring that the online system does not unfairly discriminate against students takes into account a diversity of circumstances and backgrounds and ensures that the course materials are easily accessible by all students.
3. Guard against excess: Ensuring that only necessary information about students is gathered.
4. Privacy and security: Ensuring that the teacher and institution take all reasonable steps to keep private and secure all information gathered about students and patients and maintain their anonymity.
5. Do no harm: Taken from Hippocrates (Hippocrates 1957), this is a common guiding principle in medicine; modern-day interpretations cover physical harm and psychological stress.
6. Possibility: Ensuring that the institution requires an ethical standard from all that is possible to achieve.

The guide also discusses on several laws which are different in each region a country to be taken into account in designing courses and also the training of instructors in these laws.

### 6.3.1 Confidentiality and Digital Privacy

Online education exposes the data of not only students but the instructors and institute vulnerable if there are no policies of data protection and handling breeches if any. Some of these risks include unauthorized access to sensitive data, like medical records and patient identifiers, recorded therapy sessions, or student related records like assessments. Unsecure, freely available versions of many online platforms, weaker and casual passwords, shared accounts can result in vulnerabilities. Phishing attacks like impersonating authorities, fake communications or malicious links and attachments in the place of study content, malwares and ransomwares may put the users at risk and loss of valuable data. Even if these are met, data breeches even in well-structured courses may result in compromise of personal and other data. This may be relevant in Psychiatric online education as it involves highly sensitive content like discussions on suicidality, trauma and abuse, private matters of the patients' life, etc. Hence, it is of paramount importance when we deal with such sensitive data being generated during the learning process and has well planned strategies and clauses defined for the preservation of confidentiality and digital privacy of the stakeholders.

### 6.3.2 Cybersecurity Risks and Data Protection

There are many laws pertaining to cybersecurity and data protection, to name a few like Health Insurance Portability and Accountability Act of 1996 HIPAA (CDC, 2024) in US, The General Data Protection Regulation (GDPR) (European Commission, 2018) in EU, IT act and recent one DPDP act 2023 (Government of India, 2023) in India regulates the handling of collected data and norms. Online courses, as they, come under the purview of these acts at one or the other point. Online learning programmes not only involve considerable exchange, handling, or generation of healthcare data but also involve sensitive data of learners and hence come under the purview of these data protection and privacy acts for which compliance certificates have to be obtained with laws relevant to locale.

### 6.3.3 Technology-Facilitated Abuse

Abuse in education, may it be medical or otherwise is not unfamiliar. Online education, due to its relative anonymity and lack of immediate access to help, may pose challenges in regulating behaviours that may amount to abuse. Some of the possible technology-facilitated abuses that need to be kept in mind during a course of online educative process can be in the following forms:

Non-consensual recording and distribution—Like covert recording or screenshots, dissemination or sharing through various social media and other platforms. The content may be patient related or student/instructor related or copyright violations of reserved content.

Cyberbullying and harassment—Offensive chats, emails, or comments during online interactions, or on public or academic platforms can amount to bullying and may result in considerable stress or attrition. It may be ethnic, linguistic, or any other area that vulnerable person may be subjected to the abuse during the course.

Privacy invasions—Just as simple as forcing a person to keep cameras or audio on inappropriately at their homes or private places can be both a form of bullying and an ethical question.

Inappropriate Content—Misuse of authority, unrealistic expectations are all possible and to be considered under this area.

### 6.3.4 Legal Issues Involved in Online Teaching-Learning, Assessment, and Certification

Online education involves content delivery, assessment, certification, and accreditation processes which involve legal matters in many ways. These issues can be divided into five key areas, namely, legal issues involved in teaching content, data privacy and protection, integrity and validity of online assessments, validity of online certification and finally accreditation, licencing and validity beyond borders.

The content related to teaching involves sharing of many learning resources which may be in the form of documents, images, audio or video content. Many of these may be subject to copyright and sharing the material without due permissions or access may result in copyright infringement. Unauthorized contents like medical records, patient related data if shared without due consents and masking the identities may result in breach of privacy and confidentiality laws and these may come under purview of many laws depending upon the region and locale.

Other important legal accountability is the validity of online assessment and the integrity. Proctoring in online assessments is a challenge and involves multiple strategies. However, lower levels of proctoring or un-proctored assessments are cheaper and perhaps more common. Malpractice during assessments may occur in the form of impersonation using various technologies, use of unauthorized aids, smartphones and accessing information through search engines, AI platforms, social media, etc. Accessibility and equity issues may also arise where less privileged students from low-resource settings may have more glitches and interruptions during assessment leading to unfair outcomes.

Another area of possible issues is accreditation and licencing of an online course or programme which may be accepted in a region or locale and not accepted in other. This may result in considerable hardships for students after having spent their time and resources. Some agencies for higher studies, industries, and licencing bodies may not accept online only modules of learning. Hence it becomes important for the course managers and faculty to have knowledge on regional laws pertaining to the content, its delivery and assessment to maintain the validity. When it comes to online psychiatric education, it further creates challenges in the above areas as discussed in relevant sections above.

# 7 Best Practices for Effective Online Teaching-Learning in Psychiatry

Which Psychiatry teacher does not want to put the best in their profession? When we start this section with reflective question, it would be easier to digest the heaps of literature we get. Most of the articles discussing online teaching-learning invariably discuss on evaluating and opining about what best can be done. The accounts vary from personal experiences and qualitative studies to systematic reviews. But one always has to understand the need and then the challenges within their setting and then design or blend the online learning into the curriculum. Overall, we can proceed with discussion on the following headings.

Online learning, especially in its classical formats or online only formats poses unique challenges in medical education. It may be beneficial in cognitive domain but has its drawbacks in psychomotor and affective domains where skill acquisition requires face-to-face interaction with patients and teachers. Many strategies have evolved to continually bridge the gaps and make the learning experience as closer to the conventional learning but yet, it can never be truly matched. Psychiatry is a clinical branch whichrequires clinical reasoning, keen observational and communication skills, empathy and emotional intelligence apart from scientific knowledge. This poses further challenges as described in previous sections. Hence, it requires optimal utilization of as many elements of online education and technology to exploit the best.

## *7.1 Optimizing Course Design and Delivery*

Psychiatry is a subject that involves sensitive matters, high observational and interactive components, emotional engagement and ethical nuances and dilemmas. Hence, optimizing online course designs becomes necessary to blend the elements of technology and teaching-learning methods which can utilize the resources more effectively in meeting these demands. All learners may not be from a similar background or endowed with the same learning styles and technical skills. Poorly designed or optimized programmes may run the risk of poor learner engagement and motivation, ethical lapses, and ineffective understanding of concepts pertaining to diagnostics, stigma, and empathy. Some of the important aspects of optimization may involve

1. Clearly defining learning objectives and aligning with regional and global standards.
2. Effective pedagogical strategies and sequencing of modules.
3. Scaffolded engagement strategies like starting with basic concepts before progressing into complex topics requiring higher integration of knowledge and analytical skills.

4. Utilization of appropriate TL strategies depending upon the domain. E.g., Basic sciences may involve cognitive predominant learning and TL methods like recorded lectures, animated videos and graphics, reading material may be used while understanding psychopathology may require observation, interactive components, and demonstration along with the above methods. Clinical topics and skills may be better learnt through case-based or problem-based learning, virtual patients or simulation, roleplays and strategies like spiral learning where learner revisits the key themes at increasing complexity. Ethical aspects and empathy are better learnt by reflective practice, discussion forums, roleplays, and psychodrama that can be suitably adapted into online methods.
5. An optimal mix of synchronous, asynchronous, and blended delivery of content can be planned to effectively utilize resources and time. The content delivery may require the use of LMS, videoconferencing tools, and simulation platforms integrated into the learning environment. Assessment and feedback may involve appropriate technology to assess all the domains of learning. Continuous improvement opportunities with regular feedback loops (polls, mid-course surveys), course dashboard with analytics (completion progress bar, time on task, performance metrics, access to feedbacks, etc.), peer interaction & reviews, and learner feedback to suggest improvements result in a better delivery of the course and outcomes. Ethical aspects discussed above must be kept in mind.
6. Evidence-based, culturally relevant, updated content, high forum participation, response rates reflected in learner metrics, easily accessible, mobile-friendly, bandwidth-adapted delivery, with equitable and ethical assessment coupled with prompt and constructive feedback resulting in a measurable outcome of knowledge, skill, and attitude gain are the quality indicators of an optimally designed and delivered course.

### 7.1.1 Strategies for Active Learning

Active learning is a process where learners are actively engaged rather than passively receiving information. A book on active learning (Bonwell, 1991) describes it as a method of learning in which students are actively or experientially involved in the learning process and where there are different levels of active learning, depending on student involvement. Learning, especially in an environment that lacks social presence and liveliness of classroom, is more prone to student disengagement and extra efforts need to be put in place to ensure active involvement. Elements of active learning across the domains may be very much required in online learning. Some of the models of active learning may be worth mentioning here.

The ICAP framework (Chi & Wylie, 2014) describes four modes of cognitive engagement in active learning: Interactive (I), Constructive (C), Active (A), and Passive (P). Learning achievement is lowest at P and increases in the order of A, C, and I. Another review describing ICAP framework (Lim et al., 2019) discusses the adaptation of this framework in health education. A review article discussing on Strategies for beginning implementation of active learning in medical education

(Graffam, 2007) synthesized and discussed active learning methods in medical education is made up of three interrelated components, namely, intentional engagement, purposeful observation, and critical reflection. This review also suggests breaks as action moments consisting of paused procedures and bulleted breaks wherein learners are encouraged to think and reflect. It also describes questioning techniques like targeted questioning, follow-up targets, and connection questions strategy to engage, orient, and retain the material. A study on Experiential Learning of Active Learning Strategies in a mixed method approach(Chauhan et al., 2024) discusses about using active learning strategies in web-based mentor–student discussions and it was perceived as effective in fostering critical thinking and developing collaborative learning among students. The study discussed various challenges such as lack of skilled faculty and resources which necessitated robust faculty development initiatives. It also discussed various possible active learning strategies that can be used in online and blended modes.

To summarize, structuring Interactive and Engaging Content in Online Psychiatric Education, following Principles may be considered.

1. Active learning over passive consumption
2. Clinical relevance and emotional resonance
3. Multimodal delivery to suit varied learning styles
4. Scaffolded engagement from simple to complex interactions

### 7.1.2 Use of Multimedia, Discussion Forums, and Flipped Classroom Models

These methods are often described and used to enhance learner engagement in both conventional and online learning settings. Of particular interest is flipped classroom models popularly described by King (1993) as "from the sage on the stage to the guide on the side!" to emphasize student-centric model. A review on Active Learning in Psychiatry Education (Sandrone et al., 2020) discusses active learning strategies and particularly flipped classroom model. The flipped classroom, also labelled as reverse, inverse, or backwards classroom, is probably the most used among the active learning approaches. The learners are free to review the materials at their own pace and must be engaged in their learning process. While time at home is spent being initially exposed to the teaching material, face-to-face class time is dedicated to student-centred activities promoting active learning, under the supervision of a facilitator. An article describing the flipped classroom in health professions education (McLaughlin et al., 2014) describes this strategy as a method of offloading the content which encouraged students to explore the material and develop new skills on their own, with the understanding that they would apply this new knowledge through various active learning exercises during class.

### 7.1.3 Structuring Interactive and Engaging Content

Use of interactive tools can enable the effective use of case-based learning and other active learning strategies effectively into online methods. A review article (Blackley & Sheffield, 2015) revisits the term 'andragogy' and develops a new concept called 'digital andragogy'. The authors recommend that instructors should be aware of profiles of their learners and seek to create learning spaces that best suit their needs and wants in order to engage and retain students and revitalize education courses by optimizing digital affordances. A study (Kassim et al., 2025) which reviewed various online-based and technology-assisted educational methods used in psychiatric training reported five important methods used, namely, videoconference, online modules/e-learning, virtual patients, software/applications, and social media. Embedding interactive content in recorded videos enhances the engagement, like quizzes, pauses, and annotations. Well-structured online programmes have good LMS and technical support and team to create such interactive content. When such facilities are not adequate, several tools that are available online for free and subscription can be tried. Some of the most commonly used tools are Vimeo, H5P, Mind Stamp, Adobe, and other newer AI-integrated platforms. However, the user discretion has to be exercised in using free-to-use online tools. Simulation and virtual patients are other two commonly used interactive and engagement techniques. Branching scenarios or storyline creation to mimic real-world decision-making can be used where the learner can have an option of choosing the alternatives, learning from the feedback received by their choices, yet in a safe environment. Many LMS platforms have integrated options for this method and some online tools like Articulate storyline 360 may be made use in creating such content. Virtual patients (VP) and the interaction with feedback in safe environment may enhance confidence of learners and engage them. Mainly two types of virtual patients are used, namely, Rule based VP and AI based VPs. Some studies like Rakofsky et al. (2020), Parsons et al. (2008), and Pataki et al. (2012) discuss on VPs as teaching tools in psychiatric education. One study on Evaluation of Branched-Narrative Virtual Patients for Interprofessional Education of Psychiatry Residents (Wilkening et al., 2017) used a branched-narrative VP resulting in high satisfaction and improvements in knowledge of advanced psychopharmacology. VP, however, is resource-intense and may be difficult to interact when speech recognition is difficult due to many possible factors like dialects and language barriers. Other engagement strategies are live pools, word clouds, using breakout rooms, forums, roleplay which can be innovatively used as per the resource available and learning objectives. Virtual reality is another modality which is coming up in recent days and will be discussed later.

### 7.1.4 Metrics of Student Engagement

A review on measurement of student engagement in health professions education (Kassab et al., 2023) states that methods of measuring student engagement in face-to-face learning environments may not be suitable for use in online environments.

Measuring behavioural engagement of students in an online environment may need to rely on other measures such as self-report surveys, data analytics, and log files. It describes User Engagement Scale-20 (UES-20) (O'Brien & Toms, 2010), Technology-Enhanced Learning (TEL) engagement scale (Pickering & Swinnerton, 2020), and Online Student Engagement (OSE) scale (Dixson, 2015). Apart from these scales, Kassab et al. (2023) list various real-time measures of behavioural, cognitive, and emotional engagement which are measurable which is worthwhile to refer to further understand the importance and types of metrics. It is not elaborated here in view of space and scope constraints. These engagement metrics fall under level 1 (Reaction) and 2 (learning) of the Kirkpatric's evaluation of the learning process (Kirkpatrick, 2007).

### 7.1.5 Gamification and Interactive Assessments

Gamification tools are other important and innovative engagement strategies in online education that can be discussed here. Merriam-Webster dictionary defines gamification as the process of adding games or game-like elements to something (such as a task) so as to encourage participation. There are many elements of game like points, levels, badges, leader boards, challenges/tasks/quests, progress bars, rewards, narrative storylines, sharing the success, etc., that can be engaged very effectively in online learning. Platforms like Kahoot! Quizizz, Quizlet Live, and Mentimeter are popular and widely used for creating interactive quizzes and games. Many LMS platforms have readily integrated these elements and available for use. A chapter in the book related to gamification in education discusses (Landers et al., 2015) gamification and psychological theories related to learning and motivation to enhance engagement. Gamification involves classical and operant conditioning, token economy, expectancy theory of motivational processes, namely, expectancy, instrumentality and valence, goal setting theory, and self-determination theory. A review on gamification and mental health (Chandran et al., 2018) describes various models used in management of various psychiatric conditions like depression, schizophrenia, autism spectrum disorders, etc. It also discusses using gamification models to teach Psychiatry to undergraduate and postgraduate students which improve motivation, interest, and engagement in learning. Currently, there are many gamification-based LMSs available on subscription basis. Existing LMS platforms which are widely used like Moodle allows extensions(Moodle Plugins Directory, 2025) that can help creating gamification content to be integrated into the course. Some of the popular plugins are level up, Interactive Content—H5P, Quizventure, and Incentli. Gamification has potential to transform the learning environment into captivating, engaging, and motivating manner so that learners are drawn into an immersive experience. Another advantage is that it can be used in assessment as well along with learning. Though gamification can be practically integrated into many forms of conventional learning in both face-to-face and online learning, it can be distracting as well. Learning has to be in the top priority and care must be taken that fun or game does not supersede the learning. It requires considerable research and development in technical aspects and hence the prices may be premium at times, especially in more sophisticated models. It can be started as integration of simple elements in a smaller scale rather than going high profile in low-resource settings.

## 7.2 *Effective Mentorship and Feedback Mechanisms*

### 7.2.1 Virtual Mentorship Models

Medical education is increasingly incorporating online and blended elements of education where students and learners may not be always in physical proximity or able to regularly meet face-to-face for the typical mentoring process to happen. Hence, the virtual mentorship concept is evolving parallelly to online medical education. It fosters the holistic overall development of mentees especially in low resource and places which are disadvantaged geographically and technologically.

Most of the mentoring models, types, and best practices equally apply to virtual mentorship as well, but with added responsibilities to make up for the disadvantages of virtual mentoring, primarily being unable to have the face-to-face interaction and nuances that are typically conveyed in nonverbal expressions. A review article on Virtual Mentoring (Junn et al., 2023) recommends a toolkit for fostering virtual mentorship that includes three essential components: (1) a method of easy asynchronous communication, (2) a reliable method of synchronous communication, and (3) a repository to share information. Many studies described above in the section of online mentoring have reported positive results in virtual mentorships. A qualitative study done on senior mentors (Riley et al., 2024) reported some advantages being flexibility, time efficiency, building rapport informally by “getting a glimpse into their personal lives”, mentees benefiting from multiple mentors who hail from different institutions, increased demographic and geographic diversity of mentees while disadvantages being less engagement, harder to gauge someone’s emotional state. It suggests methods such as creating an “onboarding” or “getting started” webinar for mentors and mentees within the same institution that provides background information, overarching goals, contacts, resources, and expectations as mentees enter a new training programme, video conference working sessions and writing retreats to augment ongoing mentoring programmes. Regarding meeting structuring, respondents suggested considering meeting options beyond videoconferencing, offering hybrid meeting choices such as email, texting, phone, and walking phone meetings to ‘minimize zoom fatigue’, mentoring meetings should include a social and emotional check-in, virtual meetings need to spend even more time on compassion and empathy, a practice that can be reciprocal and extend beyond the mentoring dyad. The increased importance of tele-empathy in virtual mentoring is included in a new concept called digital soft skills which was described in a Forbes article (Craig, 2020). In a pre-COVID review article on online mentoring in medical education (Walsh, 2016), the author has opined that, as with other technologies, in time digital natives will see it as no different from other forms of mentoring and what makes for good face-to-face mentoring will be second nature in online mentoring.

### 7.2.2 Timely and Constructive Feedback Methods

While online feedback may not be significantly different from existing models or techniques of feedback, to name a few like SBI model, Pendleton's model, and sandwich method, it is the mode of delivery that needs to be planned and integrated. Lack of physical presence, like any other aspects of learning, is a drawback even in online learning but technology has enabled that feedbacks may be integrated in LMS platforms and delivered timely and effectively through synchronous and asynchronous modes. The effectiveness of feedback and learning outcomes may be assessed using Kirkpatrick's model (Kirkpatrick, 2007; Kirkpatrick & Kirkpatrick, 2016) at the higher levels (level 3—behaviour and level 4—results) using various metrics of student behaviour changes and impact in the work-place or real world.

## *7.3 Ensuring Ethical and Confidentiality Standards*

In continuation of what was discussed under challenges in ethical aspects of online education, before planning or designing an online programme, one needs to look through the lens of ethical principles which we all know, namely, autonomy, beneficence, non-maleficence, justice, and confidentiality. These can be translated in simple terms as respecting and acknowledging that the learners and patients' privacy and confidentiality of the information that is involved in the learning process needs to be safeguarded. Many standards for compliance to these ethical standards and liability to data security standards exist across the globe. Some of the prominent laws which are worth mentioning are HIPAA—Health Insurance Portability and Accountability Act, CCPA—California Consumer Privacy Acts in US, General Data Protection and Regulation GPDR for European Union, The Information Technology Act, 2000 (IT Act); Information Technology (Reasonable Security Practices and Procedures and Sensitive Personal Data or Information) Rules, 2011 (Privacy Rules), Digital Personal Data Protection Act, 2023 (DPDP Act) in India, Protection of Personal Data (PDPL) 2024 of UAE, The General Data Protection Law (Lei Geral de Proteção de Dados Pessoais, LGPD) in Brazil, and The Act on the Protection of Personal Information (APPI) in Japan. The protection of personal data in health information systems- principles and processes for public health (World Health Organization, Regional Office for Europe, 2021) is a document that might help readers to know more about the data protection and privacy in health information systems that many compliance standards mention above adopt. The learner's benefits and career improvement need to be considered above anything else in the objectives of the programmes. This is important than ever because of the academic incentivization and monetization aspects that are involved in the fast-developing education market and edutech industry. During the course, psychological stress, well-being and possible harms to mental health, physical health and well-being of learners, teachers, and patients are important. Principle of no harm necessitates us to look into potential harm and making suitable provisions to prevent the same at the best interests of stakeholders should be made. Lastly, the principle of justice in terms of equitable access, content, and assessment has to be considered in every stage of the programme.

### 7.3.1 Ethical Conduct in Online Education

Professional boundaries, gender, and cultural sensitivity are important in online interactions where participants may be from diverse ethno-cultural groups and gender preferences. Language is another important aspect which may act as barrier. It is ethical to make learners choose the convenience of the alternate language availability in the user interface, subtitles, translations of the contents are made available. Adequate care has to be taken to accommodate these aspects and upholding of dignity and human values should be of utmost importance along with learning as the main objective. Etiquettes in the conduct during online programme should be laid out and defined during the planning and agreed upon the onboarding. Plans for handling situations arising in online teaching learning like refraining from unnecessary discussions over irrelevant matters, using trigger warnings when discussing sensitive and distressing content during interactions (like suicide, abuse, or trauma) has to be kept in mind. Respecting the copyrights and intellectual properties of the content by avoiding recording, plagiarism, and curbing other academic malpractices has to be ensured. Regular refresher courses on ethical practice and standards may need to be conducted to all those involved in planning, designing, and implementing the online programmes.

## *7.4 Leveraging Technology for Skill Development*

### 7.4.1 Use of Telepsychiatry as a Learning Tool

Telepsychiatry is a mode of delivery of mental health services via remote telecommunications which includes interactive consultative and diagnostic services. Telepsychiatry is predominantly involved in mental health care delivery to improve access and equitable distribution, causing a huge impact in the low resource and high need regions and countries. South East Asia has a dense population and a high urban rural divide where the ratio of mental health professionals is severely low. Recruiting primary care physicians and other health care professionals in delivering primary mental health care has been ongoing and fruitful. Many countries have their models of telepsychiatry beginning as early as the 1960s, growing along with available technology. It is only recently that this area is being explored as a tool for training and skill development as it invariably involves some orientation and learning. A review article (Hilty et al., 2004) discusses various clinical and educational telepsychiatry applications. It had already listed telemedicine can be used for provider education, clinical consultation and supervision. It can also link academic centres with rural areas for continued medical education. India perhaps is the most ideal place having all the criteria mentioned above suiting the need for a telemedicine project to be made available. A study on telepsychiatry previously cited (Manjunatha et al., 2018) describes experiences of an innovative digitally driven primary care psychiatry programme in India for the Primary Care Doctors (PCDs). It contains five modules named as orientation module, basic module, advanced module [Tele-psychiatric 'On-Consultation Training' (Tele-OCT)], videoconference-based continuing skill development module, and collaborative video consultation modules which covers all essential areas of primary care psychiatry for practicing PCDs. Last three modules are fully designed digital modules in hub and spoke model of Tele Medicine. It was opined that it has a potential for higher clinical translational value. Telepsychiatry serves as both clinical exposure and simulation training and involves all three domains of learning plus digital literacy as well. It can also incorporate live supervision and observational learning in real time. Project Echo (ECHO, 2008) of India is a step ahead in telemedicine which is used as a tele-mentoring and learning tool.It is a guided practice model where the participating care provider participants become part of a knowledge-sharing platform for building capacity and sharing best practices through case-based learning. The four pillars described in ECHO model, namely, amplification, case-based learning, best practices, and monitoring programmes. Telepsychiatry is bound by telemedicine and related laws and guidelines specific for each locale and region and is revised periodically. Ethical and legal issues described elsewhere are equally applicable here. After reviewing many existing guidelines, World Psychiatric Association telepsychiatry has come up with global guidelines (Mucic et al., 2024) and provides a clearer picture in this area. It is not discussed or elaborated here for the fear of increasing the bulk but it may be worthwhile for interested readers going through it.

### 7.4.2 Simulation-Based Medical Education (SBE)

Simulation-based medical education (SBE) is a familiar technique in Psychiatric education. SBE employs standardized patients, simulated patients, voice simulation, roleplays, OSCEs, and manikins in teaching learning process. Recently, virtual and mixed realities are also being tried under SBE. A review (Piot et al., 2021) elaborately discusses on use of simulation in training in Psychiatry. However, there are many controversies that exist on the use of simulated patients and the learning outcomes achieved particularly over the validity of assessment. The empathy that is developed during these simulation based interactions, understanding nuances in phenomenological experiences, acquiring complex communication and psychotherapeutic skills is often questioned by critics. Nevertheless, this review opines that SBE is a powerful pedagogical tool where clinical educators within psychiatry can greatly benefit from and contribute to the field of SBE, with their clinical experience focusing on intrapersonal, interpersonal, and relational dimensions of care, alongside expert communication skills, that can be transferred from clinical work to the educational setting. Another similar but a systematic review by the same author (Piot et al., 2020) discusses on existing research on SBE and reports a threefold increase in research over the past 10 years. The emergence of high-quality research, the diversity of countries starting to develop simulation, and recent innovations (such as Voice Stimulation—VS and Virtual Reality—VR) indicate the growing potential in implementing simulation training in psychiatry to support and improve clinical care delivery for patients with mental health conditions. What particularly interests is the use of AI and VR to circumvent some difficulties that are faced in conventional SBE can be discussed briefly here and in the next section.

### 7.4.3 Virtual Patient Encounters and AI-Driven Simulations

Efforts in medical education are being done for more than a decade to replace the real humans in the form of simulated or standard patients by using computer programs. A systematic review in 2010 on Computerized Virtual Patients in Health Professions Education (Cook et al., 2010) describes Virtual Patients (VPs) as computer simulations of virtual humans within clinical situations used for teaching, education, or assessment in the health professions. A systematic review on Virtual Patient Simulations in Health Professions Education (Kononowicz et al., 2015) reports a wide heterogeneity in the definition and contexts where VPs are used. This article attempts to classify VPs based on the adaptation from Talbot et al. (2012) which describes the role, contexts, and technology used in various levels of VPs starting from text and multimedia based VPs to advanced VPs using VR technology, dialogue AI and Natural Language Processing (NLP). Interactive virtual patients powered by AI allow learners to engage in branching conversations, ask questions, and make clinical decisions. Clinical reasoning and decision-making are the most important skills that are acquired by learners, in a safe environment. VPs just like any other online methods, have its own ethical considerations, especially when the design and the creation is biased based on many aspects like race, ethnicity, religion, language, and geographical locations. Another review on Emerging Roles of Virtual Patients in the Age of AI by Combs and Combs (2019) discusses these aspects as perils of VP and poses the following questions adapted from a policy briefing on Ethical issues in AI in healthcare and research (Nuffield Council on Bioethics, 2018) that we need to keep in mind when evaluating VPs in training.

- What is the danger of VPs providing incorrect feedback?
- Who is responsible when the feedback is flawed?
- What is the potential for the malicious use of VPs?
- Will VPs diminish in-person interactions among teachers and learners?
- What impact does the growing use of VPs have on teaching and learning?

# 8 Future Directions and Innovations in Online Psychiatry Education

## *8.1 Role of VR, AI, and Machine Learning in Psychiatric Training*

Perhaps one of the most prevailing challenges in psychiatric training, regardless of traditional and online methodologies is providing an adequate and uniform clinical exposure in various areas in a world of unequitable opportunities and without compromising safety and quality. SBE is complemented to fulfil the gap. While this is valuable and perceived as beneficial, it has its own limitation in scalability, consistency, and the range of clinical scenarios they can effectively simulate. These methods often struggle to replicate the complexity and variability of real-world psychiatric presentations, particularly when it comes to rare disorders or complex comorbidities (Cook et al., 2010). With the advent of VR and AI, these challenges are being addressed to create a consistent and immersive learning environments which are reproducible, have got high fidelity, scalable, and close to reality. A recent review on AI in psychiatric education by Ajluni (2025) examines the role of AI-powered simulations in enhancing clinical competence within psychiatric education, addressing the longstanding challenge.

Possible challenging contexts where VR and AI in psychiatric training which are difficult to be simulated in other areas are hallucination simulations and other simulations to bring the experiential understanding of psychotic experiences, VR experiences in emergency psychiatry to have an immersive experience close to real-world scenarios, and empathy training by various methods of branched narratives and embodied VPs. Conventional training and even SPs offer only observational level leaving the experiential and empathy as a skill that have to be developed based on the sophistication of mentalizing capacity of learners.

Digital extended reality termed as XR includes all those of immersive technologies that blend physical and digital worlds. At one end, there is augmented reality where there is an overlay of digital content on real world and at another end, there is virtual reality which is a fully immersive virtual world and mixed reality being the blend of both which allows users to interact with digital objects in the physical surroundings. Another recent review on Virtual Reality Training as Enhanced Experiential Learning (Riches & Kaleva, 2025) discusses on various advanced technology used in VR such as head mounted displays and Cave Automated Virtual Environment (CAVE). It also broadly categorizes educational applications into Skill-Based Practical Virtual Reality Training and Interpersonal Virtual Reality Training. A review on virtual and augmented reality for biomedical applications by Venkatesan et al. (2021) provides a perspective on XR in current biomedical applications such as biomedical education, medical training, surgical guidance, and molecular data visualization to enhance trainees' and students' learning, medical operation accuracy, and the comprehensibility of complex biological systems. The article also lists various available models in both research and commercial domains and not elaborated here. The field is fast developing and it is possible that several new models may have been added by the time this chapter goes to print! By creating immersive, interactive environment and experience to the users, XR can affect better engagement of emotions, increased sense of spatial awareness, improving spatial organization and memory. VR simulations may range from dialoguing, controlling, and manipulating with virtual elements enhancing the presence, motivation, ease of control, and enjoyment in the process (Makransky & Lilleholt, 2018). Currently XR has many challenges that one should be aware. These can be categorized into limitations to technology and hardware, software development resources and costs, privacy-security & ethical challenges, user related challenges including the side effects, harm to physical and more importantly psychological health. The reviews such as (Venkatesan et al., 2021)and Riches and Kaleva (2025) discuss on the limitations and challenges of VR in medical education.

## *8.2 Expanding Online Continuing Medical Education (CME) and Certification Programmes*

Mental health is being perceived as an essential need and there is a shift in perception especially post-COVID. Psychiatry is being considered as one of the most sought specialities for higher training as well as research. This has resulted in an increased need for developing training infrastructure and programmes. Traditional training programmes like specialist and superspeciality training have their limitations of having to go through stringent norms and guidelines due to which the opportunities are not expected to cater the need for the demand of training. However, with the online certification programmes and enrichment options, especially after the basic training in specific fields is completed, learners can have the option of pursuing in their field of their interests which can provide a wide range of opportunities. Almost every major society or organization in Psychiatry worldwide is offering its online continued medical education or professional development courses and the list becomes exhaustive. A simple google search provides many online learning options in both commercial and university or academic domains in the fast-developing edutech industry. Overall, the courses are generally categorized based on the stake of the learning outcome from a brief CPD/CME course to certification course with beginner to advanced levels, PG diplomas and Masters courses offering various levels of skill development. Advanced levels of courses invariably have some offline elements or on-site exposure. Many universities have collaborated with edutech providers handling the online and LMS component and chains of hospitals convenient to the learners' geographical area which provide clinical exposure (Hybrid or blended models explained in next section) while providing academic resources through their faculty. Cost-wise, low stake CPD/CME courses and some certification programmes generally are priced lower. While many of them are open and free, there are many pricing slabs such as free/discount for members, fee only for assessment and/or certification and paid courses ranging from average $50 to $500. PG diploma and other advanced master's course may range anywhere in few thousand to 10,000 dollars. These are of longer duration, lesser intake, competitive, and more structured with certification being valid in most of the places globally. It requires some guidance and mentorship in the form of informal or peer mentorship in selecting these courses and navigating application processes to effectively manage learning in one's area of interests. This section highlights some important online programmes offered by reputed universities, organizations, and commercial platforms. Only links to the organizations are provided in the references while the exact course details can be explored by visiting the relevant website.

NIMHANS Digital Academy (NIMHANS, 2025a) with its initiatives such as Virtual Knowledge (NIMHANS, 2025b), NIMHANS ECHO (What We Do—VKN NIMHANS, n.d.) is one of the leading online course platforms of India offering numerous courses and continuing medical education in Psychiatry and its subspecialities, for a wide range of audiences covering health care workers. Other few reputed and popular courses are

- IACAM online courses (IACAM Academy, 2025)
- American Psychiatric Association online CME courses (American Psychiatric Association, 2025)
- Harvard University courses (Courses | Harvard University, 2025)
- Massachusetts General Hospital courses (MGH Institute of Health Profession, 2025)
- European Psychiatric Association courses (European Psychiatric Association, 2025)
- RCPsych online courses (Royal College of Psychiatrists, 2025)
- World Psychiatric Association courses (World Psychiatric Association, 2019)
- Queensland Centre for Mental Health Learning courses (The Queensland Centre for Mental Health Learning, 2025)
- The Mental Health Commission, Western Australia online courses (Mental Health Commission, 2025)
- Coursera (Coursera, 2025)
- NPTEL-Swayam (Swayam, 2025)

## *8.3 Hybrid Models Integrating Online and In-Person Learning*

Completely online courses, especially those with brief duration, self-paced, with no/less synchronous methodologies, may result in apply-pay-finish the course-certification process in most of the CME/CPD programmes and develop a 'course shopping' mindset in learners without developing much of teacher-learner bonding. Due to various factors like enormous investment in development of edutech industry, higher norms and benchmarks required for universities to fare higher in rankings at their accreditation bodies, competitive know-all, CV decoration mindset in younger generation, many universities and faculty may be compelled to develop such courses regardless of the true learning outcomes and real-world impact. Grants and other funding may not be optimized if certain benchmarks are not met. The growing trend of micro-credentialing is discussed in the next section which is a topic of debate between the generational mindsets and needs of advanced medical education. The whole scenario of online learning, not just in Psychiatry but generally, has started to look more commercial and glamorous with metrics, reviews, and testimonies boasting about the successes. It may not be surprising to find a substandard course after 'purchasing' and hence choosing a proper platform and offering is very important. It may be vaguely comparable to online shopping of commodities in e-commerce websites, when we do not really receive a product as seen in the picture. In a critique, Ralston (2021) expresses similar idea on the new craze that has caught up in recent years. This is discussed in next section. If this is on one end, on the other hand, harnessing the true potential of online learning on bridging the gaps in equity and accessibility, some capacity building and focussed courses inviting students over different regions, with a brief in-person teaching–learning interaction over contact sessions, exchange programmes, travel fellowships, etc., have the capacity to mitigate the shortcomings of the global divide in resources, geographical and ethno-cultural aspects, and economy. This blended method of online–offline teaching-learning methods retains the learning culture and environment with meaningful interaction and bonding between teachers and learners and sustain lifelong learning. This may be particularly effective when the topics involve competencies that require real-world skills like patient care and not just enhancement of knowledge. The list is again exhaustive and deliberately not given fearing the ethical lapse of inadvertent advertising!

## 8.4 *Trends of Micro-Credentials and Certificate Stacking*

As the generations change, learning needs, methods, and trends keep changing along with generational mindsets. With the rapid advancement of medical field, education has to keep up the pace, where the so-called revised editions of text books, methods, skills, and knowledge keep getting outdated faster than the ever before. A learner has to keep abreast of the same and 'remain' in the race. Often it does not take the full structured programme such as a post-graduate or post-doctoral diploma or a degree to enhance to achieve this but smaller, focussed, and intense learning on a skill or area makes the learner more confident and competent as well. This smaller focussed learning and certifications are termed as micro-credentials and has caught up the trend among the new generation learners, especially gained impetus post-COVID era. European Union (EU) defines (A European approach to micro-credentials—European education area, 2024) a micro-credential as the record of the learning outcomes that a learner has acquired following a small volume of learning. These learning outcomes have been assessed against transparent and clearly defined standards. Courses leading to micro-credentials are designed to provide the learner with specific knowledge, skills, and competences that respond to societal, personal, cultural, or labour market needs. Micro-credentials are owned by the learner, can be shared, and are portable. They may be standalone or combined into larger credentials. They are underpinned by quality assurance following agreed standards in the relevant sector or area of activity. This document cited above contains a brochure on approach of EU towards micro-credentialing, its mandatory elements, quality, transparency and how to design micro-credentials.

A systematic review of the opportunities and challenges of micro-credentials for multiple stakeholders by Varadarajan et al. (2023) describes the alternate terminologies used for this, namely, online qualifications, online certificates, digital badges for MOOCs, microlearning, alternative credentials, open badges, micro-masters, and nano-degrees. The review article discusses learners', employers', institutional, and governmental perspectives on opportunities and challenges of micro-credentialing. Key findings revealed that implementing micro-credentials can be disruptive in the higher education sector and present several challenges. However, these challenges are likely to be mitigated by increased collaboration among stakeholders. A critical review on micro-credentialing (Ralston, 2021) describes this trend as 'micro credentialing craze' or could be no more than a fad, marketing hype, or another case of 'learning innovation theatre'. It reflects (1) administrative urgency to unbundle higher education curricula and degree programmes for greater efficiency and profitability and (2) a renascent movement among industry and higher education leaders to reorient the university curriculum towards vocational training. In another review providing an Australian perspective Desmarchelier and Cary (2022) provide a counterargument by opining that micro-credentialing will allow universities to respond quickly to changing worker educational needs rather than only offering full degrees that may not be economically viable or personally desirable for individuals. It also suggests the potential of micro-credentials lies in their pathways and potential to enhance lifelong learning and suggest that micro-credentials do not stand outside of the pedagogical ethical imperative that learning experiences should be positive and inclusive.

## 9 Summary

Online teaching-learning is not unfamiliar in psychiatric and medical education. It dates back to as long as the constant curiosity of human to supersede the sensory and physical limits and a thirst to learn. The visible start was seen at dawn of communication technology and real impetus was derived by the advent of Internet. Innovations have constantly taken pace and especially taken a leap after the COVID pandemic drove the need on an emergency basis. Psychiatry is a branch of medical science needing an art of keen observation, communication skills, and high degree of empathy and mentalization to understand experiences and needs of mentally ill. Hence, there is a special need of integrating various additional online tools and methods requiring the 'presence' close to the in-person experience. This means, integrating outer and inner senses in the right blend during the process of training and practice. Videoconferencing has been the holding ground of online tools. Introduction of simulations, virtual and extended realities, AI that can create and enable these technologies to seamlessly integrate with degrees that can simulate and even complement the reality with those elements which go unnoticed even in reality, has revolutionized the edutech ecosystem to a great extent. Efforts of using these technologies in various methods of teaching, creating a blend of online and traditional elements along with adaptive learning and learning analytics are helping students to create personalized path of learning, accessing to major and minor skills, micro-credentialing, and venturing into new areas of health care and research. However, there exists high disparity of resources, a global and digital divide in important areas like funding, policy making, budgeting, technical competencies of faculty and learners, learning ecosystem creating an inequitable distribution of the online learning. The edutech industry involved in research, development, and delivery of platforms enabling online education is rapidly evolving and equally commercialized attracting huge investments. Universities have either deliberately or invariably adopted blended learning models and collaborated with various agencies to create online courses which forms one of the main sources of their excellence, reputation, and, of course, the revenues. These are increasingly being monitored and assessed for the quality and integrity by accreditation bodies. A learner has to carefully choose after being thoroughly informed about the course structure and recognition before taking up. Online Psychiatric learning has special ethical issues mainly pertaining to accessibility and data privacy and protection. Many laws like HIPAA, GDPR, and DPDP are applicable in their respective regions, and the online course has to maintain strict compliance to these laws. Considering purely traditional and online only methods at each end, blended or hybrid learning systems are evolving at a rapid rate which tend to exploit the advantages of both methods and mitigating disadvantages. The next era of medical education is moving towards a blended mode incorporating elements from online methods and investing considerably in future technology like AI, VR-XR, and simulation-based education. Curriculum and policy making need to consider this trend, accommodate and incorporate the blended methods into the updating of curriculum to enhance learning outcomes and real-world impact with an attempt to bridge the global divide and mindful of ethical aspects.

## 10 Recommendations for Educators and Institutions

Designing curriculum and pedagogical strategies—Adopting frameworks recommended by various accreditation bodies and aligning the competencies with their standards, being locally and globally relevant. Incorporating blended elements to maximize the learning and impact.

Development of online learning infrastructure—Investment in stable and scalable LMS platforms preferably with smart device access like mobiles and tablet pc, use of AI enhanced tools in teaching and assessment (like virtual OSCEs), simulation-based education, VR and XR technology.

Funding—Seeking institutional grants, corporate social responsibility funds, philanthropic funding, and public–private partnership apart from government aids and grants would enhance the sustainability of the online programmes.

Collaboration—Within universities, extramural collaborations with technology providing institutes including technical universities in research, development, joint implementation of online learning, collaborating with industries and commercial partners of edutech industry and other intermediaries which can integrate academia, health care, and technology. Partnering with regional, national, and international societies like WPA can enhance global participation and standardization of curricula and methods with resource sharing and valid credentialing.

Continuous faculty development and training—in digital pedagogy, adaptive learning, and learning analytics

Assessment and credentialing—Use of valid and reliable assessment tools and ensuring transparency and integrity. Clear policies and transparency in credentials which are valid across the world.

Considering data privacy, ethical and legal aspects in designing and practice of online education, incorporating policies to ensure compliance to these norms and standards with periodic training of faculty in these aspects are essential. Content quality and relevance should ensure inclusion of vulnerable population, be sensitive to linguistic, cultural and ethnical aspects, gender sensitive and inclusive.

Monitoring, Evaluation, and Improvement—Multilevel feedback and assessment (Kirkpatrick model), learning analytics and establishing key performance indicators for online modules, regular peer and expert reviews, promoting research in psychiatric and medical education.

## 11 Conclusion

The fast-paced technological development and the rate of expansion of knowledge is revolutionizing the trend of learning. Learning habits and behaviour of newer generation have moved away from the typical four walls bound by traditional book-journal-classroom-laboratory to virtual world interacting with their physical world with endless opportunities to experience beyond the conventional ways. With psychiatric and medical education in this juncture, we have to don new hats yet retain the true academic attire to ensure comprehensive learning of the subject happens but in newer methods and tools and embrace technology-enabled learning. Hybrid learning with the right blend of online elements and conventional learning results in optimized learning mitigating each other's disadvantages but posing a new challenge to gear up to this new mode which is going to be the future way and norm of psychiatric training and medical education. Globally valid credentials, continued lifelong learning with micro-credentialing and skill enhancement, adoption of newer technologies in learning have the potential to make the psychiatric education better. Policy makers, universities, and industry need to have a long-term view in planning to make this closer and equitable. The beneficiaries of the new way of learning will be the new generation of technologically and academically competent psychiatrists who can propagate and innovate in this field. The ultimate benefit will be to the increasing population of mentally ill that need intervention and upliftment of mental health status across the world without a great divide.

## References

A European approach to micro-credentials—European education area. (2024, December 19). https://education.ec.europa.eu/education-levels/higher-education/micro-credentials

Aivaz, K. A., & Teodorescu, D. (2022). College students' distractions from learning caused by multitasking in online vs. face-to-face classes: A case study at a public university in Romania. *International Journal of Environmental Research and Public Health, 19*(18), 11188. https://doi.org/10.3390/ijerph191811188

Ajluni, V. (2025). Artificial intelligence in psychiatric education: Enhancing clinical competence through simulation. *Industrial Psychiatry Journal, 34*(1), 11. https://doi.org/10.4103/ipj.ipj_377_24

Almeheyawi, R., Alsini, A., Aljadrawi, B., Alshehri, L., Algethami, R., Althobaiti, R., Alrubeai, A., Alzahrani, H., Alshehri, F., & Alshehre, Y. (2024). Impact of online learning on physical activity during COVID-19 lockdown period among female undergraduate students in Saudi Arabia: A cross-sectional study. *PeerJ, 12*, e16579. https://doi.org/10.7717/peerj.16579

Ameen, D. S. (2015, January 22). *Brief course in psychiatric research—Home*. Brief Course in Psychiatric Research. https://bcpr.in/.

American Psychiatric Association. (2025). *Psychiatry online*. https://www.psychiatryonline.org/.

Anthology Inc. (2025). *Experience the Power of Together™ | Anthology*. Anthology. https://www.anthology.com/.

Arora, S., Kalishman, S. G., Thornton, K. A., Komaromy, M. S., Katzman, J. G., Struminger, B. B., Rayburn, W. F., & Bradford, A. M. (2017). Project ECHO: A telementoring network model for continuing professional development. *The Journal of Continuing Education in the Health Professions, 37*(4), 239–244. https://doi.org/10.1097/CEH.0000000000000172

Baessler, F., Sartorius, N., Javed, A., Tasman, A., Coskun, B., Frydecka, D., Kazakova, O., Sampogna, G., Zhabenko, O., Koelkebeck, K., Hepdurgun, C., Zafar, A., & Fiorillo, A. (2021). Training the trainers: Finding new educational opportunities in the virtual world. *Asia-Pacific Psychiatry, 13*(4), e12499. https://doi.org/10.1111/appy.12499

Barche, A., Nayak, V., Pandey, A., Bhandarkar, A., Nayak, S. G., & Nayak, K. (2022). Student perceptions towards online learning in medical education during the COVID-19 pandemic: A mixed-methods study. *F1000Research, 11*, 979. https://doi.org/10.12688/f1000research.123582.1

Basavarajappa, C., Grover, S., Dalal, P. K., Avasthi, A., Kumar, C. N., Manjunatha, N., Sahoo, S., Saha, G., Mehra, A., Singh, O. P., Tripathi, A., Gangadhar, B. N., & Math, S. B. (2022). Perceived advantages and disadvantages of telepsychiatry—An online survey of psychiatrists in India. *Indian Journal of Psychiatry, 64*(1), 93. https://doi.org/10.4103/indianjpsychiatry.indianjpsychiatry_332_21

Basu, A., Duvall, J., & Kaplan, R. (2019). Attention restoration theory: Exploring the role of soft fascination and mental bandwidth. *Environment and Behavior, 51*(9–10), 1055–1081.

Beatty, B. (2019). *Hybrid-flexible course design*. EdTech Books. https://www.hkmu.edu.hk/wp--content/uploads/sites/33/2022/10/Hybrid-Flexible-Course-Design.pdf

Blackley, S., & Sheffield, R. (2015). Digital andragogy: A richer blend of initial teacher education in the 21st century. *Issues in Educational Research, 25*(4), 397–414.

Bonwell, C. C. (with Bonwell, C. C., Eison, J. A.). (1991). *Active learning: Creating excitement in the classroom*. School of Education and Human Development, George Washington University. https://eric.ed.gov/?id=ED336049.

CDC. (2024, September 10). *Health Insurance Portability and Accountability Act of 1996 (HIPAA)*. Public Health Law. https://www.cdc.gov/phlp/php/resources/health-insurance-portability-and-accountability-act-of-1996-hipaa.html

Chakrabarti, S. (2024). Digital psychiatry in low-and-middle-income countries: New developments and the way forward. *World Journal of Psychiatry, 14*(3), 350–361. https://doi.org/10.5498/wjp.v14.i3.350

Chalmers, K. J., Wilson, A., Rossetto, A., Kelly, C. M., Lyons, J. N., Sabo, A. V., Baillie, S. E., & Reavley, N. J. (2024). Instructors' experience and acceptance of online mental health training: Implementation considerations. *Advances in Mental Health,* 22(3), 268–285. https://doi.org/10.1080/18387357.2024.2341064

Chandran, S., Prakrithi, S. N., & Kishor, M. (2018). Gamifying Education and Mental Health. *Archives of Medicine and Health Sciences, 6*(2), 284. https://doi.org/10.4103/amhs.amhs_92_18

Charoenporn, V., Hanvivattanakul, S., Jongmekwamsuk, K., Lenavat, R., Hanvivattanakul, K., & Charernboon, T. (2024). Zoom fatigue related to online learning among medical students in Thailand: Prevalence, predictors, and association with depression. *F1000Research, 13*, 617. https://doi.org/10.12688/f1000research.146084.2

Chauhan, A., Begum, J., Lavanya, K. M., Gupta, A., Ghosh, S., & Kulkarni, S. (2024). Experiential learning of active learning strategies in mentor learner web-based discussions: A perceptions study. *International Journal of Applied and Basic Medical Research, 14*(4), 258. https://doi.org/10.4103/ijabmr.ijabmr_277_24

Chen, Y., & Zhou, S. (2023). Impacts of video communication on psychological well-being and cosmetic surgery acceptance. *Computers in Human Behavior, 141*, 107625. https://doi.org/10.1016/j.chb.2022.107625

Chi, M. T., & Wylie, R. (2014). The ICAP framework: Linking cognitive engagement to active learning outcomes. *Educational Psychologist, 49*(4), 219–243.

Chu, K., & Sathanandan, S. (2023). The virtual Clinical Assessment of Skills and Competence: The impact and challenges of a digitised final examination. *BJPsych Bulletin, 47*(2), 110–115. https://doi.org/10.1192/bjb.2021.112

Chu, Y.-H., & Li, Y.-C. (2022). The impact of online learning on physical and mental health in university students during the COVID-19 pandemic. *International Journal of Environmental Research and Public Health, 19*(5), 2966. https://doi.org/10.3390/ijerph19052966

Combs, C. D., & Combs, P. F. (2019). Emerging roles of virtual patients in the age of AI. *AMA Journal of Ethics, 21*(2), 153–159. https://doi.org/10.1001/amajethics.2019.153

Cook, D. A., Erwin, P. J., & Triola, M. M. (2010). Computerized virtual patients in health professions education: A systematic review and meta-analysis. *Academic Medicine, 85*(10), 1589. https://doi.org/10.1097/ACM.0b013e3181edfe13

Coursera. (2025). *Best Psychiatry Courses & Certificates [2025] | Coursera Learn Online*. Coursera. https://www.coursera.org/courses?query=psychiatry.

Courses | Harvard University. (2025, November 14). https://pll.harvard.edu/catalog.

Craig, R. (2020, September 18). What the work from home revolution means for higher education. *Forbes Media LLC*. https://www.forbes.com/sites/ryancraig/2020/09/18/what-the-work-from-home-revolution-means-for-higher-education/.

Csikszentmihalyi, M. (1990). *Flow: The psychology of optimal experience* (Vol. 1990). Harper & Row.

de Oliveira Kubrusly Sobral, J. B., Lima, D. L. F., Lima Rocha, H. A., de Brito, E. S., Duarte, L. H. G., Bento, L. B. B. B., & Kubrusly, M. (2022). Active methodologies association with online learning fatigue among medical students. *BMC Medical Education, 22*(1), 74. https://doi.org/10.1186/s12909-022-03143-x

Desai, V., Lee, D. J., Lin, R. J., Alvinia, M., MacNeill, H., & Chan, Y. (2024). Assessing educator burnout in online synchronous teaching in surgical disciplines. *Journal of Surgical Education, 81*(10), 1409–1417. https://doi.org/10.1016/j.jsurg.2024.06.017

Desmarchelier, R., & Cary, L. J. (2022). Toward just and equitable micro-credentials: An Australian perspective. *International Journal of Educational Technology in Higher Education, 19*(1), 25. https://doi.org/10.1186/s41239-022-00332-y

Dixson, M. (2015). Measuring student engagement in the online course: The online student engagement scale (OSE). *Online Learning, 19*(4).

ECHO. (2008). *ECHO India*. Project ECHO. https://echoindia.in/about/.

European Commission. (2018). *Legal framework of EU data protection—European Commission*. https://commission.europa.eu/law/law-topic/data-protection/legal-framework-eu-data-protection_en.

European Psychiatric Association. (2025). *EPA Congress Courses*. European Psychiatric Association. https://www.europsy.net/epa-courses/.

Fauville, G., Luo, M., Queiroz, A. C. M., Bailenson, J. N., & Hancock, J. (2021). Zoom exhaustion & fatigue scale. *Computers in Human Behavior Reports, 4*, 100119. https://doi.org/10.1016/j.chbr.2021.100119

Fredricks, J. A., Blumenfeld, P. C., & Paris, A. H. (2004). School engagement: Potential of the concept, state of the evidence. *Review of Educational Research, 74*(1), 59–109. https://doi.org/10.3102/00346543074001059

Gasteratos, K., Spyropoulou, G.-A., & Suess, L. (2021). "Zoom dysmorphia": A new diagnosis in the COVID-19 pandemic era? *Plastic and Reconstructive Surgery, 148*(6), 1073e. https://doi.org/10.1097/PRS.0000000000008559

Government of India, The Gazette of India. (2023, November 8). *The Digital Personal Data Protection Act, 2023*. The Controller of Publications. https://www.meity.gov.in/static/uploads/2024/06/2bf1f0e9f04e6fb4f8fef35e82c42aa5.pdf.

Graffam, B. (2007). Active learning in medical education: Strategies for beginning implementation. *Medical Teacher, 29*(1), 38–42. https://doi.org/10.1080/01421590601176398

Grover, S., Goyal, S. K., Sahoo, S., Goyal, S., & Mehra, A. (2021). Views of medical students about online classes started during the COVID-19 pandemic: An online exploratory survey from India. *Journal of Mental Health and Human Behaviour, 26*(1), 62–67. https://doi.org10.4103/jmhhb.jmhhb_43_21

Henrie, C. R., Halverson, L. R., & Graham, C. R. (2015). Measuring student engagement in technology-mediated learning: A review. *Computers & Education, 90*, 36–53. https://doi.org/10.1016/j.compedu.2015.09.005

Hilty, D. M., Marks, S. L., Urness, D., Yellowlees, P. M., & Nesbitt, T. S. (2004). Clinical and educational telepsychiatry applications: A review. *The Canadian Journal of Psychiatry, 49*(1), 12–23. https://doi.org/10.1177/070674370404900103

Huang, L., & Pricer, L. (2024). How video conferencing promotes preferences for self-enhancement products. *International Journal of Research in Marketing, 41*(1), 93–112. https://doi.org/10.1016/j.ijresmar.2023.09.001

IACAM Academy. (2025, April). https://iacamacademy.com/.

Indian Teachers of Psychiatry (IToP). (2024). *STEPS & MUST—Indian Teachers of Psychiatry*. https://indianteachersofpsychiatry.com/scolarship/.

Junn, J. C., Whitman, G. J., Wasnik, A. P., Wang, M. X., Guelfguat, M., Goodman, E. D., & Middlebrooks, E. H. (2023). Virtual mentoring: A guide to navigating a new age in mentorship. *Academic Radiology, 30*(4), 749–754. https://doi.org/10.1016/j.acra.2022.08.014

Kallivayalil, R. A., & Enara, A. (2020). Undergraduate education in psychiatry in India. *Global Psychiatry Archives, 3*(1), 9–16. https://doi.org/10.52095/gpa.2020.1313

Kaplan, R., & Kaplan, S. (1989). *The experience of nature: A psychological perspective*. Cambridge University Press.

Kar, S. K., Dere, S. S., Mishra, D. K., & Das, G. (2022). Training of psychiatry teachers on teaching skills: Needs, innovations and initiatives. *Asian Journal of Psychiatry, 72*, 103108. https://doi.org/10.1016/j.ajp.2022.103108

Kassab, S. E., Al-Eraky, M., El-Sayed, W., Hamdy, H., & Schmidt, H. (2023). Measurement of student engagement in health professions education: A review of literature. *BMC Medical Education, 23*(1), 354. https://doi.org/10.1186/s12909-023-04344-8

Kassim, M. A. M., Shah, S. M. Y. A., Lim, J. T. Y., & Daud, T. I. M. (2025). Online-based and technology-assisted psychiatric education for trainees: Scoping review. *JMIR Medical Education, 11*(1), e64773. https://doi.org/10.2196/64773

King, A. (1993). From sage on the stage to guide on the side. *College Teaching, 41*(1), 30–35. https://doi.org/10.1080/87567555.1993.9926781

Kirkpatrick, D. (2007). *The four levels of evaluation: Measurement and evaluation*. American Society for Training & Development.

Kirkpatrick, J. D., & Kirkpatrick, W. K. (2016). *Kirkpatrick's four levels of training evaluation*. Association for Talent Development.

Kishor, M., Menon, V., Vinay, H. R., Shah, H., Isaac, M., & Arun, M. (2023). The IToP-STEPS: A unique scholarship program to upskill teachers of psychiatry. *Indian Journal of Psychiatry, 65*(3), 381–384. https://doi.org/10.4103/indianjpsychiatry.indianjpsychiatry_428_22

Kononowicz, A. A., Zary, N., Edelbring, S., Corral, J., & Hege, I. (2015). Virtual patients—What are we talking about? A framework to classify the meanings of the term in healthcare education. *BMC Medical Education, 15*(1), Article 1. https://doi.org/10.1186/s12909-015-0296-3

KPMG International. (2025). *KPMG International | Home*. KPMG. https://kpmg.com/xx/en.html.

Lagera, P. G. D., Chan, S. R., & Yellowlees, P. M. (2023). Asynchronous technologies in mental health care and education. *Current Treatment Options in Psychiatry*, 1–13. https://doi.org/10.1007/s40501-023-00286-6

Landers, R. N., Bauer, K. N., Callan, R. C., & Armstrong, M. B. (2015). Psychological theory and the gamification of learning. In T. Reiners & L. C. Wood (Eds.), *Gamification in education and business* (pp. 165–186). Springer. https://doi.org/10.1007/978-3-319-10208-5_9

Lim, J., Ko, H., Yang, J. W., Kim, S., Lee, S., Chun, M.-S., Ihm, J., & Park, J. (2019). Active learning through discussion: ICAP framework for education in health professions. *BMC Medical Education, 19*(1), 477. https://doi.org/10.1186/s12909-019-1901-7

MacNeill, H., Masters, K., Nemethy, K., & Correia, R. (2024). Online learning in health professions education. Part 1: Teaching and learning in online environments: AMEE Guide No. 161. *Medical Teacher, 46*(1), 4–17.

Makransky, G., & Lilleholt, L. (2018). A structural equation modeling investigation of the emotional value of immersive virtual reality in education. *Educational Technology Research and Development, 66*(5), 1141–1164.

Manjunatha, N., Kumar, C. N., Math, S. B., & Thirthalli, J. (2018). Designing and implementing an innovative digitally driven primary care psychiatry program in India. *Indian Journal of Psychiatry, 60*(2), 236. https://doi.org/10.4103/psychiatry.IndianJPsychiatry_214_18

Massachusetts Institute of Technology. (2025). *MIT OpenCourseWare | Free online course materials*. MIT OpenCourseWare. https://ocw.mit.edu/.

Masters, K., Taylor, D., Loda, T., & Herrmann-Werner, A. (2022). AMEE Guide to ethical teaching in online medical education: AMEE Guide No. 146. *Medical Teacher, 44*(11), 1194–1208. https://doi.org/10.1080/0142159X.2022.2057286

McLaughlin, J. E., Roth, M. T., Glatt, D. M., Gharkholonarehe, N., Davidson, C. A., Griffin, L. M., Esserman, D. A., & Mumper, R. J. (2014). The flipped classroom: A course redesign to foster learning and engagement in a health professions school. *Academic Medicine, 89*(2), 236. https://doi.org/10.1097/ACM.0000000000000086

Mental Health Commission, Government of Western Australia. (2025). *Training for professionals*. Mental Health Commission. https://www.mhc.wa.gov.au/training-for-professionals.

MGH Institute of Health Profession. (2025). *Courses | MGH Academy*. https://lms.mghcme.org/course--catalog-list?f%25255B0%25255D=field_course_format%3A7&f%255B0%255D=field_

course_format%3A7&f%5B0%5D=field_course_format%3A7&f%25255B0%25255D=field_course_format%3A7&f%255B0%255D=field_course_format%3A7

Mind Garden, Inc. (2025). *Maslach Burnout Inventory—Educators Survey (MBI-ES)—Assessments, Tests | Mind Garden—Mind Garden*. https://www.mindgarden.com/316-mbi-educators-survey.

Mittal, A. (2021). Opportunities and challenges of E-learning in South Asia: An analytical study of India as an emerging market. In B. Khan, S. Affouneh, S. Hussein Salha, & Z. Najee Khlaif (Eds.), *Challenges and opportunities for the global implementation of E-learning frameworks* (Advances in educational technologies and instructional design) (1st ed., p. 328). Information Science Reference. IGI Global. https://doi.org/10.4018/978-1-7998-7607-6.ch007

Moodle Plugins directory: Set: Gamification | Moodle.org. (2025, May 13). https://moodle.org/plugins/browse.php?list=set&id=88.

Moore, M. G. (1989). Editorial: Three types of interaction. *American Journal of Distance Education, 3*(2), 1–7. https://doi.org/10.1080/08923648909526659

Morris, N. P., Johansen, S. L., May, M., & Gold, J. A. (2018). Media-related education in psychiatry residency programs. *Academic Psychiatry: The Journal of the American Association of Directors of Psychiatric Residency Training and the Association for Academic Psychiatry, 42*(5), 679–685. https://doi.org/10.1007/s40596-018-0973-8

Mosalanejad, L., Karimian, Z., Ayaz, R., Maghsodzadeh, S., & Sefidfard, M. (2024). Zoom dysmorphia in medical students: The role of dysmorphic concern and self-efficacy in online environments amidst COVID-19 pandemic. *BMC Medical Education, 24*(1), 1330. https://doi.org/10.1186/s12909-024-06300-6

Mucic, D., Shore, J., & Hilty, D. M. (2024). The world psychiatric association telepsychiatry global guidelines. *Journal of Technology in Behavioral Science, 9*(3), 572–579. https://doi.org/10.1007/s41347-023-00339-w

Nadler, R. (2020). Understanding "Zoom fatigue": Theorizing spatial dynamics as third skins in computer-mediated communication. *Computers and Composition, 58*, 102613. https://doi.org/10.1016/j.compcom.2020.102613

Naskar, C., Cheung, G., Pinto da Costa, M., & Ramalho, R. (2022). Online academic mentoring—Experiences from a virtual international exchange program for early career psychiatrists. *Asian Journal of Psychiatry, 78*, 103287. https://doi.org/10.1016/j.ajp.2022.103287

National Medical Commission (NMC). (2019). *UG curriculum | NMC*. https://www.nmc.org.in/information-desk/for-colleges/ug-curriculum/.

National Medical Commission (NMC). (2020). *Module on online learning and assessment*. NMC. https://www.nmc.org.in/wp-content/uploads/2020/11/Module-8-Online-learning-and-assessment-17-11-20-version-final-for-uploading-converted.pdf.

NIMHANS. (2025a). *Certificate courses*. NIMHANS Digital Academy (NDA). https://nda.nimhans.ac.in/certificate-courses/.

NIMHANS. (2025b). *VKN NIMHANS—Empowering providers, transforming lives*. https://vknnimhans.in/.

Nuffield Council on Bioethics. (2018, May). *AI in healthcare and research*. Nuffield Council on Bioethics. https://www.nuffieldbioethics.org/publication/ai-in-healthcare-and-research/.

O'Brien, H. L., & Toms, E. G. (2010). The development and evaluation of a survey to measure user engagement. *Journal of the American Society for Information Science and Technology, 61*(1), 50–69. https://doi.org/10.1002/asi.21229

Orsolini, L., Jatchavala, C., Noor, I. M., Ransing, R., Satake, Y., Shoib, S., Shah, B., Ullah, I., & Volpe, U. (2021). Training and education in digital psychiatry: A perspective from Asia-Pacific region. *Asia-Pacific Psychiatry, 13*(4), e12501. https://doi.org/10.1111/appy.12501

Parsons, K., Parsons, T., Pataki, C., Paton, M., St George, C., Sugar, J., & Rizzo, A. (2008). Virtual Justina: A PTSD virtual patient for clinical classroom training. *Annual Review of Cybertherapy and Telemedicine, 6*.

Pataki, C., Pato, M. T., Sugar, J., Rizzo, A. S., Parsons, T. D., George, C. S., & Kenny, P. (2012). Virtual patients as novel teaching tools in psychiatry. *Academic Psychiatry, 36*(5), 398–400. https://doi.org/10.1176/appi.ap.10080118

Pickering, J. D., & Swinnerton, B. J. (2020). *Technology-Enhanced Learning Engagement Scale* [Dataset]. https://doi.org/10.1037/t77387-000.

Pinto da Costa, M., Cheung, G., Larnaout, A., Ramalho, R., Palavra, I. R., Shalbafan, M., & Costa, T. (2023). The World Psychiatry Exchange Program: Expanding the world of early career psychiatrists. *World Psychiatry, 22*(3), 490–491. https://doi.org/10.1002/wps.21131

Piot, M.-A., Attoe, C., Billon, G., Cross, S., Rethans, J.-J., & Falissard, B. (2021). Simulation training in psychiatry for medical education: A review. *Frontiers in Psychiatry, 12*, 658967. https://doi.org/10.3389/fpsyt.2021.658967

Piot, M.-A., Dechartres, A., Attoe, C., Jollant, F., Lemogne, C., Layat Burn, C., Rethans, J.-J., Michelet, D., Cross, S., Billon, G., Guerrier, G., Tesniere, A., & Falissard, B. (2020). Simulation in psychiatry for medical doctors: A systematic review and meta-analysis. *Medical Education, 54*(8), 696–708. https://doi.org/10.1111/medu.14166

Prabhakar, R. R. C. (2024). Adaptive learning systems in medical education: Personalization through AI-driven data analytics. *IJIRMPS—International Journal of Innovative Research in Engineering & Multidisciplinary Physical Sciences, 12*(3). https://doi.org/10.5281/zenodo.14850966

Rajesh, E., Subramaniam, S., Pasupathy, P., Suresh, T., & Gopichandran, V. (2024). Lived experiences of medical students of online learning: Lessons for adopting virtual learning in medical education. *BMC Medical Education, 24*(1), 982. https://doi.org/10.1186/s12909-024-05953-7

Rakofsky, J. J., Talbot, T. B., & Dunlop, B. W. (2020). A virtual standardized patient-based assessment tool to evaluate psychiatric residents' psychopharmacology proficiency. *Academic Psychiatry, 44*(6), 693–700. https://doi.org/10.1007/s40596-020-01286-x

Ralston, S. J. (2021). Higher education's microcredentialing craze: A postdigital-Deweyan critique. *Postdigital Science and Education, 3*(1), 83–101. https://doi.org/10.1007/s42438-020-00121-8

Ravichandran, K., Virgin, D. B. A., Edwin, D. M. R. S., Morris, D. V. S., & Milton, D. B. J. (2024). Moving towards a blended tomorrow: The evolution of EdTech in education. *Library Progress International, 44*(3), Article 3. https://doi.org/10.48165/bapas.2024.44.2.1

Riches, S., & Kaleva, I. (2025). Virtual reality training as enhanced experiential learning. *Journal of Technology in Behavioral Science*. https://doi.org/10.1007/s41347-024-00477-9

Riley, E. D., Chur, E., Gandhi, M., Fuchs, J. D., Sauceda, J. A., Sterling, L. A., & Johnson, M. O. (2024). Lessons for expanding virtual mentoring in academic medical institutions: A qualitative study among senior mentors. *BMC Medical Education, 24*, 934. https://doi.org/10.1186/s12909-024-05852-x

Royal College of Psychiatrists. (2025). *eLearning Hub*. https://elearninghub.rcpsych.ac.uk/.

Sandrone, S., Berthaud, J. V., Carlson, C., Cios, J., Dixit, N., Farheen, A., Kraker, J., Owens, J. W. M., Patino, G., Sarva, H., Weber, D., & Schneider, L. D. (2020). Active learning in psychiatry education: Current practices and future perspectives. *Frontiers in Psychiatry, 11*, 211. https://doi.org/10.3389/fpsyt.2020.00211

Sharma, N., Doherty, I., & Dong, C. (2017). Adaptive learning in medical education: The final piece of technology enhanced learning? *The Ulster Medical Journal, 86*(3), 198–200.

Suhas, S., Chougule, A., Innamuri, R., Nayok, S. B., Sheth, S., Nagendrappa, S., Patel, K. G., Shetty, S. B., Nagendra, B., Bhaumik, U., Pugalenthi, S., Uppal, G., Babu, G. N., Rao, N. P., & Behere, R. V. (2022). Training initiative for psychiatry post-graduate students (TIPPS)—A unique early career psychiatry training initiative in India and its response to the COVID-19 Pandemic. *Academic Psychiatry, 46*(6), 763–768. https://doi.org/10.1007/s40596-021-01570-4

Swayam, Ministry of Education (Govt of India). (2025). *Swayam Central*. https://swayam.gov.in/nc_details/NPTEL.

Talbot, T. B., Sagae, K., John, B., & Rizzo, A. A. (2012). Sorting out the virtual patient: How to exploit artificial intelligence, game technology and sound educational practices to create engaging role-playing simulations. *International Journal of Gaming and Computer-Mediated Simulations (IJGCMS), 4*(3), 1–19. https://doi.org/10.4018/jgcms.2012070101

The Queensland Centre for Mental Health Learning. (2025). *Learning Centre: eLearning*. https://www.qcmhl.qld.edu.au/course/index.php?categoryid=2.

Varadarajan, S., Koh, J. H. L., & Daniel, B. K. (2023). A systematic review of the opportunities and challenges of micro-credentials for multiple stakeholders: Learners, employers, higher education institutions and government. *International Journal of Educational Technology in Higher Education, 20*(1), 13. https://doi.org/10.1186/s41239-023-00381-x

Venkatesan, M., Mohan, H., Ryan, J. R., Schürch, C. M., Nolan, G. P., Frakes, D. H., & Coskun, A. F. (2021). Virtual and augmented reality for biomedical applications. *Cell Reports Medicine, 2*(7), 100348. https://doi.org/10.1016/j.xcrm.2021.100348

Verma, N., Gupta, S., & Shatadal, P. (2024). Research in psychiatry medical education through "MUST Enrich Grant": A scoping review. *Indian Journal of Psychological Medicine, 46*(5), 382–390. https://doi.org/10.1177/02537176241265742

Walsh, K. (2016). Online mentoring in medical education. *South African Family Practice, 58*(sup1), S7–S8. https://doi.org/10.1080/20786190.2015.1059020

Wang, C. (2022). Comprehensively summarizing what distracts students from online learning: A literature review. *Human Behavior and Emerging Technologies, 2022*(1), 1483531. https://doi.org/10.1155/2022/1483531

Warren, N., Parker, S., Khoo, T., Cabral, S., & Turner, J. (2020). Challenges and solutions when developing online interactive psychiatric education. *Australasian Psychiatry, 28*(3), 359–362. https://doi.org/10.1177/1039856220901477

Wegge, J. (2006). Communication via videoconference: Emotional and cognitive consequences of affective personality dispositions, seeing one's own picture, and disturbing events. *Human-Computer Interaction, 21*(3), 273–318.

What we do—VKN NIMHANS. (n.d.). Retrieved May 21, 2025, from https://vknnimhans.in/nimhansecho/.

Wilkening, G. L., Gannon, J. M., Ross, C., Brennan, J. L., Fabian, T. J., Marcsisin, M. J., & Benedict, N. J. (2017). Evaluation of branched-narrative virtual patients for interprofessional education of psychiatry residents. *Academic Psychiatry, 41*(1), 71–75. https://doi.org/10.1007/s40596-016-0531-1

World Health Organization, Regional Office for Europe. (2021). *The protection of personal data in health information systems—Principles and processes for public health* (No. WHO/EURO:2021-1994-41749-57154). World Health Organization. Regional Office for Europe. https://iris.who.int/handle/10665/341374.

World Psychiatric Association. (2019). *Education*. WPA. https://www.wpanet.org/education.

Zimmer, T. (2014, October, 22). Rethinking higher ed: A case for adaptive learning. *Forbes*.

# Chapter 18
# Psychiatry Education in the Digital World

**Shubhangi S. Dere, Dhvani Satija, and Rupinder Gill Das**

**Abstract** The digital era has brought significant transformations to psychiatry training, reshaping traditional methods of education and clinical practice. With the increasing integration of technology in mental health care, psychiatry trainees must now navigate a landscape enriched with digital tools. These innovations offer expanded access to psychiatry knowledge, enhanced opportunities for remote mentorship, and global collaboration. Virtual learning platforms and simulation-based training modules further enable interactive and flexible educational experiences, which have proven their effectiveness, especially in the wake of global disruptions like the COVID-19 pandemic. However, the digital shift also presents challenges. Trainees must develop competencies in digital literacy, ethical data handling, and managing online professional boundaries. Furthermore, disparities in access to digital resources can widen gaps in training quality across different regions and institutions. Ensuring the development of empathy and communication skills in virtual environments remains a pedagogical concern. Psychiatry educators must therefore adapt curricula to include structured training on digital tools, cybersecurity, and their psychological impact. Ultimately, psychiatry training in the digital era necessitates a hybrid approach that balances technological proficiency with core clinical skills. This transformation, though challenging, holds the promise of creating a more accessible, efficient, and responsive future.

**Keywords** Psychiatry · Medical education · Distance education · Curriculum · Mentors

S. S. Dere (✉) · R. G. Das
Department of Psychiatry, MGM Medical College, Nerul, Navi Mumbai, India

D. Satija
Department of Psychiatry, Era's Lucknow Medical College & Hospital, Lucknow, India





S. K. Kar et al. (eds.), *Teaching and Training in Psychiatry in South Asia*, South Asian Perspectives in Mental Health and Psychology,
https://doi.org/10.1007/978-981-95-1845-6_18

# 1 Introduction

The teaching-learning (T-L) methods and educational tools in the field of medicine are rapidly evolving. It is recommended that the T-L methods suit the learner's demands and capacity. The current educational system in medicine, including the field of psychiatry, needs upgradation of the traditional teaching-learning methods to digital learning tools, which can better suit the technologically oriented millennial learners (Bairy et al., 2019). The novel situation of the COVID-19 pandemic has also demanded digital involvement in psychiatry education globally.

In recent decades, worldwide, web-related services have penetrated widely into the healthcare system, catering both to training and offering interventions. Internet services are accessible to a wider population and provide easy, economical access to knowledge and information. With the wide use of smartphones and Internet facilities, digital learning has become an unmatched solution for most curricula in a modern learning environment, especially for higher education (Azat M et al., 2021).

Digital evolution in the field of higher education carries better acceptance due to many factors like ease of access and reachability, being time-saving, cost-effectiveness, and the one that allows self-paced learning (Zisook S et al., 2007; Dhir SK et al., 2017). E-learning also collaborates with the broad competency described by the National Medical Council to be a "lifelong learner" (*Vision 2015 Medical Council of India*, 2011).

# 2 Status of Psychiatry Education in the Digital World

A major portion of the psychiatry curriculum is designed using traditional teaching-learning methods like didactic lectures, bedside clinics, seminars, and grand rounds. However, studies observe that e-learning has comparable outcomes in comparison to traditional educational systems. While e-learning is penetrating other medical specialties, its use is thought to be restricted in the subject of psychiatry due to some inherent limitations, like a lack of face-to-face interaction with patients, difficulty in simulating empathy and communication skills, and teaching severe mental health scenarios. However, it has been proven that e-learning can be successfully incorporated in psychiatry. Improved outcomes can be achieved when digital learning is integrated with traditional methods. A study in Chhattisgarh, India, compared blended and fully digital training modes in primary care psychiatry for 941 doctors using NIMHANS modules. The blended group showed significantly higher engagement, more completed KAP forms, assessments, case presentations, and certifications. They also had greater improvement in knowledge, attitude, and practice (KAP) scores, even after adjusting for years of experience, and consistently identified more patients with mental illness over 8 months (Gajera et al., 2022).

It can be proposed that while e-learning attracts students' interest, several critical factors, like appropriate time management, efficient and optimum use of educational materials and techniques, self-motivation, and adequate online participation, demand consideration (Caputo et al., 2018).

## 3 Scope of Digital Training in Psychiatry Education

The digital learning tools can be used in both undergraduate and postgraduate psychiatry training, as well as training of psychiatry skills to paramedical staff and primary care physicians. In undergraduate medical training, integrating digital technology in the curriculum is essential to improve the broad competency "Lifelong learner committing to continuous improvement of skills and knowledge" (Ruben et al., 2022).

Studies on students' perception of effective medical education highlighted the role of innovative T-L tools used. In the current scenario, students depend on "multimedia slides" as an effective teaching tool to deliver information rather than other aids. As digital education has evolved, it has been proven that multimedia slides facilitate easy learning by simplifying complex concepts with the help of pictures, animations, graphs, and simulations (Kussmaul & Dunn, 1996). Multimedia slides are effective for students belonging to different cultural backgrounds (Nantz & Lundgren, 1998). Various T-L methods, such as psychiatric case studies from movies, online lectures, and animations using media to summarize the subject, are welcomed by the learners. The use of audio-visual aids in distance education is observed to improve the effectiveness of the course (Tel et al., 2022; Govindan et al., 2024).

Postgraduate training in psychiatry also needs adaptation by the inclusion of digital learning methods blended with traditional teaching. Online training and curriculum help the postgraduate trainee receive knowledge from distant mentors, which would not be possible in traditional training. In the modern era, digital psychiatry is an upcoming field of psychiatry. Digital psychiatry is the application of technology in the prevention, evaluation, and management of mental health illnesses. The scope of digital psychiatry continues to grow. However, postgraduate psychiatry trainees receive minimal or no formal education in this domain.

The practice of application of health technologies in psychiatry can be implemented and incorporated into traditional residency didactics. Such exposure has proved to significantly improve in learners' comfort level in navigating newer technologies, including digital therapeutics and smartphone apps, involved in clinical care (Noori et al., 2024).

The participants in distance education find the blended mode more effective as compared to the fully digital mode (Gajera et al., 2022). The Lancet Global Mental Health Group has recommended quality mental health training of primary care physicians as an important strategy to scale up mental health services in the community and to reduce the mental health treatment gap (Murthy, 2017; Lancet Global Mental Health Group, 2007).

Blended or hybrid learning is a popular teaching method in the field of online education. This requires technologies that integrate the physical and virtual worlds.

This way of learning is based on key concepts that the learners can easily share information, and based on the knowledge gathered from online resources, collaborative work among learners can be encouraged, enriching the overall learning experience (Mallikarjun Rao Sagi et al., 2017).

To make digital education successful, students also need to have specific characteristics like agreeableness, neuroticism, conscientiousness, and openness. The presence of these qualities in them positively influences their satisfaction with online teaching models (Mustafa et al., 2022).

The inclusion of technology in psychiatry training has been instrumental in improving the attitude of students toward psychiatry. Effective innovative e-tools can positively influence their perceptions about the field of psychiatry as a modern medical specialty. The technologies could facilitate learners' mastery over core concepts of psychiatry (Zhang et al., 2015).

## 4 Digital Tools in Psychiatry Training

Modern technology, such as Internet-enabled smartphones, software for video conferencing, and Learning Management Software (LMS), can enhance the quality of psychiatry training in medical and allied professionals. The following tools can be of particular use in digital learning:

### *4.1 Massive Open Online Course*

Massive Open Online Courses (MOOCs) are a popular platform that offers a wide range of courses designed for psychiatry training, covering topics ranging from basics of mental health to specialized domains like child and adolescent psychiatry or addiction psychiatry. These courses can be useful for a diverse audience, including medical and allied professionals, educators, and lay people interested in understanding mental health and diseases. Open platforms like Coursera, Stanford Online, National Program on Technology Enhanced Learning (NPTEL), and My MOOC offer various certification courses related to mental health (Wikipedia Contributors, 2019; Hoy, 2014).

The National Medical Council (NMC), India, has mandated completion of the Basic Course in Biomedical Research (BCBR) in NPTEL as a part of PG curriculum. This course focuses on the fundamental concepts in research methodology, is being offered through SWAYAM programme of Ministry of Education, Government of India, through SWAYAM-NPTEL (Basic Course in Biomedical Research (BCBR) | NMC, 2019) https://nie.gov.in/icmr_sph/BCBR.html

The following are the types of MOOCs in Psychiatry:

- Introductory Courses: This provides a basic overview of mental health. These are usually suitable for those who are new to the field.
- Specialized Courses: Caters to a learner who wants to explore specific areas like child and adolescent psychiatry, addiction psychiatry, or positive psychology.
- Focused Disorder Courses: These MOOCs target specific conditions like schizophrenia or psychosis.
- Skill-Building Courses: Some of the MOOCs can also help with practical skills building, with a focus on communication skills while working with patients or on practicing psychological first aid.

Being an open-access platform with simple content demonstrated in short sessions, a wide variety of learners, such as healthcare professionals, medical students, educators, and the general public, including parents of children with mental health issues, can benefit.

Here are a few examples of MOOCs available in Psychiatry:

1. International Association for Child and Adolescent Psychiatry and Allied Professions (IACAPAP) MOOC on child and adolescent mental health. https://iacapap.org/
2. University of Melbourne's MOOC on the foundations of international psychiatry or Coursera. https://www.coursera.org/learn/international-psychiatry
3. A MOOC on Positive Psychiatry and Mental Health by the University of Sydney on Coursera. https://www.coursera.org/learn/positive-psychiatry
4. NPTEL offers a free online course on the "basics of mental health and clinical psychiatry." https://onlinecourses.nptel.ac.in/noc23_ge19/preview
5. "Psychology of Addiction and Recovery" by Stanford Online. https://online.stanford.edu/courses/som-xche0005-psychology-addiction-and-recovery
6. "The Addicted Brain" on Coursera explores the neuroscience of addiction, emphasizing its biological and behavioral aspects. https://www.coursera.org/learn/addiction-and-the-brain

MOOCs hold popularity due to its accessibility as they are freely available to wider audience are flexible, and allow learners to study at their own pace and availability, offer variety of courses for diverse needs and interests of the learners, are cost-effective as the courses are more affordable if not free as compared to traditional classroom courses (Online Courses – Learn Anything, on Your Schedule | Udemy, 2025; Ebben & Murphy, 2014; Reich & Ruipérez-Valiente, 2019).

## *4.2 E-learning*

It is a learning system that uses technologies to extract educational curriculum out of the traditional classroom (Vivek Benegal et al., 2007). Teaching can take place inside or outside classrooms with the help of digital technology. It includes web-based learning, computer-based learning, virtual classrooms, and digital collaboration.

Examples of E-learning are:

1. American Society of Addiction Medicine: Providing an e-learning center (e-LC) with over 300 h of online Continuing Medical Education (CME), study resources for self-paced learning, round-the-clock, on-demand available LIVE webinars which are compatible with most smartphones (*Vision 2015 Medical Council of India*, 2011).
2. The Association of Faculties of Medicine of Canada (AFMC), along with the Palix Foundation, has designed a set of e-learning tools on early childhood development, epigenetics, and biological development and treatment strategies in addictions. The available resources include a primer, virtual patients, and podcasts (Dhir et al., 2017).

## 4.3 *Virtual Reality*

Virtual reality (VR) refers to creating a simulated environment with the use of computerized technology. VR places the user at the center of a simulated experience, unlike conventional user interfaces. Concepts such as Epson Moverio, Google Cardboard, and Samsung Gear VR are popular technologies in this domain (Wikipedia Contributors, 2024). VR and related technologies could be useful to teach assessment, diagnostic skills, as well as psychoeducation of patients with the help of simulated patients (Hoy, 2014).

## 4.4 *Simulations*

Simulation is a method used in education to replace real patient experiences with scenarios that are specifically designed to replicate real-life health encounters, with the use of computers and digital technologies. This is a comprehensive problem-solving technique with a focus on the affective, cognitive, and social aspects of learning. Simulation-based learning in medical education enables learners to acquire knowledge and skills safely and effectively. It facilitates the learning of procedure-based skills, communication skills, leadership, and teamwork skills. It also has the potential to be used as a reliable mode of certification for becoming an independent practitioner. Kognito provides interactive virtual humans that facilitate trainees to learn screening, assessment, brief intervention, and referral practice. Conversational simulation can be set up in various clinical settings, like emergency rooms, hospital settings, and educational settings. Simulation is easy to use, and learners can access it anytime. Throughout the process, the simulation offers feedback to the learner and provides valuable tips to improve their techniques. Nowadays, video simulation is increasingly used in psychiatry board exams by the American Board of Neurology and Psychiatry, where case-based video vignettes now make up 40–50% of the test and are often followed by related questions (Mitra & Fluyau, 2023).

Traditional methods like role-modeling often face limitations in replicating the actual complexity and variability observed in real-world psychiatric presentations, particularly in complex comorbidities or rare disorders (Ajluni, 2025). Simulation-Based Education (SBE) using Psychodrama allowed mental health workers to experience profound transformations through simulated interactions with therapists and patients, extending beyond traditional one-on-one consultations (Piot MA et al., 2021).

## 4.5 *Artificial Intelligence*

Artificial Intelligence (AI)-powered simulations provide a promising solution to these challenges. With the use of natural language processing, advanced algorithms, and machine learning, these systems can create dynamic and realistic patient encounters that adapt to the learner's dialogues (Chan & Zary, 2019). Especially in psychiatry education, this adaptability is crucial, in which the details of patient communication and the ability to pick up subtle cues are essential skills to develop in students. A key benefit of AI simulations is that they provide a safe learning environment for learners to practice diagnostic and therapeutic skills, particularly for sensitive and high-stakes scenarios like acute psychosis management and suicide risk assessment (Lok, 2006). Given these high-risk scenarios, the ability to practice multiple times without endangering real patients is invaluable. Unlike standardized human patients, AI simulations can consistently represent the same case scenarios across multiple interactions, ensuring uniform and equal training experiences (Kononowicz et al., 2015). This consistency in learning allows for standardized evaluation of student performance and enables educators to track progress over the period of training. A randomized controlled trial at the Yale School of Medicine showed that students who trained with AI-simulated patients experienced less anxiety and greater confidence during their psychiatry rotations with real patients (Ajluni V., 2025). Similarly, a study at Massachusetts General Hospital found that residents using AI-driven interactive case studies showed better diagnostic accuracy and treatment planning than those using traditional methods alone (Ben-Zeev D et al., 2019).

## 4.6 *Flipped Classroom*

It is an innovative teaching tool where students first engage with lecture material, preferably in an online format beforehand, outside of class, and the class time is utilized for activities and discussions like problem-solving and collaborative work.

This approach can offer flexibility, enabling students to understand the topic at their own pace and revisit content material as needed. This also ensures more individualized attention by the teachers during class time, as they can focus on individual student's needs and give targeted support. This learning reverses the traditional method of having didactic teacher-centric learning in class and unsupervised practice or homework after the class. The effectiveness of online resources can be enhanced by using videos, podcasts, and online quizzes. The relaxed, facilitating classroom attention can lead to better team-building skills, creativity, peer communications, and collaborative learning (*Flipped Classroom > Course for Teachers (2020-2021)*, n.d.).

## 4.7 Learning Management System

It is a software application useful for carrying out, documenting, tracking, delivering, and reporting various educational courses or online training programs. It encompasses various tools and techniques which are made available to collect, analyze, and display the data representing the participation and performance of the students. Based on this data, the institute or trainer can easily track the student's progress. Examples of smartphone-compatible LMS include Google Classroom, Talent LMS, Edmodo, Blackboard, etc. Several open-access digital platforms facilitate remote psychiatric mentorship and supervision. Video conferencing tools like Zoom, Microsoft Teams, and Google Meet enable real-time discussions, case presentations, and academic meetings (Bairy et al., 2019; Iftakhar, 2016,.

Most of these tools are very user-friendly for both the trainer and the trainee. They enable the trainer to streamline the process of training by sharing, uploading the lessons, attaching resource materials like photos, links, and scheduling the exams. They can also be useful for implementing innovative formative assessment methods like online quizzes and opinion polls to track their progress, along with the course-end summative assessment. This can be a completely paperless process and allows teachers to give individual comments and feedback. The trainee can access it anytime and learn the courses at their own pace, which can facilitate a non-pressurized environment. At the same time, they can interact and discuss to get handholding from their teachers.

## 4.8 Social Networks and Communities

Social media and online communities have transformed psychiatry by promoting mental health awareness, facilitating education, and expanding access to care. Social groups can allow an individual to get "benefit from one another's knowledge and actions." Various social communities like WhatsApp, Facebook, YouTube,

Academia, LinkedIn, ResearchGate, and X/Twitter, etc., are being used in medical education (Raiman et al., 2017; Pander T et al., 2014; Jalali et al., 2015).

Social media hosts webinars, live discussions, and case-based learning, bridging gaps in formal training. Online communities allow psychiatrists to share research, discuss clinical cases, and stay updated on emerging trends. Digital tools such as podcasts and infographics simplify complex psychiatric concepts for wider audiences. For instance, the website of the American Psychiatric Association offers useful information to patients and doctors alike (Tang & Helmeste, 2000).

**Example of Digital Learning in Psychiatry in an Indian Scenario**
An example of digital learning in Psychiatry in the Indian scenario is that of the Virtual Knowledge Network – Extension of Community Healthcare Outcomes (VKN-ECHO) project at the National Institute of Mental Health and Neurosciences (NIMHANS). NIMHANS, in collaboration with the Project ECHO, University of New Mexico, USA, has been running weekly tele-ECHO sessions (with local adaptation) since 2014. The main objective of this training is to reduce variations in the quality and standard of care, and to share the "best practices" model, "wisdom," and "clinical practice guidelines" by the use of technology to leverage limited mental health care resources in India. The core of the ECHO model is a "hub and spoke" knowledge-sharing network which links a team of expert interdisciplinary specialists located at an academic medical institute (hub) with those who are Primary Care Providers (i.e., mental health professionals like psychiatrists, psychologists, counselors, non-psychiatrist doctors, public health expert, etc.) in underserved areas (spokes) majorly "virtually" through tele-ECHO clinics (Arora et al., 2007; Chand et al., 2014).

## 5 Remote Supervision and Mentorship in Psychiatry in South Asia

Remote supervision and mentorship in psychiatry involve guiding trainees and early-career professionals through digital platforms. In South Asia, where psychiatric services face challenges such as workforce shortages and geographic disparities, remote mentorship serves as a vital tool for professional development. The increasing availability of Internet-based communication tools has made it easier for experts to mentor students, residents, and early-career psychiatrists across different locations.

Different models of remote mentorship in psychiatry training are one-on-one mentorship and a blended model, which caters to the varied training needs of the mentor and mentee. In places where in-person training may be limited due to logistical constraints, adopting these models ensures that trainees receive continuous supervision, feedback, and support, fostering professional growth in the field of psychiatry. Training should be provided to residents to assist them in finding and using local resources, getting comfortable in a range of roles and environments, building cultural competency for the community, and learning how to use system-based practice (Danilewitz et al., 2020; Coleman et al., 2022). Remote mentorship fosters interdisciplinary collaboration by connecting psychiatrists, psychologists, and researchers globally. Furthermore, trainees gain exposure to diverse case studies, enhancing their clinical knowledge. By integrating remote supervision into psychiatric training, institutions can bridge gaps in education, ensuring that learners receive continuous guidance despite geographical and infrastructural limitations.

Few such programs have been run recently in India, mentoring young psychiatrists and those with a keen interest in psychiatry training to upskill their teaching, teamwork, and leadership skills (M Kishor et al., 2023), (Certificate Course in Child & Adolescent Psychiatry for General Psychiatrists (Batch 1) – IACAM ACADEMY, 2025).

## 6 Ethical Concerns in Digital Psychiatry Training

In South Asia, where psychiatric training faces challenges due to shortages of manpower and geographical barriers, digital platforms provide an effective alternative to traditional in-person learning. However, the shift toward digital psychiatry training raises significant ethical concerns, including issues related to confidentiality, patient privacy, informed consent, data security, and the reliability of digital educational resources.

### *6.1 Confidentiality and Patient Privacy*

Maintaining confidentiality is a fundamental ethical obligation in psychiatric practice and training. Digital platforms used for supervision, case discussions, and online learning often involve patient information, raising concerns about unauthorized access and data breaches. Institutions must establish secure platforms, encrypt sensitive data, and implement strict access controls. Trainees should be educated on ethical guidelines regarding online case discussions, ensuring patient identifiers are removed before sharing clinical cases.

### *6.2 Informed Consent in Digital Training*

Informed consent is an essential aspect of ethical psychiatry practice, and it extends to digital training settings. When patient cases are discussed in online supervision or used in educational materials, explicit consent must be obtained. Patients should be made aware of how their data will be used, who will access it, and what measures are in place to protect their privacy (Sussman M & DeJong, 2018).

### 6.3 Data Security and Cybersecurity Risks

The increasing use of digital tools for psychiatry training introduces cybersecurity risks, including hacking, data leaks, and misuse of sensitive information. Training programs should educate psychiatrists and trainees on digital security best practices to minimize risks associated with online learning platforms.

### 6.4 Reliability and Quality of Digital Educational Resources

Digital psychiatry training relies on various online resources, including recorded lectures, webinars, and case studies, which lack regulatory standards. The quality and credibility of these materials vary widely, leading to concerns about misinformation and substandard education. Unlike traditional medical education, where standardized curricula and peer-reviewed materials guide training, digital psychiatry lacks universal quality control. Institutions must ensure that online content is evidence-based, reviewed by experts, and regularly updated to reflect current psychiatric practices.

### 6.5 Ethical Boundaries in Online Supervision and Training

Digital psychiatry training blurs traditional mentor–mentee boundaries. Virtual supervision, online discussions, and social media interactions can lead to ethical dilemmas regarding professionalism and appropriate engagement. Maintaining formal communication channels, establishing clear guidelines for virtual interactions, and avoiding informal or inappropriate digital exchanges are essential ethical considerations. Psychiatrists involved in digital training must ensure that online mentorship follows professional standards and respects hierarchical structures in education.

To address ethical concerns in digital psychiatry training, institutions and policymakers should implement structured guidelines, including:

- Developing standardized ethical protocols for online case discussions and patient data sharing.
- Strengthening cybersecurity measures to protect sensitive information.
- Ensuring informed consent when using patient data for educational purposes.
- Promoting digital literacy among psychiatry trainees to enhance ethical online engagement.
- Bridging the digital divide by increasing access to online training for underserved areas.
- Ensuring quality control in digital educational resources through peer review and expert validation.

## 7 Advantages of Digital Education in Psychiatry

Digital education has transformed psychiatric training by providing innovative, flexible, and cost-effective learning opportunities. With advancements in technology, digital platforms offer psychiatrists and trainees easy access to educational resources, virtual mentorship, and global collaboration (Torous & Roberts, 2017).

A few of the notable advantages of digital education are:

- Increased accessibility and flexibility
- Cost-effectiveness and resource efficiency
- Exposure to global expertise and opportunity for collaboration
- Interactive and innovative learning methods
- Standardization and consistency in training
- Integration of artificial intelligence and data analytics
- Bridging the digital divide in psychiatry training

## 8 Challenges in Digital Learning

The major challenges in digital learning are engaging the learners and increasing the level of interest in continuing education. So, before creating a curriculum, we must understand the current technology trends and challenges among clinicians and patients.

A reasonable interpretation of the relative lag in technology curriculum can be attributed to the ambivalent feelings toward the rapid advancement and infiltration of technology in multiple domains of life, including the field of psychiatry (Bairy et al., 2019). Online learning programs come with challenges of the convenience of the participants and trainers in the use of technology, availability of high-speed Internet, making plans to re-engage the drop-outs, etc. Also, there is the challenge of changing the capabilities and roles of classical teachers to modern digital trainers.

## 9 Future Directions and Recommendations

To maximize the advantages of digital education in psychiatry, institutions should:

- Expand online training programs that align with standardized psychiatric curricula.
- Promote blended learning approaches that combine digital education with hands-on clinical training.
- Invest in AI-driven learning platforms to enhance personalized education.
- Strengthen cybersecurity measures to ensure safe and ethical digital learning environments.

- Encourage digital literacy initiatives to bridge access gaps in underserved regions.
- To conduct regular Continuing Medical Education (CME) and workshops relevant to the field of basic as well as specialty psychiatry through digital platforms.
- To establish Hubs at various centers in India a wide base for training and collaboration.
- To develop an open online forum for discussion where questions can be posted to the experts by postgraduates and early-career psychiatrists for discussion and guidance.

## References

Ajluni, V. (2025). Artificial intelligence in psychiatric education: Enhancing clinical competence through simulation. *Industrial Psychiatry Journal*. https://doi.org/10.4103/ipj.ipj_377_24

Arora, S., Geppert, C. M. A., Kalishman, S., Dion, D., Pullara, F., Bjeletich, B., Simpson, G., Alverson, D. C., Moore, L. B., Kuhl, D., & Scaletti, J. V. (2007). Academic health center management of chronic diseases through knowledge networks: Project ECHO. *Academic Medicine: Journal of the Association of American Medical Colleges, 82*(2). https://doi.org/10.1097/ACM.0b013e31802d8f68

Azat, M., Norair, A., Aelita, S., Azat, G., Gulchachak, G., Albina, G. (2021). *Students' attitude to e-learning*. SHS Web of Conferences 97, 01042. TEDUVIS 2020.

Bairy, B. K., Ganesh, A., Govindraj, D., & Chand, P. K. (2019). Role of digital learning in addiction psychiatry. *Digital Psychiatry, 2*(1), 25–33. https://doi.org/10.1080/2575517x.2019.1622983

Basic Course in Biomedical Research (BCBR) | NMC. (2019). Nmc.org.in. https://www.nmc.org.in/information-desk/for-students-to-study-in-india/online-research-methods-course

Ben-Zeev, D., Buck, B., Chu, P. V., Razzano, L., Pashka, N., & Hallgren, K. A. (2019). Transdiagnostic mobile health: Smartphone intervention reduces depressive symptoms in people with mood and psychotic disorders. *JMIR Mental Health, 6*(4), e13202. https://doi.org/10.2196/13202

Benegal, V., et al. (2007). *Proposal to the Indian Psychiatric Society for adopting a specialty section on addiction medicine (alcohol and other substance abuse)*. https://doi.org/10.4103/0019-5545.37669

Caputo, F., Merlotti, E., Andlauer, O., & Galderisi, S. (2018). Opportunities of e-learning in education in psychiatry. *Mental Health and Illness Worldwide*, 1–19. https://doi.org/10.1007/978-981-10-0866-5_22-1

*Certificate Course in Child & Adolescent Psychiatry for General Psychiatrists (Batch 1) – IACAM ACADEMY*. (2025). Iacamacademy.com. https://iacamacademy.com/courses/certificate-course-in-child-adolescent-psychiatry-for-general-psychiatrists-batch-1

Chan, K. S., & Zary, N. (2019). Applications and challenges of implementing artificial intelligence in medical education: Integrative review. *JMIR Medical Education, 5*(1), e13930. https://doi.org/10.2196/13930

Chand, P., Murthy, P., Gupta, V., Kandasamy, A., Jayarajan, D., Sethu, L., Benegal, V., Varghese, M., Komaromy, M., & Arora, S. (2014). *Technology enhanced learning in addiction mental health: Developing a virtual knowledge network: NIMHANS ECHO*. https://doi.org/10.1109/t4e.2014.14

Coleman, M., Amos, A., Hoimes, J., & Ridley, K. (2022). Remote supervision in psychiatry training: Unlocking capacity and technology. *Australasian Psychiatry, 30*(6), 768–770. https://doi.org/10.1177/10398562221127825

Danilewitz, M., Docherty, C., & Bahji, A. (2020). How to serve the underserved: Making the case for rural and remote mental health training for psychiatry residents. *Academic Psychiatry*. https://doi.org/10.1007/s40596-020-01274-1

Dhir, S. K., Verma, D., Batta, M., et al. (2017). E-learning in medical education in India. *Indian Pediatrics, 54*, 871–877. https://doi.org/10.1007/s13312-017-1152-9

Ebben, M., & Murphy, J. S. (2014). Unpacking MOOC scholarly discourse: A review of nascent MOOC scholarship. *Learning, Media and Technology, 39*(3), 328–345. https://doi.org/10.1080/17439884.2013.878352

*Flipped Classroom > Course for Teachers (2020-2021)*. (n.d.). Europass Teacher Academy. Retrieved November 5, 2020, from https://www.teacheracademy.eu/course/flipped-classroom/

Gajera, G. V., Pandey, P., Malathesh, B. C., Lakshmi Nirisha, P., Hari, K., Ibrahim, F. A., Suhas, S., Manjunatha, N., Kumar, C. N., Suresha, B. M., & Jain, S. (2022). Effectiveness of blended versus fully digital training in primary care psychiatry: A retrospective comparison from India. *Journal of Neurosciences in Rural Practice, 14*, 91–97. https://doi.org/10.25259/jnrp-2022-4-20

Govindan, R., Gandhi, S., Nattala, P., Ramu, R., & Marimuthu, P. (2024). Effectiveness of digital learning in community mental health care among nurses in India. *Indian Journal of Community Medicine/Indian Journal of Community Medicine, 49*(2), 334–341. https://doi.org/10.4103/ijcm.ijcm_619_22

Hoy, M. B. (2014). MOOCs 101: An introduction to massive open online courses. *Medical Reference Services Quarterly, 33*(1), 85–91. https://doi.org/10.1080/02763869.2014.866490

Iftakhar, S. (2016). GOOGLE CLASSROOM: WHAT WORKS AND HOW? *Journal of Education and Social Sciences, 3*. https://www.jesoc.com/wp-content/uploads/2016/03/KC3_35.pdf

Jalali, A., Sherbino, J., Frank, J., & Sutherland, S. (2015). Social media and medical education: Exploring the potential of Twitter as a learning tool. *International Review of Psychiatry, 27*(2), 140–146. https://doi.org/10.3109/09540261.2015.1015502

Kishor, M., Menon, V., Vinay, H. R., Shah, H., Isaac, M., & Arun, M. (2023). The IToP-STEPS: A unique scholarship program to upskill teachers of psychiatry. *Indian Journal of Psychiatry, 65*(3), 381–384. https://doi.org/10.4103/indianjpsychiatry.indianjpsychiatry_428_22

Kononowicz, A. A., Zary, N., Edelbring, S., Corral, J., & Hege, I. (2015). Virtual patients – what are we talking about? A framework to classify the meanings of the term in healthcare education. *BMC Medical Education, 15*(1). https://doi.org/10.1186/s12909-015-0296-3

Kussmaul, C., & Dunn, J. (1996). Using technology in education. *College Teaching, 44*(4), 123. https://doi.org/10.1080/87567555.1996.9932338

Lancet Global Mental Health Group. (2007). Scale up services for mental disorders: a call for action. *The Lancet, 370*(9594), 1241–1252. https://doi.org/10.1016/s0140-6736(07)61242-2

Lok, B. (2006). Teaching communication skills with virtual humans. *IEEE Computer Graphics and Applications, 26*(3), 10–13. https://doi.org/10.1109/mcg.2006.68

Medical Council of India. (2011). *Vision 2015*. Medical Council of India. https://www.nmc.org.in/wp-content/uploads/2018/01/MCI_booklet.pdf

Mitra, P., & Fluyau, D. (2023). The current role of medical simulation in psychiatry. In *StatPearls*. StatPearls Publishing.

Murthy, R. S. (2017). National M Mental Health Survey of India 2015–2016. *Indian Journal of Psychiatry, 59*(1), 21. https://doi.org/10.4103/psychiatry.indianjpsychiatry_102_17

Mustafa, S., Qiao, Y., Yan, X., Anwar, A., Hao, T., & Rana, S. (2022). Digital students' satisfaction with and intention to use online teaching modes, role of big five personality traits. *Frontiers in Psychology, 13*. https://doi.org/10.3389/fpsyg.2022.956281

Nantz, K. S., & Lundgren, T. D. (1998). Lecturing with technology. *College Teaching, 46*(2), 53–56. https://doi.org/10.1080/87567559809596235

Noori, S., Khasnavis, S., DeCroce-Movson, E., Blay-Tofey, M., & Vitiello, E. (2024). A curriculum on digital psychiatry for a US-based psychiatry residency training program: Pilot implementation study. *JMIR Formative Research, 8*, e41573. https://doi.org/10.2196/41573

*Online Courses – Learn Anything, On Your Schedule | Udemy*. (2025). Udemy. https://www.udemy.com/courses/search/?src=ukw&q=addiction

Pander, T., Pinilla, S., Dimitriadis, K., & Fischer, M. R. (2014). The use of facebook in medical education – a literature review. *GMS Zeitschrift Fur MedizinischeAusbildung, 31*(3). https://doi.org/10.3205/zma000925

Piot, M. A., Attoe, C., Billon, G., Cross, S., Rethans, J. J., & Falissard, B. (2021). Simulation training in psychiatry for medical education: A review. *Frontiers in Psychiatry, 12*, 658967. https://doi.org/10.3389/fpsyt.2021.658967

Raiman, L., Antbring, R., & Mahmood, A. (2017). WhatsApp messenger as a tool to supplement medical education for medical students on clinical attachment. *BMC Medical Education, 17*(1). https://doi.org/10.1186/s12909-017-0855-x

Reich, J., & Ruipérez-Valiente, J. A. (2019). The MOOC pivot. *Science, 363*(6423), 130–131. https://doi.org/10.1126/science.aav7958

Ruben, J.-P., Shah, H., Sreedaran, P., Chandran, S., Selvam, S., & Kurpad, S. S. (2022). Effective and innovative teaching methods in psychiatry for the medical undergraduates in South India: An exploratory study of teachers' and students' perspectives. *Indian Journal of Psychiatry, 64*(6), 545. https://doi.org/10.4103/indianjpsychiatry.indianjpsychiatry_954_21

Sagi, M. R., Chand, P., Narasimha, V. L., Murthy, P., Mamatha, M., Karthick, C., Shetty, M., Kubenthiran, N., Aurobind, G., Prabhakara, & Arora, S. (2017). *A pilot from the virtual knowledge network (VKN) nimhans ECHO*. https://doi.org/10.1109/eleltech.2017.8075000

Sussman, N., & DeJong, S. M. (2018). Ethical considerations for mental health clinicians working withadolescents in the digital age. *Current Psychiatry Reports, 20*(12), 113.https://doi.org/10.1007/s11920-018-0974-z. PMID: 30317406.

Tang, S., & Helmeste, D. (2000). Digital psychiatry. *Psychiatry and Clinical Neurosciences, 54*(1), 1–10. https://doi.org/10.1046/j.1440-1819.2000.00628.x

Tel, H., Kelleci, M., & Kısaoğlu, Ö. (2022). Teaching and student attitudes in an online psychiatric nursing course. *American Journal of Distance Education*, 1–12. https://doi.org/10.1080/08923647.2022.2137355

Torous, J., & Roberts, L. W. (2017). The ethical use of mobile health technology in clinical psychiatry. *The Journal of Nervous and Mental Disease, 205*(1), 4–8. https://doi.org/10.1097/NMD.0000000000000596

Wikipedia Contributors. (2019, March 14). *Massive open online course*. Wikipedia, Wikimedia Foundation. https://en.wikipedia.org/wiki/Massive_open_online_course

Wikipedia Contributors. (2024, December 18). *Massive*. Wikipedia, Wikimedia Foundation.

Zhang, M. W. B., Ho, C. S. H., Cheok, C. C. S., & Ho, R. C. M. (2015). Bringing smartphone technology into undergraduate and postgraduate psychiatry. *British Journal of Psychiatry Advances, 21*(4), 222–228. https://doi.org/10.1192/apt.bp.114.013649

Zisook, S., Balon, R., Björkstén, K. S., et al. (2007). Psychiatry residency training around the world. *Academic Psychiatry, 31*(4), 309–325. https://doi.org/10.1176/appi.ap.31.4.309

# Chapter 19
# Evolution of Psychiatric Subspecialties in South Asia

**Amit Singh**

**Abstract** Psychiatry in South Asia has undergone significant transformation, evolving from a subject heavily focused on severe mental illnesses within institutional settings to a specialized field with distinct subspecialties addressing diverse mental health needs. Increasing mental health awareness, enhanced understanding of the subject, and evolving mental health needs of the population have prompted select academic institutions to initiate subspecialty courses in the niche areas, including addiction psychiatry, child and adolescent psychiatry, forensic psychiatry, and geriatric psychiatry. Despite progress, the development across the region remains inconsistent, as nations such as Afghanistan, Bhutan, Nepal, and the Maldives still lack specialized training programs. Challenges to the initiation of subspecialty programs include a shortage of trained faculty, limited funding, a lack of standardized curricula, and poor integration into national health policies. The evolution of psychiatric subspecialties in South Asia reflects the broader global trend toward comprehensive mental health care. Continued efforts to enhance the quality of mental health care through improved training of psychiatrists will be essential in addressing the unique mental health challenges of the region.

**Keywords** Specialty boards · Teaching · Psychiatry · Curriculum · South Asia

## 1 Introduction

Psychiatry in South Asia has undergone significant changes. Historically, there was a strong emphasis on managing severe mental illnesses in institutional settings, and this is where students used to undergo their training in psychiatry (Isaac, 2011). In 1941, the postgraduate MD (Doctor of Medicine) psychiatry program was started at the Medical College at Patna in India, the first such program in South Asia. The

A. Singh (✉)
King George's Medical University, Lucknow, Uttar Pradesh, India



S. K. Kar et al. (eds.), *Teaching and Training in Psychiatry in South Asia*, South Asian Perspectives in Mental Health and Psychology,
https://doi.org/10.1007/978-981-95-1845-6_19

initial growth in institutes providing postgraduate psychiatry training was relatively slow. Till about two decades after the independence of India from British occupation in 1947, only six institutes used to offer MD degrees in psychiatry (Sharma, 2010) However, this trend changed gradually, and there occurred remarkable developments in the field of psychiatry training in India, with psychiatry becoming increasingly diversified and specialized (Sharma, 2010). In other nations of the region, the postgraduate psychiatry training course in psychiatry started years later. In Sri Lanka, the first MD examinations were conducted in 1952 (Chandradasa & Champika, 2019). However, the teaching programs were not systematic. In 1980, Sri Lanka started offering a 5-year MD course in Psychiatry at the Postgraduate Institute of Medicine (PGIM) of the University of Colombo (Gambheera, 2011). In Pakistan, the College of Physicians and Surgeons of Pakistan (CPSP), the examining body of postgraduate medical education, included psychiatry in its list of specialties in 1975 (Naeem & Ayub, 2004). Bangladesh started fellowship (Fellow of Bangladesh College of Physicians and Surgeons; FCPS) in psychiatry in 1979 (Arafat, 2020). Those completing this program successfully, which runs for 3 years before the MD (Psychiatry) examination and an additional 2 years as Senior Registrars, were certified as specialists in psychiatry. In Nepal, a 3-year residency program started in the Institute of Medicine (IOM) in 1997 (Sharma, 2011). Recently, Bhutan also started a 4-year postgraduate residency training in psychiatry at the Khesar Gyalpo University of Medical Sciences of Bhutan (KGUMSB) in 2019 (Dorji, 2023). Afghanistan and the Maldives are yet to start a postgraduate psychiatry course. Thus, compared to global standards, South Asia continues to lag behind in producing an adequate number of trained psychiatrists to meet the mental health needs of its population.

Despite considerable disparities across the region, recent years have seen meaningful progress in psychiatric education and training. This includes improvements in the quality of training, an increase in the number of institutions offering postgraduate programs, and a gradual rise in the mental health workforce to population ratio. Advancements in psychiatric knowledge continue at a rapid pace. The understanding related to mental illnesses, their neurobiological, psychological, and social underpinnings and management strategies has remarkably augmented, necessitating a more specialized approach to psychiatric training. Several South Asian nations recognized the need to develop and implement intensive and domain-specific subspecialty training programs. This approach is of particular relevance to South Asia, owing to the presence of a broad spectrum of disorders and substantial mental health burden, often with prevalence rates exceeding global averages due to socio-economic stressors, conflict, political instability, and under-resourced health systems.

## 2 Need for Specialization Courses in Psychiatry

The need arises from the increasing complexity, diversity, and specificity of mental health conditions across different populations. The psychiatric subspecialties are vital for delivering high-quality, person-centered care, fostering innovation, and addressing evolving mental health challenges across populations and systems.

### *2.1 Complexity of Psychiatric Disorders*

Psychiatric disorders often have multifactorial causation and present with overlapping symptoms. Also, co-occurring psychiatric (e.g., substance use with mood disorders) and physical illnesses (e.g., diabetes mellitus with depression) are common. Thus, a nuanced understanding of the subject is required to appropriately and effectively manage the issues. The subspecialty training allows psychiatrists to develop advanced assessment and management skills tailored to specific conditions.

### *2.2 Enhancing Quality of Care*

Specialists contribute to improved patient outcomes through evidence-based, targeted interventions. The experiential knowledge garnered through dealing with a specific set of disorders, especially their severe forms, is invaluable in providing care. It thus enhances the quality of care received by the patients and reduces the illness burden.

### *2.3 Diverse Patient Populations*

Different population groups (e.g., children, the elderly, women, and people using drugs) have unique psychological, social, and biological needs. The specialty training in areas like child and adolescent psychiatry, geriatric psychiatry, and perinatal psychiatry equips psychiatrists to address age- and gender-specific challenges effectively.

### 2.4 Bridging Gaps in Care

Specialized training helps fill service gaps in underdeveloped areas like child and adolescent psychiatry, addiction psychiatry, forensic psychiatry, or consultation-liaison psychiatry, where general training may be insufficient. It ensures comprehensive and interdisciplinary approaches to patient care through a heightened understanding of patient needs that may extend beyond medical ones to include legal, social, financial, and vocational aspects.

### 2.5 Academic and Research Advancements

Sub-specialization fosters academic excellence and research in niche areas, promoting innovation and a deeper understanding of mental health disorders. Specialists have a crucial role to play in building mental health systems and training mental healthcare professionals in developing nations. The graduates and postgraduates trained under specialists in a domain can be expected to have a better understanding of the subject, perform better academically and clinically. Also, the research evidence generated helps in validating or amending the general understanding of a subject. Thus, it contributes to the development of clinical guidelines, novel therapies, and policy frameworks fitting the locoregional needs and advocating for policy changes.

### 2.6 Career Development

Specialty training enables psychiatrists to pursue interests aligned with their passion and strengths. It helps them create career paths in clinical care, teaching, leadership, and advocacy.

## 3 Psychiatry Subspecialty Training in Developed Nations

Several developed nations, including the United States (US), the United Kingdom (UK), many European nations, as well as Australia and New Zealand, offer higher specialty training programs in psychiatry to keep psychiatry students conversant with the advancements in the respective fields.

In the United States, the American Board of Medical Specialties (ABMS) approved subspecialty certificates were first issued for child psychiatry in 1959 (Cannon et al., 2022). It was followed by the approval of geriatric psychiatry and addiction psychiatric courses in 1989 and 1991, respectively (American Board of Medical Specialties, 2023). Subsequently, many other subspecialty courses were

**Table 19.1** Specialty and subspecialty courses in various countries

| Country | Subject | Approved by |
|---|---|---|
| USA | 1. Addiction Medicine<br>2. Addiction Psychiatry<br>3. Brain Injury Medicine<br>4. Child and Adolescent Psychiatry<br>5. Consultation-Liaison Psychiatry<br>6. Forensic Psychiatry<br>7. Geriatric Psychiatry<br>8. Hospice and Palliative Medicine<br>9. Sleep Medicine | American Board of Medical Specialties (ABMS) |
| UK | Specialty<br>1. General Adult Psychiatry<br>2. Child and Adolescent Psychiatry<br>3. Forensic Psychiatry<br>4. Old Age Psychiatry<br>5. Medical Psychotherapy<br>6. Psychiatry of Intellectual Disability<br>Subspecialty<br>1. Addictions Psychiatry (Substance Misuse)<br>2. Liaison Psychiatry<br>3. Rehabilitation Psychiatry | General Medical Council (GMC) |
| Australia and New Zealand | 1. Addiction Psychiatry<br>2. Adult Psychiatry<br>3. Child and Adolescent Psychiatry.<br>4. Consultation-Liaison Psychiatry<br>5. Forensic Psychiatry<br>6. Neuropsychiatry<br>7. Old Age Psychiatry<br>8. Psychotherapies | Royal Australian and New Zealand College of Psychiatrists (RANZCP) |

approved by the ABMS (Table 19.1). After the 4-year General Psychiatry Residency program, psychiatry residents have the opportunity to pursue various subspecialty fellowships evaluated and accredited by the Accreditation Council for Graduate Medical Education (ACGME). The ACGME emphasizes transforming medical education by fostering competency-based, customized professional development, guided by inspiring faculty and grounded in evidence-based, data-driven, and humanistic environments. It attempts to ensure that the training serves the local and regional community needs and produces doctors dedicated to lifelong learning and prioritizing patients and communities. These fellowships typically span 1–2 years and provide advanced training in specific areas of psychiatric practice. The ACGME and the ABMS developed six core competencies necessary for practicing physicians, including (1) Patient Care and Procedural Skills, (2) Medical Knowledge, (3) Practice-Based Learning and Improvement, (4) Interpersonal and Communication Skills, (5) Professionalism, and (6) Systems-Based Practice. Most ACGME-accredited courses are 12-month fellowship programs. However, the duration may vary depending on the goals and complexity of the specialty. For example, the child and adolescent psychiatry fellowship in the USA spans 2 years (ACGME, 2025).

In the United Kingdom, following the establishment of the Royal College of Psychiatrists in 1971, the Joint Committee on Higher Psychiatric Training (JCHPT) was formed to ensure the adequacy of training programs for higher trainees, such as senior registrars and lecturers. The committee operated through specialist subcommittees that oversee various psychiatric disciplines, including general psychiatry, child and adolescent psychiatry, forensic psychiatry, learning disabilities (previously termed mental handicap), and psychotherapy (Brook, 1982). The JCHPT was responsible for maintaining and enhancing training standards by publishing guidance on objectives and methods, as well as by inspecting and approving training schemes. It also worked to adapt training programs in response to changes in the organization and delivery of psychiatric services (Hersov, 1986). Currently, the psychiatric training is structured into core and higher specialty training phases. After completing Core Training (CT1–CT3), doctors progress to Higher Specialty Training (ST4–ST6), where they can specialize in six General Medical Council (GMC) approved specialties of at least 36 months duration, including general psychiatry, child and adolescent psychiatry, forensic psychiatry, psychiatry of learning disability, old age psychiatry, and medical psychotherapy (NHS England, 2024). The Royal College of Psychiatrists (RCPsych) oversees the curricula and training standards for these specialties (Table 19.1). Trainees may also pursue dual training in approved combinations of these specialties. Within General Adult and Old Age Psychiatry, trainees can obtain endorsements in specific subspecialties by completing additional training. These endorsements typically require 12 months of whole-time equivalent training in the subspecialty area.

Psychiatric subspecialty training in other countries in Europe is diverse, reflecting varying national standards, healthcare systems, and educational structures. While some countries offer formal subspecialty certifications, others provide specialized training through clinical rotations, endorsements, or continuing medical education (CME) programs. The French medical system does not formally recognize subspecialties in psychiatry as separate qualifications. However, the French universities offer various University and Inter-University Diplomas programs that provide in-depth training in specific psychiatric fields. The subspecialties commonly recognized and offered across European countries are General Adult Psychiatry, Child and Adolescent Psychiatry (CAP), Old Age Psychiatry (Geriatric Psychiatry), Forensic Psychiatry, Addiction Psychiatry, Consultation-Liaison Psychiatry, Psychotherapy, and Intellectual Disability Psychiatry.

Similarly, Australia and New Zealand offer advanced training in the final 24 months of the psychiatry fellowship training program in distinct areas, including adult psychiatry, child and adolescent psychiatry, addiction psychiatry, forensic psychiatry, consultation-liaison psychiatry, psychiatry of old age, and psychotherapies.

# 4 Status of Psychiatry Subspecialty in South Asia

## 4.1 Afghanistan

Despite the psychiatric services beginning in Afghanistan as early as 1933 with a custodial inpatient unit at Ali Abad Hospital in Kabul, the country has lagged when it comes to providing psychiatry postgraduate and subspecialty training (Rahimi & Azimi, 2012). As of now, there is no formal, accredited psychiatric subspecialty program. Limited infrastructure and ongoing conflict have hindered the development of comprehensive psychiatry training programs.

## 4.2 Bangladesh

The first mental hospital in the country was established in Pabna in 1957. The first postgraduate psychiatry course in the form of Diploma in Psychological Medicine (DPM) was introduced in 1975 at the Institute of Postgraduate Medicine and Research (Arafat, 2020). The Doctor of Medicine (MD) in psychiatry was started at Bangladesh Medical University (formerly Bangabandhu Sheikh Mujib Medical University, BSMMU) in 1995. Postgraduate programs in Child and Adolescent Psychiatry were introduced, aimed at building capacity in this specialty. Child and adolescent psychiatry specialty course of 5 years duration runs at Bangladesh Medical University (MD in Child Psychiatry) and Bangladesh College of Physicians and Surgeons (BCPS) (Fellowship of the College of Physicians and Surgeons (FCPS). In 2016, the MD residency course in child and adolescent psychiatry was started at BSMMU (Arafat, 2020). Though postgraduate training provides exposure to multiple key domains of psychiatry, accredited specialty training programs are lacking.

## 4.3 Bhutan

The mental health infrastructure is limited in Bhutan, with a shortage of trained professionals and facilities dedicated to psychiatry. A 4-year postgraduate residency training program in psychiatry was started in 2019 in the Faculty of Post Graduate Medicine, Khesar Gyalpo University of Medical Sciences of Bhutan (KGUMSB) (Dorji, 2023). The need for specialty services is apparent from the increasing trend in mental health issues, including adolescent suicide and substance use disorders. With the establishment of PEMA Centre as the apex referral, research and training center, mental health training and services can be expected to pick up pace in the near future.

## 4.4 India

India has been the nation leading in psychiatry subspecialty courses in South Asia. Over the past two decades, several subspecialty training programs encompassing various domains of psychiatry have been introduced. While the Doctorate of Medicine (DM) programs (of 3 years duration) are limited, a range of postdoctoral fellowship (PDF) courses of 1 year duration encompassing diverse domains of psychiatry were started in public sector and private medical institutions (Table 19.2). The National Medical Commission has recently renamed the 1-year course as post postdoctoral certificate course, while only the 2 year courses can now be referred to as the postdoctoral fellowships course. Research reported that a substantial number of psychiatrists and psychiatry residents express a need for additional training and specialization in various subspecialties within the field (Singh et al., 2024). Participants not only opted for the available specialty course options but also proposed several additional ones, reflecting a wide range of interests.

The DM program in geriatric mental health was started in 2011 at the King George's Medical University, Lucknow. Subsequently, DM program in child and adolescent psychiatry was initiated at the National Institute of Mental Health and Neurosciences (NIMHANS), Bengaluru, in 2011, followed by another at the Post-Graduate Institute of Medical Education and Research (PGIMER, Chandigarh) in

**Table 19.2** Psychiatry subspecialty courses in India

| Course | Specialty |
|---|---|
| DM (3 year) | Addiction Psychiatry<br>Child & Adolescent Psychiatry<br>Forensic Psychiatry<br>Geriatric Psychiatry<br>Psychosomatic Medicine |
| PDF (1 year) | Acute care and emergency psychiatry<br>Addiction medicine<br>Child and adolescent psychiatry<br>Clinical neuropsychology<br>Clinical neurosciences & therapeutics in schizophrenia<br>Cognitive behavior therapy<br>Community mental health<br>Consultation-liaison psychiatry<br>Forensic psychiatry<br>Geriatric psychiatry<br>Integrative psychiatry<br>Molecular psychiatry<br>Neuropsychiatry<br>Non-invasive brain stimulation/neuromodulation<br>Obsessive compulsive disorder and related disorders<br>Psychiatric rehabilitation<br>Psychosexual medicine<br>Tele-psychiatry<br>Women's mental health |

*PDF* Postdoctoral fellowship, *DM* Doctorate of Medicine

2014. The first DM program in addiction medicine/psychiatry was started at PGIMER, Chandigarh, in 2014, which was followed by programs at NIMHANS (since 2015), National Drug Dependence Treatment Centre (NDDTC), All India Institute of Medical Sciences (AIIMS) New Delhi (since 2016), and AIIMS Gorakhpur (since 2024). In 2019, AIIMS Rishikesh also introduced DM in addiction psychiatry. However, due to a subsequent shortage of trained faculty, the program was discontinued. The other DM programs in the psychiatry subspecialty are in forensic Psychiatry at NIMHANS and in psychosomatic medicine at AIIMS, New Delhi.

Several 1-year specialty courses are available at multiple institutions in India in both the public and private sectors. The child and adolescent psychiatry fellowship course is offered at NIMHANS, Jawaharlal Institute of Postgraduate Medical Education and Research (JIPMER) Puducherry, King George's Medical University (KGMU) Lucknow, Christian Medical College (CMC) Vellore, Asha Hospital (Hyderabad), St. John's Medical College in Bengaluru, Indlas Hospitals, Vijayawada, Andhra Pradesh, and Sri Aurobindo University, Indore (Kommu & Jacob, 2020). Similarly, a 1-year specialty course in addiction psychiatry is available at NIMHANS, KGMU Lucknow, Lokopriya Gopinath Bordoloi Regional Institute of Mental Health (LGBRIMH), Tezpur, and Grant Government Medical College, Mumbai. The NIMHANS also offers PhD in several areas of psychiatry, including child and adolescent psychiatry, clinical neurosciences and clinical psychopharmacology and neurotoxicology.

## *4.5 The Maldives*

The Maldives currently lacks a formal postgraduate psychiatry residency program. However, the country has been actively working to enhance its mental health services through various initiatives and collaborations. The Human Resource Division, Ministry of Health, has identified the need for long-term training (PhD) in psychiatry subspecialties, including addiction psychiatry, child and adolescent psychiatry, and forensic psychiatry (Ministry of Health, 2023). The National Mental Health Strategic Action Plan (2025–2029), launched in February 2025, also emphasized on specialty training of health officers (Ministry of Health, 2025). However, the ground-level implementation of the plan will need concerted efforts of stakeholders and initiation of postgraduate psychiatry residency programs to begin with.

## *4.6 Nepal*

Nepal has made strides in general psychiatry education. Postgraduate psychiatry training has been in existence for over two decades, with multiple institutes providing education. However, the development of subspecialty training programs remains a significant area for growth. At present, psychiatry specialty training programs are not available in Nepal. Addressing this gap is crucial to meet the diverse mental health needs of the population. A significant number of psychiatrists express interest in a 1-year neuropsychiatry training program post-MD (Rai et al., 2020). Similarly, another study highlighted the willingness of psychiatrists to undergo higher training in child and adolescent psychiatry and psychotherapy (Karki et al., 2020; Rai et al., 2021). The only full-time CAP outpatient clinic operates at Kanti Children's Hospital in Kathmandu. The absence of specialized training programs and limited resources hinders the development of psychiatry subspecialties in Nepal.

## 4.7 Pakistan

The Jinnah Postgraduate Medical Centre was the first fully accredited institution to offer a psychiatry residency training program in 1965 (Malik et al., 2021). Since then, psychiatry postgraduate courses have been available at various institutions. In 2014, the College of Physicians and Surgeons Pakistan (CPSP) approved the Child and Adolescent Psychiatry fellowships, making it the only subspecialty currently recognized by CPSP. The Aga Khan University (AKU) was the first to start a structured fellowship program in Child and Adolescent Psychiatry in 2016, focusing on addressing mental health disorders prevalent in the pediatric population (Younus, 2017). In 2022, the child psychiatry subspecialty fellowship was also started at the King Edward Medical University, Lahore. However, considering the treatment gap, more psychiatrists should be trained to handle child and adolescent psychiatric issues. Also, there is a need for specialty training in other domains like geriatric psychiatry, addiction psychiatry, etc., however, other accredited psychiatry specialty training programs are unavailable in the country. The patients falling in these domains are being managed by general practitioners or adult psychiatrists. Despite the widespread recognition of growing substance use-related problems in Pakistan, education and training in this specialty are lacking. Organizations like the International Society of Substance Use Professionals (ISSUP) Pakistan Chapter continue to organize training sessions in addiction (Saima Asghar, 2023). Similarly, despite the 1999 National Policy emphasizing the development of a workforce of healthcare professionals equipped to address the needs of older adults, including geriatricians and mental health specialists, its implementation has been insufficient. This has resulted in a pronounced shortage of specialized practitioners, with only a limited number of geriatricians and clinicians receiving formal training in old age psychiatry (Murad & Siraj, 2024).

## 4.8 Sri Lanka

In Sri Lanka, the Postgraduate Institute of Medicine (PGIM), operational since 1980 at the University of Colombo, is the primary institution responsible for postgraduate medical education, including psychiatry and its subspecialties (Gambheera,

**Table 19.3** Summary of specialty programs in Sri Lanka

| Domain | Program |
|---|---|
| Forensic Psychiatry | Board Certification in Forensic Psychiatry |
| Child and Adolescent Psychiatry | Board Certification in Child and Adolescent Psychiatry |
| Old Age Psychiatry (Geriatric Psychiatry) | Board Certification in Old Age Psychiatry |
| Addiction Psychiatry | Board Certification in Addiction Psychiatry |

2011). A comprehensive 5-year Doctor of Medicine (MD) in Psychiatry program leading to board certification as a specialist in psychiatry is designed to equip medical professionals with the necessary skills and knowledge to specialize in various areas of psychiatry, addressing the mental health needs of diverse populations in Sri Lanka. Board certification programs in the subspecialties, namely, forensic psychiatry, child and adolescent psychiatry, old age psychiatry (geriatric psychiatry), and addiction psychiatry, are in place (Table 19.3). It requires 24 months of local training in Sri Lanka and 12 months of training at an approved overseas center. Carrying out a research project, directly relevant to the concerned subject, is a mandatory requirement for certification. In order to meet international examination standards, the panel of examiners for the specialty psychiatry examination is constituted by the Board of Study in Psychiatry, a body sanctioned by the university senate. This panel comprises senior consultants and includes at least one examiner from either the Royal College of Psychiatrists (United Kingdom) or the Royal Australian and New Zealand College of Psychiatrists (Kathriarachchi et al., 2019).

## 5 Challenges in the Development of Psychiatry Subspecialty Courses in South Asia

There are multiple hurdles to the development of psychiatry subspecialty courses in South Asia. The foremost is the shortage of trained faculty and mentors, especially in small nations like the Maldives and Bhutan. Prolonged war and geopolitical turmoil have created an even direr situation in Afghanistan. Similar shortages of trained specialists and experts are evident throughout the region, particularly given the vast population they must serve (Tripathi et al., 2020). A substantial number of specialists often migrate to developed nations like the UK, the USA, or Australia, looking for better career prospects, resulting in a brain drain of skilled psychiatrists (Chandradasa & Champika, 2019). The training programs are thus confined to a few urban academic institutions. The other major issue is a lack of resources and infrastructure. Subspecialty training requires dedicated units with trained support staff, quality instruments, and a supply of medicines and other consumables, the availability of which is often limited or absent in public hospitals. It can severely limit the research and academic opportunities provided by the specialty training programs. The situation in South Asia presents a challenging reality, as the majority of countries in the region are classified as low and middle-income. Owing to limited mental health infrastructure, the government's efforts have predominantly been directed toward narrowing the mental health treatment gap by implementing training initiatives to develop a workforce of general psychiatrists. As a result, subspecialty training remains a matter of lower priority. Besides, psychiatry services in South Asia are overwhelmed by high patient loads, leaving little room for training in niche areas. In order to meet demand, most psychiatrists practice general psychiatry and have a limited time or incentive to pursue sub-specialization.

The lack of a standardized curriculum and its non-uniform implementation pose another crucial challenge. For instance, in India, the different institutes offering DM courses in addiction psychiatry have their own curricula. A uniformity in the training curricula, defined competencies, and evaluation patterns will help standardize the training and make it easier and simpler for other institutes to adopt and initiate programs. Also, licensing and recognition of subspecialties are not formalized in many national medical councils. In India, the postdoctoral fellowship courses in psychiatry subspecialties, offered by many institutes, are not yet recognized by the regulatory body, National Medical Commission (NMC).

Mental health policies often lack a roadmap for academic subspecialties. The emanating uncertainties regarding academic advancement and financial sustainability may deter those willing to pursue subspecialty courses (Narasimha et al., 2024). When health systems prioritize seniority over specialized qualifications in determining professional benefits and career advancement, psychiatrists may be less inclined to invest time in pursuing subspecialty training (Chandradasa & Champika, 2019).

## 6 Way Forward

The specialty programs should be based on the needs of the population and the healthcare system, and the evolving demands in the field of psychiatry. The institutes should be promoted to train specialists in the domains where there is an increased need for them, so that treatment gaps can be promptly reduced. The health policies and programs should endorse specialty training efforts through manpower and resource support. The relevant psychiatric societies and other stakeholders should advocate for the development of subspecialties, which is likely to benefit all in future. Aligning with the evidence-based approaches, competency-based training should be integral to the psychiatry subspecialty training programs. The national medical boards formalizing the training and certification in subspecialties will enhance the quality of training and implementation of the training programs in new institutes. Providing incentives for trained specialists to pursue and remain in academic careers could help expand the pool of qualified experts capable of leading and sustaining specialty training programs.

# 7 Conclusion

Psychiatry has evolved from a branch of medicine into a distinct and complex specialty, driven by advances in research and clinical insights. This growth has led to the emergence of subspecialties, including child and adolescent psychiatry, addiction psychiatry, forensic psychiatry, and geriatric psychiatry. In South Asia, countries like India and Sri Lanka have made progress in developing subspecialty training, while others face challenges due to resource constraints, inadequate infrastructure, and a shortage of trained professionals. Thus, the development of structured subspecialty training programs is both timely and essential, as general psychiatrists can no longer cover the full spectrum of mental health conditions. Such initiatives are critical to building a skilled, responsive, and sustainable mental health workforce capable of meeting the region's diverse and growing needs.

# References


ACGME. (2025). *Overview—Psychiatry*. Accreditation Council for Graduate Medical Education. https://www.acgme.org/specialties/psychiatry/overview/

American Board of Medical Specialties. (2023). *ABMS Board Certification Report 2022-2023*. American Board of Medical Specialties. https://www.abms.org/abms-board-certification-report/

Arafat, S. M. Y. (2020). The current status of psychiatric education in Bangladesh. *Asian Journal of Psychiatry, 52*, 102108. https://doi.org/10.1016/j.ajp.2020.102108

Brook, P. (1982). The British model of postgraduate training in general psychiatry. *Academic Psychiatry, 6*(3), 131–143. https://doi.org/10.1007/BF03399848

Cannon, M., Power, E., Cotter, D., & Hill, M. (2022). Youth psychiatry: Time for a new subspecialty within psychiatry. *World Psychiatry, 21*(1), 2–3. https://doi.org/10.1002/wps.20923

Chandradasa, M., & Champika, L. (2019). Subspecialisation in postgraduate psychiatry and implications for a resource-limited specialised child and adolescent mental health service. *Academic Psychiatry, 43*(1), 135–139. https://doi.org/10.1007/s40596-018-0920-8

Dorji, C. (2023). Addressing mental health in Bhutan. *The Druk Journal, 9*(1), 4–14.

Gambheera, H. (2011). The evolution of psychiatric services in Sri Lanka. *South Asian Journal of Psychiatry, 2*(1), 25–27.

Hersov, L. (1986). Child psychiatry in Britain--the last 30 years. *Journal of Child Psychology and Psychiatry, 27*(6), 781–801. https://doi.org/10.1111/j.1469-7610.1986.tb00201.x

Isaac, M. (2011). Mental health services in South Asia: Past, present and future. *South Asian Journal of Psychiatry, 2*(1), 4–11.

Karki, U., Rai, Y., Dhonju, G., Sharma, E., Jacob, P., Kommu, J. V. S., & Seshadri, S. P. (2020). Child and adolescent psychiatry training in Nepal: Early career psychiatrists' perspective. *Child and Adolescent Psychiatry and Mental Health, 14*(1), 13. https://doi.org/10.1186/s13034-020-00319-5

Kathriarachchi, S. T., Seneviratne, V. L., & Amarakoon, L. (2019). Development of mental health care in Sri Lanka: Lessons learned. *Taiwanese Journal of Psychiatry, 33*(2), 55. https://doi.org/10.4103/TPSY.TPSY_15_19

Kommu, J. V. S., & Jacob, P. (2020). Specialty training in child and adolescent psychiatry in India. *European Child & Adolescent Psychiatry, 29*(1), 89–93. https://doi.org/10.1007/s00787-019-01407-4

Malik, W. A., Arnold, C., Vithiananthan, A., & Hassan, T. (2021). Forensic psychiatry in Pakistan: An update. *International Journal of Risk and Recovery, 4*(2), 42–50. https://doi.org/10.15173/ijrr.v4i2.4622

Ministry of Health. (2023). *Training Requirement 2024-2026*. Ministry of Health, Republic of Maldives. https://health.gov.mv/en/publications/training-requirement-2024-2026

Ministry of Health. (2025). *National Mental Health Strategic Action Plan 2025-2029*. Ministry of Health. https://health.gov.mv/storage/uploads/7wzEkvoW/bwjwjfot.pdf

Murad, S., & Siraj, S. (2024). Bridging the void: Unraveling mental health policies for the older adults in Pakistan's tapestry – A literature review. *Journal of Clinical Psychology and Neurology, 2*(2), 1–4. https://doi.org/10.61440/JCPN.2024.v2.17

Naeem, F., & Ayub, M. (2004). Psychiatric training in Pakistan. *Medical Education Online, 9*(1), 4369. https://doi.org/10.3402/meo.v9i.4369

Narasimha, V. L., Suhas, S., Kishor, M., Dixit, A., & Murthy, P. (2024). Advances in psychiatry training and faculty development in India. *Indian Journal of Psychological Medicine, 46*(5), 391–399. https://doi.org/10.1177/02537176241284348

NHS England. (2024, April 27). *Overview of Higher Training | Workforce, training and education | NHS England*. NHS England | Workforce, Training and Education | Medical Hub. https://medical.hee.nhs.uk/medical-training-recruitment/medical-specialty-training/psychiatry/higher-psychiatry-training/overview-of-higher-psychiatry-training/overview-of-higher-training

Rahimi, Y. A., & Azimi, S. (2012). War and the crisis of mental health in Afghanistan. *International Psychiatry, 9*(3), 55–57.

Rai, Y., Karki, U., & Pinto da Costa, M. (2021). Psychotherapy training in Nepal: Views of early career psychiatrists. *BJPsych International, 18*(2), E6. https://doi.org/10.1192/bji.2020.50

Rai, Y., Karki, U., Thapaliya, S., & Molina, R. (2020). Neuropsychiatry training in Nepal: Experiences of trainees and psychiatrists. *Journal of Psychiatrists' Association of Nepal, 9*(1), 23–28. https://doi.org/10.3126/jpan.v9i1.31312

Saima Asghar. (2023, February 27). *Training on UTC-1 "An Introduction to the Science of Addiction" organized by ISSUP Pakistan Chapter and Subhan Trust on February 2nd-4th, 2023 at the Institute of Souther Punjab/University, Multan-Pakistan. | Global Recovery Network*. ISSUP in Pakistan. https://www.globalrecoverynetwork.org/national-chapters/issup-in-pakistan/news/2023-02/training-utc-1-introduction-science-addiction-organized-issup-in-pakistan

Sharma, S. (2010). Postgraduate training in psychiatry in India. *Indian Journal of Psychiatry, 52*(Suppl 1), S89. https://doi.org/10.4103/0019-5545.69219

Sharma, V. (2011). Mental health in Nepal. *South Asian Journal of Psychiatry, 2*(1), 23–24.

Singh, A., Kishor, M., & Kar, S. K. (2024). A survey among psychiatrists to assess the need for psychiatry sub/super-specialization courses in India. *Indian Journal of Psychological Medicine, 46*(5), Article 5. https://doi.org/10.1177/02537176241273934

Tripathi, R., Singh, S., & Bhad, R. (2020). The need, scope, challenges, and potential solutions for enhancing addiction psychiatry training in India. *Indian Journal of Psychiatry, 62*(6), 728. https://doi.org/10.4103/psychiatry.IndianJPsychiatry_355_19

Younus, S. (2017). 58.4 Child and adolescent mental health services in Pakistan. *Journal of the American Academy of Child & Adolescent Psychiatry, 56*(10), S85. https://doi.org/10.1016/j.jaac.2017.07.333

# Chapter 20
# Training for Research in Psychiatry

**Sujita Kumar Kar**

**Abstract** Psychiatry, as a discipline of medicine, is evolving rapidly. Despite the stigma, several challenges still exist as students opt for psychiatry as a career. Research in psychiatry has significantly grown in recent years across the globe. Interest in psychiatric research has also increased among medical students and researchers. However, there is a gross lack of formal training for research for undergraduate medical students from low- and middle-income countries (LAMICs) in the field of psychiatry, although this situation has been changing in recent years. This chapter provides an overview of training for research in psychiatry with a specific focus on South Asia.

**Keywords** Research · Psychiatry · Psychiatry training · Psychiatry teaching · Medical education

## 1 Introduction

Research is an integral part of academics. In the twenty-first century, people are developing an inclination to rely on evidence. Several decades ago, research was considered to be a sophisticated need or a higher-order need in the medical education more so in south Asia. However, in recent decades, research has been considered an integral component of medical education. Good quality of research is considered an important factor to academic excellence (Ellemers, 2021). Research facilitates collaboration, development, and strengthening of an organization. It also gives an identity to the researcher, institution, and nation at large (Hall et al., 2018).

S. K. Kar (✉)
Department of Psychiatry, King George's Medical University, Lucknow, Uttar Pradesh, India
e-mail: sujitakumarkar@kgmcindia.edu



S. K. Kar et al. (eds.), *Teaching and Training in Psychiatry in South Asia*, South Asian Perspectives in Mental Health and Psychology,
https://doi.org/10.1007/978-981-95-1845-6_20

Medical education is a form of higher education in which all content related to health is developed through research. Over the past several decades, academic scientists have competed significantly to avail research funding (Edwards & Roy, 2017). There is a significant increase in research publications from the science and engineering background in recent years. Publication is considered as a marker of research output.

Every year, around 1.5 million publications in the field of biomedicine and life sciences are being added to the PubMed database (González-Márquez et al., 2024). A recent database of the United States reports that in the year 2022, about 3.3 million articles from science and engineering background were published in the *Scopus* database (NCSES, 2023). Majority of the publications (approximately 86%) are by the authors of higher-income and upper-middle-income countries; China, the United States, and India being the top three countries in terms of the research output (NCSES, 2023). A significant increase in medical students' research has been seen in recent decades (Wickramasinghe et al., 2013), indicating an increasing interest of medical students in research. Psychiatry is one of the common areas that interests medical students to pursue research (Wickramasinghe et al., 2013). This chapter aims to discuss the relevance and contexts of research in psychiatry and the scope of training in research in psychiatry.

## 2 Research in Psychiatry: Relevance

The burden of mental illnesses is high across the globe. As per a recent estimate, 16% of the global disability-adjusted life years (DALYs) are due to mental illnesses in the year 2019 (Arias et al., 2022). The causes of mental illnesses are multifactorial. For many mental illnesses, the precise causes are poorly understood. Similarly, the treatment targets for mental illnesses are multiple. Research in mental illness over the past several decades has helped in understanding the pathogenesis, treatment, and outcome of mental illnesses. Hence, there is a potential role of research in psychiatry to generate more evidence and bring more clarity to the conceptualization of mental illnesses (Abrams et al., 2003).

The awareness about mental illness and the importance of mental health are increasing significantly (Abrams et al., 2003). It is expected to increase the interest for research in mental health and mental illnesses. As stigma is a major barrier to deal with mental illnesses globally (Ahad et al., 2023; CORRIGAN & WATSON, 2002; Gaiha et al., 2020), researchin mental health will give more clarity to the understanding about mental illnesses and is expected to reduce stigma associated with mental illnesses (Ahad et al., 2023; Corbière et al., 2012; Hajizadeh et al., 2024).

Research gives an opportunity to generate more evidences that help in improvising mental healthcare (Abrams et al., 2003). For example, research in neuromodulation techniques in psychiatric disorder suggest that several neuromodulation techniques can be useful in the treatment of various psychiatric disorders and these evidences influence the treatment guidelines and finding effective and more acceptable solutions for mental illnesses (Kar & Kl, 2023; Vlaicu & Bustuchina Vlaicu, 2020).

Research is an important component of academics which gives job satisfaction, developing a research portfolio, and giving an identity or recognition to the researcher (Sinclair et al., 2025). Research is a part of the academic curriculum when people pursue higher education in psychiatry (for example: MD, DM, Fellowship, or PhD degree) (Sagar & Sarkar, 2017; Sinclair et al., 2025). Faculty promotion in medical institutions largely depends on experience and research publications. The requirement for research publications for the promotion of medical faculty is observed in the majority of countries worldwide (Fang et al., 2000; D. B. Rice et al., 2020; Xierali et al., 2021; Yeo et al., 2024).

An important domain of psychiatric research is clinical trials. Clinical trials can be researcher-initiated, agency-sponsored, or pharmaceutical industry sponsored. A significant number of drug trials in developing and underdeveloped countries were industry sponsored drug trials. Clinical trials are the researches that often target to measure safety and efficacy of drugs or devices. Additionally, these trials also explore the role of a medication or device or intervention in various psychiatric conditions (Carrier et al., 2017; Everitt & Wessely, 2008; March et al., 2005).

Research helps in developing practice guidelines and policies in mental health (Sinclair et al., 2025). Research helps in infrastructure development, enhancing collaboration and strengthening partnerships in mental health which is likely to impact the mental health service delivery (Sinclair et al., 2025). Research leads to the development of innovative technologies, effective medications, and treatment approaches for the management of psychiatric disorders.

## 3 Research in Psychiatry: Contexts

It has been seen that understanding the context is highly important in psychiatric care, as it strongly influences the outcome (Carpenter-Song, 2015). Similarly, it is important to understand the contexts of research in psychiatry, as this helps in understanding the outcome and its utility in clinical practice. A large amount of research in psychiatry is carried out to understand the psychopathologies, conceptualizing the psychopathologies, disease burden and its impact, and developing and facilitating evidence-based practices (Marková & Berrios, 2016).

Research in psychiatry generates evidence, and the level of evidence depends on the nature of research conducted (Ghaemi, 2023; Löhrs et al., 2020; M. J. Rice, 2008). A recent research attempted to evaluate the levels of evidences of various psychiatric interventions and it was found that nearly 24.5% of the evidence is labeled as level A evidence (Löhrs et al., 2020).

Research in psychiatry helps in the appropriate classification of psychiatric disorders and placement of diagnostic categories in justified places in the diagnostic system (Stein & Seedat, 2007). As evidence are emerging regarding the role of molecular and micromolecular neuronal changes in psychiatric disorder, neurogenetics, epigenetics, neuroimaging changes, and cognitive-affective-behavioral changes in psychiatric disorder, more research is being conducted in these domains to have an in-depth understanding about these aspects in psychiatric disorders (Stein & Seedat, 2007).

Certain psychiatric disorders are largely influenced by culture and are unique to a particular culture; popularly known as culture-bound syndromes (Kallivayalil et al., 2010). Research is required in these cultural contexts to understand the explanatory models of the culture-specific psychopathologies and designing culture sensitive interventions (Kar et al., 2021, 2022a).

## 4 Research Training in Psychiatry

The number of students enrolled on the medical streams has increased significantly. Recent data from India mentions that there is a significant increase in medical undergraduates and psychiatry postgraduates in the country in recent years (Kar et al., 2023). Slowly, research is entering the medical curriculum as an essential component rather than being an optional component. Understanding the relevance of research in medical education, the National Medical Commission in India has made it mandatory to pursue a Basic Course in Biomedical Research (BCBR) for all medical postgraduates and faculties (National Medical Commission, 2020). Though it is not specific to psychiatric research; but it gives an orientation to the students and teachers in basic research methodologies. Research conducted on participants who completed the BCBR course module shows that the training improved the orientation toward research, more research submissions, and ultimately increasing the research output (Joshi et al., 2024; Singh et al., 2024). The National Institute of Health (NIH) is one of the largest research agencies in the world, which facilitates biomedical research in the USA and many other countries. It provides training in research as well (Zerhouni, 2005). Other important international organizations like the National Institute of Mental Health (NIMH), National Institute of Drug Abuse (NIDA), National Institute of Alcohol Abuse and Alcoholism (NIAAA), and National Institutes of Neurological Disorders and Stroke (NINDS) invest for mental health-related research (Abrams et al., 2003).

For the research training of undergraduate medical students, an elective research training exposure has been recommended in the competency-based medical education (CBME) module, recently implemented in India (Chatterjee & Kar, 2023; Kar & Singh, 2024). Similarly, CBME modules have been implemented for medical trainees in various countries (Ai Li et al., 2023; Gupta & Menon, 2022; Harris et al., 2010). To promote research among the medical undergraduate students, the Indian Council of Medical Research (ICMR) provides the ICMR-Short-Term Studentship (ICMR-STS) grant, which provides medical undergraduate students to learn research by being associated with a faculty mentor, by conducting a research study in a short-stimulated time (ICMR, 2024). It has been found that participation in the STS initiative enhances the research learning of the students (Gore et al., 2014).

This initiative is a unique one in the region of South Asia. It gives a window to pursue psychiatry research.

As in the postgraduate (MD-Psychiatry) curriculum, dissertation/thesis is mandatory in several countries, and the students learn research under the mentorship of psychiatry teachers/guides (Sagar & Sarkar, 2017). The ICMR has also started small research grants for best postgraduate thesis work, right at the level of synopsis submission for first-year postgraduates.

Globally, training in psychiatric research is an essential part of the medical university/institution curriculum. Several reputed international medical institutes provide structured research training in psychiatry to their trainees (Harvard Medical School, 2025; Johns Hopkins School of Medicine, 2025; NYU Grossman School of Medicine, 2025; University of Pittsburgh, 2017; Washington University School of Medicine, 2025; Yale School of Medicine, 2025). The World Psychiatric Association which is one of the largest global bodies of mental health professionals also provides opportunities for training in psychiatric research, including research training in various sub-specialties of psychiatry, like child and adolescent psychiatry (Kindler et al., 2023). A unique initiative has been taken in India to enhance psychiatry teaching and research in psychiatry in recent years. Indian Teachers of Psychiatry-Minds United Scholarship for Teachers (IToP MUST) Enrich Research Grant is an initiative by a public charitable trust to empower early career psychiatry teachers in education research (IToP, 2021; Kar et al., 2022b; Kishor, 2022; Kishor et al., 2023; Verma et al., 2024). This initiative has been reviewed and appears to have given robust thrust to research in psychiatry education in recent years (Verma et al., 2024).

The psychiatry training overall (including research training) is largely affected in South Asia, due to limited hours of teaching hours of psychiatry for undergraduate students, paucity of psychiatry teachers, lack of motivation of undergraduate students to attend psychiatry teaching, insufficient teaching facilities for postgraduate trainees in psychiatry, lack of formal and uniform standards for teaching, and increased clinical workload on the psychiatry departments (Arafat et al., 2021; Isaac et al., 2018; Kallivayalil & Enara, 2021). It is not only the treatment gap for psychiatric disorders that is significant in the LMICs; the teaching and training gap in psychiatry is also substantial. Regarding the training in psychiatry research, the gap is expected to be much bigger (Isaac et al., 2018; Kallivayalil & Enara, 2021). Similar challenges in psychiatry teaching and possibly, training in psychiatry research, are being encountered in other countries as well at different levels (Hermans, 2020; Okasha & Shaker, 2020).

As the field of research is expanding, manipulations and unethical practices in research are also increasing (Edwards & Roy, 2017). Several publishing houses give a platform for fraudulent research work for publication and make huge profits. Such research contaminates evidence and are threats to the growth of science (Beall, 2012; Kurt, 2018; Nagarkar, 2024; Parker et al., 2024). The students and researchers also need to understand the research ethics and publication ethics as a part of their research training.

## 5 Future Directions

Understanding the existing challenges in psychiatry research training is an essential guiding force for framing the blueprint for psychiatry research training. The major challenges encountered in the current scenario related to psychiatry research training are:

- Research is not an integral part of undergraduate psychiatry curriculum
- Training in psychiatry research is limited to only few institutes (mostly self-initiated)
- Lack of formal, uniform, standardized training curriculum for psychiatry research
- Challenges related to human resources, infrastructures, and funding (grants)

Initiatives that need to be taken to overcome these issues in the coming days may help in enhancing psychiatry research training, which may ultimately influence psychiatry research outputs. Recently, some initiatives have been taken to enhance the teaching and training skills of the psychiatry teachers, which is expected to enhance the psychiatry research training as well (Kishor & Isaac, 2024; Narasimha et al., 2024). It has been realized that psychiatry teachers should have a good understanding of research, so that they can effectively train and teach about psychiatry research. Hence, emphasis should be also given to create good trainers for psychiatry research by enhancing the research skills of psychiatry teachers (Williams, 2024). It has been seen that involvement of resident doctors in psychiatry research also increases their research acumen and understanding (Roane et al., 2009). Good mentoring of the faculty members, departmental support, interest and initiatives taken by the psychiatry trainee enhances the output of psychiatry research (Dewan et al., 2016). So, initiatives need to be taken in enhancing these domains as well. Figure 20.1 summarizes some recommendations to facilitate training in psychiatry research.

## 6 Conclusion

The research needs in psychiatry are enormous, and the amount of research in mental health is rapidly expanding. Despite the increase in psychiatry research, there are substantial deficits in training opportunities for psychiatry research. Increasing training opportunities in psychiatry research is expected to meet the growing research needs in the field.

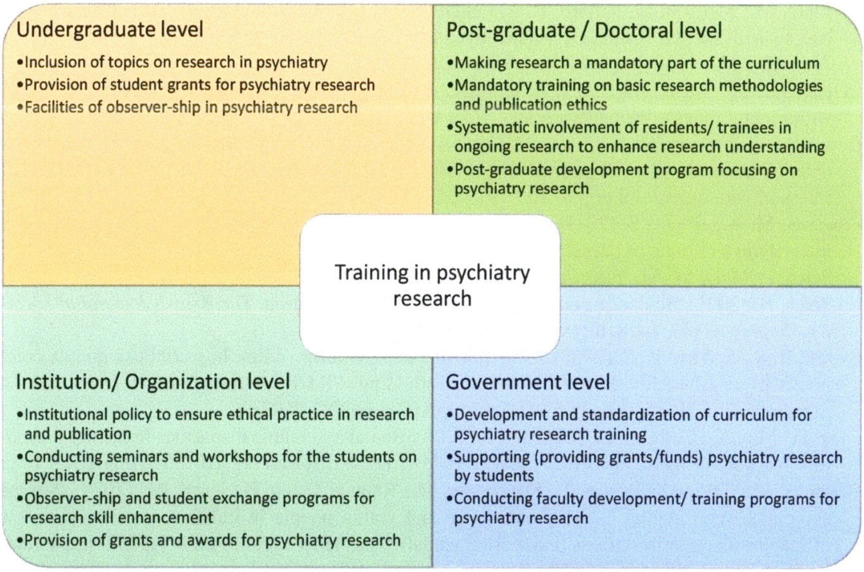


**Fig. 20.1** Recommendations to facilitate training in psychiatry research

## References


Abrams, M. T., Patchan, K., & Boat, T. F. (2003). *Research training in psychiatry residency: Strategies for reform*. National Academies Press (US). https://www.ncbi.nlm.nih.gov/books/NBK222024/

Ahad, A. A., Sanchez-Gonzalez, M., & Junquera, P. (2023). Understanding and addressing mental health stigma across cultures for improving psychiatric care: A narrative review. *Cureus, 15*(5), e39549. https://doi.org/10.7759/cureus.39549

Ai Li, E., Wilson, C. A., Davidson, J., Kwong, A., Kirpalani, A., & Wang, P. Z. T. (2023). Exploring perceptions of competency-based medical education in undergraduate medical students and faculty: A program evaluation. *Advances in Medical Education and Practice, 14*, 381–389. https://doi.org/10.2147/AMEP.S399851

Arafat, S. M. Y., Kar, S. K., Sharma, P., Marahatta, K., & Baminiwatta, A. K. A. B. (2021). A comparative analysis of psychiatry curriculum at undergraduate level of Bangladesh, India, Nepal, and Sri Lanka. *Indian Journal of Psychiatry, 63*(2), 184–188. https://doi.org/10.4103/psychiatry.IndianJPsychiatry_615_20

Arias, D., Saxena, S., & Verguet, S. (2022). Quantifying the global burden of mental disorders and their economic value. *eClinicalMedicine, 54*. https://doi.org/10.1016/j.eclinm.2022.101675

Beall, J. (2012). Predatory publishers are corrupting open access. *Nature, 489*(7415), Article 7415. https://doi.org/10.1038/489179a

Carpenter-Song, E. (2015). Putting meaning into medicine: Why context matters in psychiatry. *Epidemiology and Psychiatric Sciences, 24*(4), 292–295. https://doi.org/10.1017/S2045796015000475

Carrier, F., Banayan, D., Boley, R., & Karnik, N. (2017). Ethical challenges in developing drugs for psychiatric disorders. *Progress in Neurobiology, 152*, 58–69.

Chatterjee, S., & Kar, S. K. (2023). Undergraduate research elective under competency-based medical education (CBME) in India: Challenges and directions. *Indian Journal of Psychological Medicine, 45*(5), 548–551. https://doi.org/10.1177/02537176231165219

Corbière, M., Samson, E., Villotti, P., & Pelletier, J.-F. (2012). Strategies to fight stigma toward people with mental disorders: Perspectives from different stakeholders. *The Scientific World Journal, 2012*, 1–10. https://doi.org/10.1100/2012/516358

CORRIGAN, P. W., & WATSON, A. C. (2002). Understanding the impact of stigma on people with mental illness. *World Psychiatry, 1*(1), 16–20.

Dewan, M., Silberman, E., & Kramer, M. (2016). Psychiatric research. In N. R. Rao & L. W. Roberts (Eds.), *International medical graduate physicians: A guide to training* (pp. 171–183). Springer International. https://doi.org/10.1007/978-3-319-39460-2_12

Edwards, M. A., & Roy, S. (2017). Academic research in the 21st century: Maintaining scientific integrity in a climate of perverse incentives and hypercompetition. *Environmental Engineering Science, 34*(1), 51–61. https://doi.org/10.1089/ees.2016.0223

Ellemers, N. (2021). Science as collaborative knowledge generation. *The British Journal of Social Psychology, 60*(1), 1–28. https://doi.org/10.1111/bjso.12430

Everitt, B. S., & Wessely, S. (2008). *Clinical trials in psychiatry*. Wiley. https://books.google.com/books?hl=en&lr=&id=aE8IOfMUo9QC&oi=fnd&pg=PR5&dq=clinical+trials+psychiatric+drugs&ots=BbC7Bm5rly&sig=bN8P6zChuIpAIOxrwnjO_UYRTuY

Fang, D., Moy, E., Colburn, L., & Hurley, J. (2000). Racial and ethnic disparities in faculty promotion in academic medicine. *JAMA, 284*(9), 1085–1092. https://doi.org/10.1001/jama.284.9.1085

Gaiha, S. M., Taylor Salisbury, T., Koschorke, M., Raman, U., & Petticrew, M. (2020). Stigma associated with mental health problems among young people in India: A systematic review of magnitude, manifestations and recommendations. *BMC Psychiatry, 20*(1), 538. https://doi.org/10.1186/s12888-020-02937-x

Ghaemi, S. N. (2023). Levels of evidence. In S. N. Ghaemi (Ed.), *A clinician's guide to statistics in mental health* (2nd ed., pp. 10–13). Cambridge University Press. https://doi.org/10.1017/9781108887526.004

González-Márquez, R., Schmidt, L., Schmidt, B. M., Berens, P., & Kobak, D. (2024). The landscape of biomedical research. *Patterns, 5*(6), 100968. https://doi.org/10.1016/j.patter.2024.100968

Gore, C. R., Jadhav, S. L., Dubhashi, S. P., Buch, A. C., & Chandanwale, S. S. (2014). Assessment of the impact of short term studentship program on attitude of undergraduate medical students toward future research. *Medical Journal of Dr. D.Y. Patil Vidyapeeth, 7*(6), 696. https://doi.org/10.4103/0975-2870.144847

Gupta, S., & Menon, V. (2022). Psychiatry training for medical students: A global perspective and implications for India's competency-based medical education curriculum. *Indian Journal of Psychiatry, 64*(3), 240–251. https://doi.org/10.4103/indianjpsychiatry.indianjpsychiatry_187_22

Hajizadeh, A., Amini, H., Heydari, M., & Rajabi, F. (2024). How to combat stigma surrounding mental health disorders: A scoping review of the experiences of different stakeholders. *BMC Psychiatry, 24*(1), 782. https://doi.org/10.1186/s12888-024-06220-1

Hall, K. L., Vogel, A. L., Huang, G. C., Serrano, K. J., Rice, E. L., Tsakraklides, S. P., & Fiore, S. M. (2018). The science of team science: A review of the empirical evidence and research gaps on collaboration in science. *The American Psychologist, 73*(4), 532–548. https://doi.org/10.1037/amp0000319

Harris, P., Snell, L., Talbot, M., & Harden, R. M. (2010). Competency-based medical education: Implications for undergraduate programs. *Medical Teacher, 32*(8), 646–650. https://doi.org/10.3109/0142159X.2010.500703

Harvard Medical School. (2025). *Research Training Programs | Department of Psychiatry*. https://psych.hms.harvard.edu/research-training-programs

Hermans, M. H. M. (2020). Education in psychiatry in Western Europe. *International Review of Psychiatry (Abingdon, England), 32*(2), 133–139. https://doi.org/10.1080/09540261.2019.1657810

ICMR. (2024). *Short-Term Studentship (STS) | Indian Council of Medical Research | Government of India*. https://www.icmr.gov.in/short-term-studentship-sts

Isaac, M., Ahmed, H. U., Chaturvedi, S. K., Hopwood, M. J., Javeed, A., Kanba, S., Mufti, A. A., Maramis, A., Samaniego, R. M., Udomratn, P., Yanling, H., Zainal, N. Z., & Sartorius, N. (2018). Postgraduate training in psychiatry in Asia. *Current Opinion in Psychiatry, 31*(5), 396–402. https://doi.org/10.1097/YCO.0000000000000444

IToP. (2021). *INDIAN TEACHERS OF PSYCHIATRY.* http://indianteachersofpsychiatry.com/about/

Johns Hopkins School of Medicine. (2025). *Postdoctoral Fellowships and Research Training.* https://www.hopkinsmedicine.org/psychiatry/education/fellowships

Joshi, K. J., Singhal, S., & Gupta, S. (2024). Impact of basic course in biomedical research (BCBR) on medical teachers and postgraduate students across India: A cross-sectional survey-based study. *Cureus, 16*(6) https://www.cureus.com/articles/250431-impact-of-basic-course-in-biomedical-research-bcbr-on-medical-teachers-and-postgraduate-students-across-india-a-cross-sectional-survey-based-study.pdf

Kallivayalil, R. A., Chadda, R. K., & Mezzich, J. E. (2010). Indian psychiatry: Research and international perspectives. *Indian Journal of Psychiatry, 52*(Suppl 1), S38–S42. https://doi.org/10.4103/0019-5545.69205

Kallivayalil, R. A., & Enara, A. (2021). Education and training in psychiatry in South Asian countries. *Asia-Pacific Psychiatry: Official Journal of the Pacific Rim College of Psychiatrists, 13*(4), e12494. https://doi.org/10.1111/appy.12494

Kar, S. K., Arafat, S. M. Y., & Menon, V. (2021). A bibliometric analysis of Dhat syndrome. *Psychiatry International, 2*(4), Article 4. https://doi.org/10.3390/psychiatryint2040029

Kar, S. K., Arafat, S. M. Y., Menon, V., Sharma, P., Das, A., Perera, S., & Shankar, A. (2022a). A bibliometric analysis of Koro syndrome. *Global Psychiatry Archieves, 5*(1), 36–41. https://doi.org/10.52095/gp.2022.4460.1039

Kar, S. K., Dere, S. S., Mishra, D. K., & Das, G. (2022b). Training of psychiatry teachers on teaching skills: Needs, innovations and initiatives. *Asian Journal of Psychiatry, 72*, 103108. https://doi.org/10.1016/j.ajp.2022.103108

Kar, S. K., & Kl, V. (2023). Newer neuromodulation techniques for psychiatric disorders: A 2023 update. *Indian. Journal of Clinical Psychiatry, 3*(01), Article 01. https://doi.org/10.54169/ijocp.v3i01.70

Kar, S. K., Kumari, B., & Singh, V. (2023). Undergraduate psychiatry teaching and learning in India: A bumpy ride. *Indian Journal of Clinical Psychiatry, 3*(02), Article 02. https://doi.org/10.54169/ijocp.v3i02.96

Kar, S. K., & Singh, A. (2024). Research elective under CBME: A teacher's perspective reflections on research elective under CBME. *Indian Journal of Psychological Medicine, 46*(5), 499–500. https://doi.org/10.1177/02537176231219445

Kindler, J., Kaess, M., Eliez, S., Cosentino, M., Liebrand, M., & Klauser, P. (2023). Research training in child and adolescent psychiatry: Lack of motivation or a structural problem? *European Child & Adolescent Psychiatry, 32*(10), 1817–1820. https://doi.org/10.1007/s00787-023-02293-7

Kishor, M. (2022). A center for psychiatry education, faculty training, and research. *Indian Journal of Psychiatry, 64*(5), 518–519. https://doi.org/10.4103/indianjpsychiatry.indianjpsychiatry_170_22

Kishor, M., & Isaac, M. (2024). Can subject specific teacher's forum transform medical education in India? The IToP model. *Indian Journal of Psychiatry, 66*(12), 1081–1082. https://doi.org/10.4103/indianjpsychiatry.indianjpsychiatry_1060_24

Kishor, M., Menon, V., Vinay, H. R., Shah, H., Isaac, M., & Arun, M. (2023). The IToP-STEPS: A unique scholarship program to upskill teachers of psychiatry. *Indian Journal of Psychiatry, 65*(3), 381. https://doi.org/10.4103/indianjpsychiatry.indianjpsychiatry_428_22

Kurt, S. (2018). Why do authors publish in predatory journals? *Learned Publishing, 31*(2), 141–147.

Löhrs, L., Handrack, M., Kopp, I., Jessen, F., Wagner, E., Falkai, P., Röh, A., Strube, W., & Hasan, A. (2020). Evaluation of evidence grades in psychiatry and psychotherapy guidelines. *BMC Psychiatry, 20*, 503. https://doi.org/10.1186/s12888-020-02897-2

March, J. S., Silva, S. G., Compton, S., Shapiro, M., Califf, R., & Krishnan, R. (2005). The case for practical clinical trials in psychiatry. *American Journal of Psychiatry, 162*(5), 836–846. https://doi.org/10.1176/appi.ajp.162.5.836

Marková, I. S., & Berrios, G. E. (2016). Research in psychiatry: Concepts and conceptual analysis. *Psychopathology, 49*(3), 188–194. https://doi.org/10.1159/000447596

Nagarkar, S. (2024). 'Research paper mills': A factory outlet for dubious research. *Indian Journal of Medical Ethics, 9*(3), 222–227.

Narasimha, V. L., Suhas, S., Kishor, M., Dixit, A., & Murthy, P. (2024). Advances in psychiatry training and faculty development in India. *Indian Journal of Psychological Medicine, 46*(5), 391–399. https://doi.org/10.1177/02537176241284348

National Medical Commission. (2020). *Basic Course in Biomedical Research (BCBR) | NMC.* https://www.nmc.org.in/information-desk/for-students-to-study-in-india/online-research-methods-course/

NCSES. (2023). *Publications Output: U.S. Trends and International Comparisons* (NSB-2023-33). Article NSB-2023-33. https://ncses.nsf.gov/pubs/nsb202333/publication-output-by-region-country-or-economy-and-by-scientific-field

NYU Grossman School of Medicine. (2025). *Psychiatry Research Training*. NYU Langone Health. https://med.nyu.edu/departments-institutes/psychiatry/research/research-training

Okasha, T., & Shaker, N. (2020). Psychiatric education and training in Arab countries. *International Review of Psychiatry (Abingdon, England), 32*(2), 151–156. https://doi.org/10.1080/09540261.2019.1655717

Parker, L., Boughton, S., Bero, L., & Byrne, J. A. (2024). Paper mill challenges: Past, present, and future. *Journal of Clinical Epidemiology, 176*, 111549. https://doi.org/10.1016/j.jclinepi.2024.111549

Rice, D. B., Raffoul, H., Ioannidis, J. P. A., & Moher, D. (2020). *Academic criteria for promotion and tenure in biomedical sciences faculties: Cross sectional analysis of international sample of universities.* https://doi.org/10.1136/bmj.m2081

Rice, M. J. (2008). Evidence-based practice in psychiatric care: Defining levels of evidence. *Journal of the American Psychiatric Nurses Association, 14*(3), 181–187. https://doi.org/10.1177/1078390308321220

Roane, D. M., Inan, E., Haeri, S., & Galynker, I. I. (2009). Ensuring research competency in psychiatric residency training. *Academic Psychiatry, 33*(3), 215–220. https://doi.org/10.1176/appi.ap.33.3.215

Sagar, R., & Sarkar, S. (2017). Psychiatry research in India: Current status and future directions. *Journal of Mental Health and Human Behaviour, 22*(2), 77. https://doi.org/10.4103/0971-8990.229110

Sinclair, L. I., Ajram, L., Seneviratne, G., Tracy, D., & Critchley, H. (2025). Why does research matter to psychiatrists? *Brain and Neuroscience Advances, 9*, 23982128241305866. https://doi.org/10.1177/23982128241305866

Singh, A. P., Sayeli, V. K., Gera, S., Rao, G. H. J., & Rao, G. H. (2024). A cross-sectional study evaluating the basic course in biomedical research among medical postgraduates and teachers. *Cureus, 16*(7), e63551. https://doi.org/10.7759/cureus.63551.

Stein, D. J., & Seedat, S. (2007). From research methods to clinical practice in psychiatry: Challenges and opportunities in the developing world. *International Review of Psychiatry, 19*(5), 573–581. https://doi.org/10.1080/09540260701563536

University of Pittsburgh. (2017, December 13). *Psychiatry Research Pathway*. University of Pittsburgh, Department of Psychiatry. https://www.psychiatry.pitt.edu/research/research-training/psychiatry-research-pathway

Verma, N., Gupta, S., & Shatadal, P. (2024). Research in psychiatry medical education through "MUST Enrich Grant": A scoping review. *Indian Journal of Psychological Medicine, 46*(5), 382–390. https://doi.org/10.1177/02537176241265742

Vlaicu, A., & Bustuchina Vlaicu, M. (2020). New neuromodulation techniques for treatment resistant depression. *International Journal of Psychiatry in Clinical Practice, 24*(2), 106–115. https://doi.org/10.1080/13651501.2020.1728340

Washington University School of Medicine. (2025). Research training. *Psychiatry*. https://psychiatry.wustl.edu/education/residency-program/research-training-2/

Wickramasinghe, D. P., Perera, C. S., Senarathna, S., & Samarasekera, D. N. (2013). Patterns and trends of medical student research. *BMC Medical Education, 13*(1), 175. https://doi.org/10.1186/1472-6920-13-175

Williams, S. S. (2024). Fine-tuning postgraduate psychiatry training in South Asia. *Indian Journal of Psychological Medicine, 46*(5), 380–381. https://doi.org/10.1177/02537176241280284

Xierali, I. M., Nivet, M. A., Syed, Z. A., Shakil, A., & Schneider, F. D. (2021). Recent trends in faculty promotion in U.S. medical schools: Implications for recruitment, retention, and diversity and inclusion. *Academic Medicine, 96*(10), 1441. https://doi.org/10.1097/ACM.0000000000004188

Yale School of Medicine. (2025). *Research Training*. https://medicine.yale.edu/psychiatry/education/fellowships/resfell/

Yeo, M. M., Lim, S.-H., Kumar, A., & Thompson, A. W. (2024). Evaluation of the promotion criteria in an academic medical centre in Singapore. *BMJ Leader, 8*(3). https://doi.org/10.1136/leader-2023-000881

Zerhouni, E. A. (2005). US biomedical research basic, translational, and clinical sciences. *JAMA, 294*(11), 1352–1358. https://doi.org/10.1001/jama.294.11.1352

# Chapter 21
# Artificial Intelligence in Psychiatric Teaching and Training

**Ashlyn Tom, B. Sai Chaitanya Reddy, and Suresh Bada Math**

**Abstract** Artificial intelligence (AI) involves the development of systems or devices that simulate human intelligence. It encompasses a range of technologies which has real-world implications, including in the field of medicine. AI has also made remarkable progress in education over the past decades. The introduction of AI into medical education marks a major shift, particularly within psychiatry. This chapter aims to present a comprehensive evaluation of how AI technologies can be effectively used to enhance psychiatry teaching and training. It will examine how these tools can address current training gaps, offer scalable and adaptive learning experiences, and ultimately equip future mental health professionals to navigate the increasing complexity of modern psychiatric care. Additionally, the role of AI in assessment and medical administration will also be explored. While AI holds tremendous promise for transforming medical education, it is important to acknowledge several legal, ethical, and administrative challenges that need to be promptly addressed for its effective integration.

**Keywords** AI in medical education · AI in psychiatry · Virtual patients · Intelligent tutoring system · Chatbots in psychiatry education · Machine learning · Deep learning

A. Tom · B. S. C. Reddy (✉) · S. B. Math
Department of Psychiatry, National Institute of Mental Health and Neurosciences (NIMHANS), Bengaluru, Karnataka, India



S. K. Kar et al. (eds.), *Teaching and Training in Psychiatry in South Asia*, South Asian Perspectives in Mental Health and Psychology,
https://doi.org/10.1007/978-981-95-1845-6_21

# 1 Introduction

## *1.1 Artificial Intelligence*

The term *artificial intelligence* (AI) was first used by John McCarthy in 1955 in his Dartmouth Summer Research Project Proposal (McCarthy et al., 2006). AI deals with the theory and development of computer systems with intelligent behaviour. The field has grown exponentially over the years, with its significance becoming more prominent in the last decade. Long-term goals of AI generally include developing machines which can perform certain behaviours which are usually associated with humans. These behaviours include perception, reasoning and communication skills, learning, and the ability to act in complex environments. AI-based devices aim to emulate human intelligence, solve problems, and adapt through progressive learning algorithms, distinguishing them from traditional robotic and hardware automation. They make use of techniques that allow computers to mimic human cognition (Nilsson, 1998).

AI encompasses a range of technologies, including machine learning (ML), deep learning (DL), and natural language processing (NLP), and their interrelationships are illustrated in Fig. 21.1. NLP, a specialised branch of AI, deals with enabling

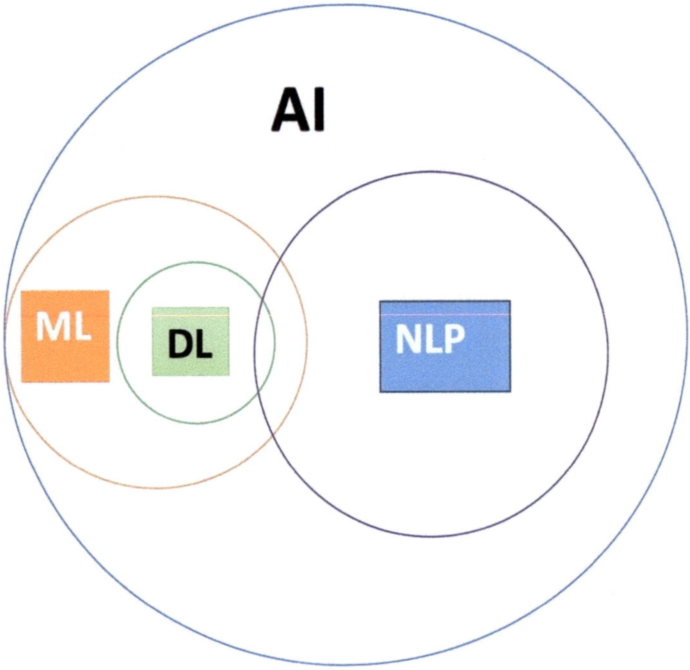


**Fig. 21.1** Relationship between Artificial Intelligence (AI), Natural Language Processing (NLP), Machine Learning (ML), and Deep Learning (DL)

machines to understand, interpret, and communicate using human language. Techniques within NLP include text mining, sentiment analysis, speech recognition, and machine translation. Large Language Models (LLMs), a type of AI algorithm, utilise deep learning and vast datasets to generate, summarise, and predict text. These models are highly effective across numerous NLP tasks, such as content creation, summarisation, rewriting, classification, and sentiment analysis.

AI has evolved significantly over the years from early rule-based systems to the current use of advanced ML and DL techniques. ML allows systems to learn from data and improve over time without being explicitly programmed. It is used to analyse data, make predictions, offer recommendations, and enhance system performance autonomously. DL, a subset of ML, is inspired by neural networks and excels at handling large volumes of unstructured data. It is capable of image classification, NLP, and outcome prediction by constructing intricate statistical models. Real-world applications of these technologies include virtual assistants, chatbots, and facial recognition systems (Alowais et al., 2023; Davenport & Kalakota, 2019).

## 2 Medical Education and AI

Medical education is a continuous process encompassing undergraduate, postgraduate, and specialisation training. It applies to a wide range of healthcare professionals, including doctors, nurses, and allied health workers (Chan & Zary, 2019). As healthcare contexts evolve, medical education must adapt to prepare future professionals for new challenges (Mir et al., 2023). The ever-expanding medical literature would require all professionals to update what they know and select the right information from the available multitude of options. Widespread and digital healthcare systems enable both doctors and patients to conveniently access biomedical data (Friedman et al., 2016). AI will be able to help in reducing the efforts required by clinicians to interpret digital data more efficiently and enhance their diagnostic capabilities.

However, in psychiatric assessments, human interaction is essential. Clinicians observe subtle nonverbal cues, facial expressions, and interpersonal dynamics that are difficult to fully replicate through technology. These human elements must be preserved in training. With the expanding use of AI in Psychiatry, the importance of these non-analytical, humanistic aspects of medicine needs to be further emphasised (Johnston, 2018).

In broader medicine, AI has reached to a point where machines can achieve radiological diagnoses with accuracy comparable to or even exceeding that of highly qualified specialists (Hamet & Tremblay, 2017). Similarly, AI has made remarkable progress in education over the past 25 years. Innovations such as "teacher bots" are being used to deliver content, provide feedback, and monitor student progress. This broader application in education shows great potential for addressing students' individual needs, identifying knowledge gaps, and enhancing personalised learning. By automating routine tasks, AI allows teachers to focus more on meaningful student engagement and improving the overall teaching process (Chan & Zary, 2019).

Future medical education must be redesigned to keep pace with these inevitable changes, considering the needs of learners who will operate within increasingly digital healthcare environments (Han et al., 2019). Identifying and implementing engaging teaching strategies is essential to capture and maintain the attention of this generation of learners (Mir et al., 2023).

## 3 AI and Psychiatry

The incorporation of AI into medical education marks a transformative shift, especially within psychiatry, where the depth of human interaction plays a critical role. Traditional training methods, such as role-play scenarios and the use of standardised patients, face challenges related to scalability, consistency, and their limited capacity to reflect the intricacies of psychiatric cases. Studies reveal that although most medical students believed that training in AI concepts would benefit their future practice, only very few of them reported receiving such training (Sami et al., 2025; Jackson et al., 2024). The PREDiCTOR (Phenotypes Reimagined to Define Clinical Treatment and Outcome Research) study, launched in September 2024, is a joint initiative by Mount Sinai Health System and International Business Machines (IBM) Research aimed at improving mental health care for young people. The study focuses on patients aged 15–30 and gathers data from clinical interviews, smartphone usage, and cognitive tests to create practical and affordable tools for predicting mental health outcomes. These tools are designed to help identify risks such as treatment dropouts, hospitalisations, and emergency room visits. By offering more precise and personalised insights, the study hopes to support better decision-making and improve the quality of care for young patients (Kahn, 2025; Raths, 2024). Early research into the use of AI simulations in psychiatric education has yielded encouraging outcomes. Although AI holds a wide range of applications in psychiatry, including machine learning for assessment, severity classification, robot-assisted interventions, and the use of avatars to enhance treatment adherence (Ray et al., 2022), this chapter aims to present a comprehensive exploration of how AI technologies can be effectively leveraged to enhance psychiatric education. It will examine how these tools can address current training gaps, offer scalable and adaptive learning experiences, and ultimately equip future psychiatrists to navigate the increasing complexity of psychiatric care with competence and confidence.

## 4 AI Tools for Teaching and Training

Studies found that residents who trained with AI-driven interactive case studies showed improved diagnostic accuracy compared to peers who used only traditional learning approaches. These findings indicate that AI simulations can play a pivotal role in bridging the gap between theoretical learning and real-world clinical practice, an essential component in the effective training of future psychiatrists (Ajluni, 2025).

AI-based tools in psychiatry education can be broadly categorised into those that facilitate direct instruction and those that support the learning process, as shown in Fig. 21.2. Intelligent Tutoring Systems (ITS) serve as virtual instructors, providing personalised and adaptive teaching experiences in a digital environment. On the other hand, supportive tools such as chatbots, virtual patients, and AI-powered educational games enhance the learning experience by fostering engagement, promoting clinical reasoning, and offering opportunities for interactive, experiential learning.

Virtual patients and augmented reality simulations enable students to engage in lifelike clinical situations safely, enhancing their practical learning without compromising patient safety, even for the rare or hard-to-find mental health conditions. Through interactive clinical cases, students can sharpen their diagnostic and problem-solving skills, and at the same time, the AI system can identify errors during these exercises, perform in-depth analysis, and guide learners towards correcting their mistakes (Mir et al., 2023).

By analysing large datasets and employing machine learning, AI can provide tailored content that aligns with each learner's pace and areas of difficulty, improving comprehension and engagement. Educators can also benefit from AI-powered analytics tools to gain insights into student performance and adjust their teaching strategies accordingly.

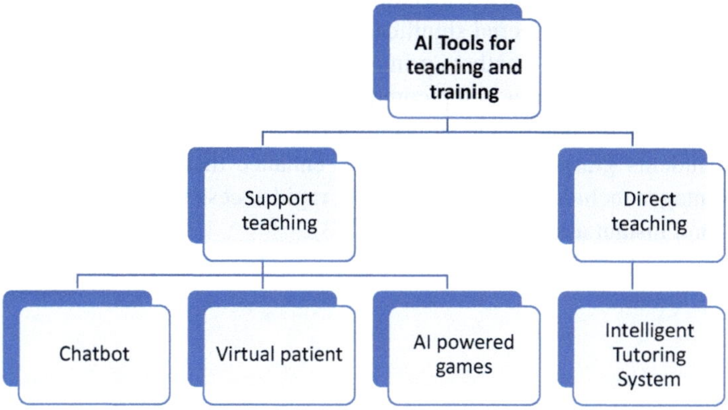


**Fig. 21.2** AI tools for teaching and training

# 5 Direct Teaching

## 5.1 Intelligent Tutoring Systems (ITS)

AI-driven ITS are adaptive educational tools designed to replicate the advantages of personalized, one-on-one human tutoring. These systems process large volumes of data related to a student's previous performance, preferences, and learning styles. Using this information, they identify areas where the student may be struggling and tailor the learning experience to fit the individual's needs and progress. In essence, ITS function like skilled human tutors by analysing student responses and guiding them through personalised, adaptive learning pathways (El Saadawi et al., 2008).

In medical education, ITS are commonly used to deliver course content, assess knowledge, strengths, and weaknesses, provide instant feedback, customise learning resources, and promote collaboration among students (Randhawa & Jackson, 2020). ITS can follow the learner in their thinking process and how they are solving problems to identify incorrect notions and additionally evaluate the learners' understanding (Mir et al., 2023).

# 6 Support Teaching

## 6.1 Chatbots

Chatbots are AI-driven systems designed to interpret, process, and respond to human queries using advanced NLP models. These systems retrieve information from online databases and generate human-like text, making them valuable tools for interactive conversations (Ghorashi et al., 2023). Given that most medical students use smartphones or tablets, chatbots can be easily deployed as web applications to support learning. Their ability to automate tasks such as summarising and analysing medical literature has garnered significant attention.

In medical education, chatbots primarily function as virtual teaching assistants, addressing students' queries and recommending study resources. They can serve as interactive tutors for preclinical subjects and as ward assistants in clinical settings, helping students grasp complex cases and enhance their decision-making skills. Key advantages include content integration, rapid access to information, multi-user support, and instant assistance (Sallam, 2023).

## 6.2 Virtual Patients

Virtual patients are computer-based simulations designed to replicate real-life clinical situations for training and educating healthcare professionals. These simulations are programmed to display realistic symptoms, react to students' clinical decisions, and offer dynamic, lifelike experiences. Learners act as healthcare providers, gathering information, forming differential diagnoses, planning treatments, and organising follow-up care. Virtual patients can simulate a wide range of medical conditions, exposing students to situations they are likely to encounter in actual practice. By interacting with these virtual scenarios, medical students can refine their communication and clinical reasoning skills within an engaging and realistic digital environment (Kononowicz et al., 2019).

AI can also simulate rare or complex psychiatric cases that may not be available in all training centres. This allows students to gain experience with a broader range of clinical presentations, enhancing their overall skills and knowledge (Ajluni, 2025).

The use of virtual reality (VR) further enhances immersion by creating a 3D simulated setting, typically experienced through head-mounted displays or specialised glasses (Kyaw et al., 2019). Meanwhile, augmented reality (AR) enriches the real world by overlaying digital elements through smartphones or other devices. The integration of VR and AR into medical training allows learners to navigate complex clinical scenarios more interactively, making the learning process both effective and engaging (Narayanan et al., 2023).

In Psychiatry, this can be used in the training of interviewing techniques as well as practicing psychotherapy techniques with real-time feedback.

## 6.3 AI-Powered Games

AI-powered educational games leverage data mining techniques to analyse player behaviour and enhance learning outcomes by building knowledge and skills. These games create personalised, immersive experiences by adapting difficulty levels and pacing based on individual performance (McCoy et al., 2016). Rewards incorporated games such as points and leader boards makes learning more enjoyable. Gamifying the educational process boosts student motivation, fosters collaboration, and leads to better academic outcomes. Additionally, these games offer a safe environment for practicing clinical decision-making and provide instant feedback, making them a valuable component of undergraduate medical training (Narayanan et al., 2023).

## 7 AI as Assistants for Students

In psychiatry, scales are standardised instruments designed to evaluate and quantify mental health symptoms, diagnoses, and treatment outcomes. Widely used in both clinical and research settings, these tools provide objective data that support accurate diagnosis, track treatment effectiveness, and assess symptom severity over time. Psychiatric scales vary in scope from brief screening questionnaires to in-depth assessments and are used to measure a broad spectrum of conditions such as depression, anxiety, psychosis, and overall psychological functioning. Utilising AI-powered tools as assistants in applying and interpreting these scales can aid in the process, thereby reducing time and effort (Weisenburger et al., 2024).

Core psychiatric competencies such as assessing the risk of suicide and violence remain heavily dependent on patient self-report. Tools widely regarded as the gold standard in suicide risk assessment are limited in scope as they rely solely on subjective accounts and do not incorporate additional data such as EMR entries, collateral information, or genetic insights. Despite its strengths, such tools have been criticised for failing to capture the full complexity of suicidal ideation and behaviour, prompting calls for a more comprehensive and data-integrated approach. AI, particularly deep learning, offers the potential to overcome these limitations by synthesising diverse data sources to make more accurate and holistic predictions.

One novel approach, known as "social suicide prevention", involves the use of AI algorithms to analyse social media activity to identify individuals at elevated suicide risk and prompt timely intervention. Similarly, current violence risk assessment tools are limited by their low to moderate predictive accuracy. Early studies suggest that AI could significantly enhance prediction in this area as well, and some researchers argue that AI-driven tools could even help reduce recidivism and violent behaviour at a broader societal level.

Together, these developments highlight the urgent need to incorporate the AI training into psychiatry, so that future clinicians are prepared to utilise these advanced tools responsibly and effectively (Weisenburger et al., 2024).

## 8 AI for Assessment of Students

AI can be applied in multiple aspects of assessment within medical education to minimise subjective bias. Its use spans the evaluation of theoretical knowledge, diagnostic and procedural competencies, as well as emergency response capabilities. AI can help in conducting exams in multiple ways, thereby reducing the time and effort required. Examples include optical mark recognition (OMR), automated essay scoring (AES), procedural skill assessment tools, prescription correction, and developing question banks (Narayanan et al., 2023).

Evaluating written answer scripts is often a labour-intensive and subjective process. However, with advancements in AI and NLP, summative assessments can now be efficiently conducted using AES systems (Ramesh & Sanampudi, 2022). Numerous studies have explored the use of AES in different contexts, and ongoing research continues to refine its effectiveness. AES can analyse entire essays, grasp the underlying concepts and mean even when grammatical errors are present. When integrated into regular assessment practices, this technology can significantly reduce the time and manpower required, while also tracking learners' study patterns and providing personalised feedback focused on areas needing improvement (Gierl et al., 2014).

OMR is another widely used and longstanding method for assessing objective-type questions, such as multiple-choice and fill-in-the-blank items. It enables the rapid evaluation of a large volume of answer sheets and facilitates the creation of a ranking system based on student performance.

Procedural skills can be effectively evaluated using VR, where learners interact with a simulated patient in a virtual setting to perform specific procedures. The system automatically assesses their performance based on the sequence and accuracy of steps taken, providing instant feedback. Medical institutions are gradually beginning to set up VR labs to support such training. Alternatively, in the absence of a virtual environment, procedural skills can be demonstrated by an instructor on a manikin, recorded, and uploaded for analysis. AI can process and store these videos as structured data. When a learner uploads a video of the same procedure, AI can compare it to the pre-recorded standard, evaluating the steps taken and offering feedback. This approach is particularly useful in settings where the student-to-teacher ratio is low (Pottle, 2019).

AI can generate multiple, diverse scenarios to evaluate a learner's understanding. This not only measures diagnostic accuracy and critical thinking but also allows for dynamic, real-time adjustments to the complexity of the case based on the learner's knowledge level, providing a personalised assessment experience that pinpoints individual learning gaps (Narayanan et al., 2023).

Medication errors, especially during transcription, prescribing, and administration, pose a major threat in healthcare. Hence, assessing prescription writing skills is crucial. AI can be used to evaluate these skills by generating data sets and algorithms that mimic real-world scenarios (Dickinson et al., 2024). Additionally, learners can be tasked with reviewing and identifying errors in intentionally flawed prescriptions, using AI-generated feedback to guide their evaluation, thus supporting safer prescribing practices (Narayanan et al., 2023).

The use of generative AI to streamline and automate the creation of medical exam questions represents a promising new frontier in medical education. Developing questions for both formative assessments and high-stakes licensing exams is traditionally a time-consuming, resource-heavy task. While there are established guidelines for effective question writing, many human authors receive minimal formal training, leading to variability in question quality and consistency. Generative AI offers a scalable solution to these challenges by rapidly generating question banks. Compared to high-stakes exams, using in-progress testing would benefit from more frequent updates and broader question sets, making it an ideal setting for leveraging AI to enhance test-enhanced learning while maintaining educational quality and reducing the burden on faculty (Pang et al., 2025)

## 9 AI for Administration in Medical Education

Administration in medical education involves the strategic management of human, financial, and physical resources to meet institutional goals. This includes activities such as curriculum design, faculty development, student evaluation, and financial planning. Administrative responsibilities often demand significant time and effort and may require the involvement of both academic and administrative personnel. AI can streamline many of these tasks, enhancing overall efficiency (Narayanan et al., 2023).

AI tools can be instrumental in admission and recruitment processes by analysing applicant data to identify individuals most likely to succeed in a programme. Using machine learning, institutions can evaluate thousands of data points, including qualifications, experiences, and even hobbies, to identify candidates who best align with institutional goals. Large language models powered by AI enable faster, more accurate candidate evaluations, resulting in well-informed hiring decisions (Narayanan et al., 2023).

AI can be applied to developing a curriculum that involves defining desired outcomes and aligning the programme to bridge the gap between current content and those outcomes (Chan & Zary, 2019).

## 10 South Asian Scenario

Post-pandemic, there is a growing demand for mental health care, coupled with a significant shortage of trained mental health professionals and services, especially in South Asian countries, leading to a substantial treatment gap (World Health Organisation, 2018). As a result, many individuals in need of psychological support remain underserved, highlighting the urgent need for scalable and innovative solutions to strengthen mental health care delivery (Choudhary et al., 2024). The magnitude of these challenges is evident even in high-income countries such as the USA, where a recent report suggested that to ensure evidence-based mental health care nationwide would necessitate the addition of approximately 4 million trained professionals, underscoring the scale of the workforce gap (Torous et al., 2021).

This challenge is multi-fold in the likes of low- and middle-income countries. There is a need to scale up resources within the constraints. This imbalance severely limits access to care for a large portion of the population. Primary Care Doctors (PCDs), who often serve as the first point of contact in rural settings, are typically not adequately trained to manage psychiatric conditions. As a result, they may provide only symptomatic treatment, which can contribute to the progression and chronicity of mental illnesses within these communities (Pahuja et al., 2020).

Similar to the treatment gap, there exists a training gap in the field of Psychiatry in most low- and middle-income countries despite continuous efforts to improve these. This remains true in most South Asian countries (Kallivayalil & Enara, 2021). Undergraduate teaching in Psychiatry in these countries is often restricted to 2–3 weeks of clinical postings and an average of 20 h of lectures during the 4–6 semesters of undergraduate training. The government expenditure on mental health is often less than 1% of the national health budget in most SAARC nations (Isaac et al., 2018).

Traditional postgraduate training programmes in South Asia focus on eliciting psychopathology to reach a clinical diagnosis based on the ICD or DSM and implementing evidence-based treatment. In the background, there is the reality of a shortage of trained manpower, facilities, and funding. Training of mental health professionals in South Asia, therefore, should not be restricted to a pattern followed in high-income Western countries. There is a need for competency-based medical education with an overarching focus on clinical skills, teaching, and leadership skills (Williams, 2024).

In recent years, several factors, including rising healthcare costs and the challenges posed by the COVID-19 pandemic, have contributed to a growing shift towards digital mental health solutions. These technologies have emerged as a promising means to bridge the treatment gap, offering accessible, scalable, and cost-effective alternatives to traditional in-person care (Choudhary et al., 2024). There is a scope for combining digital psychiatry with AI for training of available resources and teaching new batches.

In South Asian Countries, we can divide the available mental health resources into core psychiatry professionals, primary care doctors, and other mental health professionals. Core psychiatry professionals include postgraduates who are medical doctors trained in Psychiatry as a speciality. Tools such as ITS, chatbots, and virtual patients can be utilised for their training.

Primary care doctors, clinical psychologists, and psychiatric social workers who often encounter a significant number of individuals with mental illness can be trained to recognise and handle mental illness, and prescribe AI-assisted first-line treatment. Apart from the health professionals, school teachers, traditional and faith healers, and other health workers come across many individuals with mental distress and training them basic counselling techniques can be done with the use of AI-powered tools. These initiatives, which would have been resource-driven and labour-intensive, can be made practically feasible by combining digital psychiatry and artificial intelligence.

# 11 Challenges

While AI holds tremendous promise for transforming medical education, several challenges need to be addressed for its effective integration. One significant concern is ensuring the ethical use of AI. As AI becomes more widespread, issues such as algorithmic bias, data security, and patient privacy will come to the forefront. It is essential to establish robust ethical guidelines to ensure AI systems operate with transparency, fairness, and impartiality (Gerke et al., 2020).

Another key obstacle is the need for capacity building among educators and healthcare providers. For AI tools to be implemented successfully, educators must be equipped with the necessary skills and training to integrate these technologies into their teaching and assessment methods. Likewise, healthcare professionals need to understand both the capabilities and limitations of AI to make informed use of it in clinical settings (Mir et al., 2023).

## *11.1 Challenges for Faculty*

Educators and healthcare professionals need to be equipped with the necessary skills so that they can properly integrate AI technology into curriculum development, instructional delivery, and assessment procedures. Medical schools can augment the faculty preparedness by conducting focused "faculty development programs". Additionally, constant learning and collaboration between academia, industry, and regulatory agencies are essential for keeping up with the rapidly changing landscape of AI in medical education (Mir et al., 2023). AI systems to be used in psychiatric training must also be updated and refined to keep up with the advances in the field and to improve accuracy and usefulness (Ajluni, 2025).

Given the current demands of healthcare and the rapid pace of technological advancements, it is likely that nearly every clinician will incorporate AI tools into their practice soon. Rather than replacing healthcare professionals, AI systems are expected to assist with specific tasks, improving efficiency and expanding the scope of medical practice. Considering these developments, medical educators need to acknowledge the growing role of AI in healthcare. They must equip themselves with the knowledge and skills needed to train future trainees in these emerging technologies and prepare them for a tech-integrated medical environment (Çalışkan et al., 2022).

## *11.2 Challenges for Students*

A major limitation of deep learning-based AI systems is their lack of transparency often referred to as the "explainability" problem. Because of the complex and non-linear processes involved, these systems typically do not offer insight into how a specific prediction or conclusion is reached. This poses a unique challenge in medical education, where understanding the reasoning behind clinical decisions is vital. For students, especially in the medical field, access to an explicit rationale is essential to develop critical thinking and clinical reasoning skills, which are foundational to becoming competent healthcare professionals (Chan & Zary, 2019).

Current chatbot models may generate incorrect references, a phenomenon known as "hallucination", highlighting the need for cautious use. Instead of relying solely on chatbots, students should use them as supplementary tools. Future chatbot development for medical education should prioritise evidence-based resources aligned with medical science standards and ethical guidelines (Narayanan et al., 2023). Another major concern is that AI cannot fully replicate and teach human empathy, which is critical in psychiatry. Also, the long-term outcomes of AI-based training need further research and evaluation, as currently there are no studies evaluating the same or comparing outcomes with traditional teaching methods (Ajluni, 2025).

## *11.3 Ethical, Legal, and Administrative Challenges*

AI holds the potential to enhance healthcare across both affluent and underserved regions by democratising access to expert knowledge and extending services to remote areas. However, the reliability, fairness, and effectiveness of any machine learning system depend heavily on the quality and diversity of the data it is trained on. There is an inherent risk of bias and errors in AI, which can lead to discriminatory outcomes. Therefore, developers must remain vigilant and proactively address potential biases throughout every phase of AI development (Gerke et al., 2020).

Machine learning and deep learning models require large volumes of data to develop robust and accurate algorithms. External datasets are crucial for validating outcomes and minimising systemic bias. As a result, collaboration across institutions or even between nations is vital to create distinct datasets for meaningful comparison and effective learning. However, sharing data poses significant challenges, including organisational reluctance, as well as concerns related to data privacy and security (Narayanan et al., 2023). Additionally, developing cost-effective AI models is important in resource-limited settings, such as those in many South Asian Countries, to ensure equitable access to high-quality training (Ajluni, 2025).

AI systems to be used in psychiatry training must also be updated and refined to keep up with the advances in the field and to improve accuracy and clinical utility. Furthermore, medical students must recognise that informed consent in the AI era goes beyond agreeing to a procedure—it extends to the use, storage, and sharing of health data. Patients have the right to know whether their de-identified data will be used for algorithm development, who will access it, and for what purpose. This necessitates medical students to know the data policies, data laws, and effective communication. The medical students must particularly familiarise themselves with the provisions of the digital data protection acts, role of consent managers, rights of data principals (patients), and obligations of data fiduciaries (hospitals and digital health service providers) in their respective countries (Sundara & Narendran, 2023).

Cybersecurity is another paramount concern when deploying AI tools in healthcare settings. Threats such as cyber-attacks targeting hospital systems, ransomware on EHRs (Electronic Health Records), and theft of AI models pose real risks. Institutions shall appoint data protection officers to monitor for breaches, ensure compliance, and report to the relevant authorities. Effective data protection requires coordination among the clinicians, hospital administrators, and technical teams.

Lastly, while AI may support clinical decision-making, accountability for its use ultimately rests with the clinician. Therefore, healthcare professionals must apply critical judgement and take primary responsibility for any outcomes arising from AI-assisted decisions. In light of these developments, medical educators must acknowledge the growing role of AI in healthcare and equip themselves with the knowledge and skills needed to train future trainees in these emerging technologies and prepare them for a tech-integrated medical environment (Çalışkan et al., 2022).

## 12 Conclusion

AI in medical education shows great potential for addressing students' individual needs, identifying knowledge gaps, and enhancing personalised learning. Utilisation of AI tools can address current training gaps and offer scalable and adaptive learning experiences, thereby augment in the process of reaching the unreached. AI can additionally simulate the entire psychiatric process, including interviews, diagnosis, and treatment planning, providing a more complete training experience. Despite its unquestionable promise, there are several challenges which arise with the use of AI which has to be addressed adequately. Ethical concerns related to data security and patient privacy require careful consideration and have to be dealt with appropriately. It is imperative that medical educators recognise AI's growing role in healthcare and actively develop the knowledge and skills required to effectively train future clinicians in these emerging technologies.

## References

Ajluni, V. (2025). Artificial intelligence in psychiatric education: Enhancing clinical competence through simulation. *Industrial Psychiatry Journal, 34*(1), 11–15. https://doi.org/10.4103/ipj.ipj_377_24

Alowais, S. A., Alghamdi, S. S., Alsuhebany, N., Alqahtani, T., Alshaya, A. I., Almohareb, S. N., Aldairem, A., Alrashed, M., Bin Saleh, K., Badreldin, H. A., Al Yami, M. S., Al Harbi, S., & Albekairy, A. M. (2023). Revolutionizing healthcare: The role of artificial intelligence in clinical practice. *BMC Medical Education, 23*(1), 689. https://doi.org/10.1186/s12909-023-04698-z

Çalışkan, S. A., Demir, K., & Karaca, O. (2022). Artificial intelligence in medical education curriculum: An e-Delphi study for competencies. *PLoS One, 17*(7), e0271872. https://doi.org/10.1371/journal.pone.0271872

Chan, K. S., & Zary, N. (2019). Applications and challenges of implementing artificial intelligence in medical education: Integrative review. *JMIR Medical Education, 5*(1), e13930. https://mededu.jmir.org/2019/1/e13930/

Choudhary, S., Dutt, S., Torous, J., & Mehta, U. M. (2024). Bridging the mental health gap: The scope, challenges, and future of digital psychiatry in India. *Asian Journal of Psychiatry, 101*, 104215. https://doi.org/10.1016/j.ajp.2024.104215

Davenport, T., & Kalakota, R. (2019). The potential for artificial intelligence in healthcare. *Future Healthcare Journal, 6*(2), 94–98. https://doi.org/10.7861/futurehosp.6-2-94

Dickinson, H., Teltsch, D. Y., Feifel, J., Hunt, P., Vallejo-Yagüe, E., Virkud, A. V., Muylle, K. M., Ochi, T., Donneyong, M., Zabinski, J., Strauss, V. Y., Hincapie-Castillo, J. M., & Actionable AI group. (2024). The unseen hand: AI-based prescribing decision support tools and the evaluation of drug safety and effectiveness. *Drug Safety, 47*(2), 117–123. https://doi.org/10.1007/s40264-023-01376-3

El Saadawi, G. M., Tseytlin, E., Legowski, E., Jukic, D., Castine, M., Fine, J., Gormley, R., & Crowley, R. S. (2008). A natural language intelligent tutoring system for training pathologists: Implementation and evaluation. *Advances in Health Sciences Education: Theory and Practice, 13*(5), 709–722. https://doi.org/10.1007/s10459-007-9081-3

Friedman, C. P., Donaldson, K. M., & Vantsevich, A. V. (2016). Educating medical students in the era of ubiquitous information. *Medical Teacher, 38*(5), 504–509. https://doi.org/10.3109/0142159X.2016.1150990

Gerke, S., Minssen, T., & Cohen, G. (2020). Ethical and legal challenges of artificial intelligence-driven healthcare. *Artificial Intelligence in Healthcare*, 295–336. https://doi.org/10.1016/B978-0-12-818438-7.00012-5

Ghorashi, N., Ismail, A., Ghosh, P., Sidawy, A., & Javan, R. (2023). AI-powered chatbots in medical education: Potential applications and implications. *Cureus, 15*(8), e43271. https://doi.org/10.7759/cureus.43271

Gierl, M. J., Latifi, S., Lai, H., Boulais, A. P., & De Champlain, A. (2014). Automated essay scoring and the future of educational assessment in medical education. *Medical Education, 48*(10), 950–962. https://doi.org/10.1111/medu.12517

Han, E. R., Yeo, S., Kim, M. J., Lee, Y. H., Park, K. H., & Roh, H. (2019). Medical education trends for future physicians in the era of advanced technology and artificial intelligence: An integrative review. *BMC Medical Education, 19*(1), 460. https://doi.org/10.1186/s12909-019-1891-5

Hamet, P., & Tremblay, J. (2017). Artificial intelligence in medicine. *Metabolism: Clinical and Experimental, 69S*, S36–S40. https://doi.org/10.1016/j.metabol.2017.01.011

Isaac, M., Ahmed, H. U., Chaturvedi, S. K., Hopwood, M. J., Javeed, A., Kanba, S., Mufti, A. A., Maramis, A., Samaniego, R. M., Udomratn, P., Yanling, H., Zainal, N. Z., & Sartorius, N. (2018). Postgraduate training in psychiatry in Asia. *Current Opinion in Psychiatry, 31*(5), 396–402. https://doi.org/10.1097/YCO.0000000000000444

Jackson, P., Ponath Sukumaran, G., Babu, C., Tony, M. C., Jack, D. S., Reshma, V. R., Davis, D., Kurian, N., & John, A. (2024). Artificial intelligence in medical education – perception among medical students. *BMC Medical Education, 24*(1), 804. https://doi.org/10.1186/s12909-024-05760-0

Johnston, S. C. (2018). Anticipating and training the physician of the future: The importance of caring in an age of artificial intelligence. *Academic Medicine : Journal of the Association of American Medical Colleges, 93*(8), 1105–1106. https://doi.org/10.1097/ACM.0000000000002175

Kahn, R. S. (2025). PREDiCTOR study engages AI in potential to diagnose from clinical conversations. *Psychiatric Times*. https://www.psychiatrictimes.com/view/predictor-study-engages-ai-in-potential-to-diagnose-from-clinical-conversations

Kallivayalil, R. A., & Enara, A. (2021). Education and training in psychiatry in South Asian countries. *Asia-Pacific Psychiatry: Official Journal of the Pacific Rim College of Psychiatrists, 13*(4), e12494. https://doi.org/10.1111/appy.12494

Kononowicz, A. A., Woodham, L. A., Edelbring, S., Stathakarou, N., Davies, D., Saxena, N., Tudor Car, L., Carlstedt-Duke, J., Car, J., & Zary, N. (2019). Virtual patient simulations in health professions education: Systematic review and meta-analysis by the digital health education collaboration. *Journal of Medical Internet Research, 21*(7), e14676. https://doi.org/10.2196/14676

Kyaw, B. M., Saxena, N., Posadzki, P., Vseteckova, J., Nikolaou, C. K., George, P. P., Divakar, U., Masiello, I., Kononowicz, A. A., Zary, N., & Tudor Car, L. (2019). Virtual reality for health professions education: Systematic review and meta-analysis by the digital health education collaboration. *Journal of medical Internet research, 21*(1), e12959. https://doi.org/10.2196/12959

McCarthy, J., Minsky, M. L., Rochester, N., & Shannon, C. E. (2006). A proposal for the dartmouth summer research project on artificial intelligence, August 31, 1955. *AI Magazine, 27*(4), 12. https://doi.org/10.1609/aimag.v27i4.1904

McCoy, L., Lewis, J. H., & Dalton, D. (2016). Gamification and multimedia for medical education: A landscape review. *The Journal of the American Osteopathic Association, 116*(1), 22–34. https://doi.org/10.7556/jaoa.2016.003

Mir, M. M., Mir, G. M., Raina, N. T., Mir, S. M., Mir, S. M., Miskeen, E., Alharthi, M. H., & Alamri, M. M. S. (2023). Application of artificial intelligence in medical education: Current scenario and future perspectives. *Journal of Advances in Medical Education & Professionalism, 11*(3), 133–140. https://doi.org/10.30476/jamp.2023.98655.1803

Narayanan, S., Ramakrishnan, R., Durairaj, E., & Das, A. (2023). Artificial intelligence revolutionizing the field of medical education. *Cureus, 15*(11), e49604. https://doi.org/10.7759/cureus.49604

Nilsson, N. J. (1998). *Artificial intelligence: A new synthesis*. Elsevier. https://scholar.google.com/scholar?&q=Nilsson%2C%20N.J.%3A%20Artificial%20Intelligence%3A%20A%20New%20Synthesis.%20Morgan%20Kaufmann%20Publishers%20%281998%29

Pahuja, E., Kumar, T. S., Uzzafar, F., Manjunatha, N., Kumar, C. N., Gupta, R., & Math, S. B. (2020). An impact of a digitally driven primary care psychiatry program on the integration of psychiatric care in the general practice of primary care doctors. *Indian Journal of Psychiatry, 62*(6), 690–696. https://doi.org/10.4103/psychiatry.IndianJPsychiatry_324_20

Pang, H. Y. M., Meshkat, S., Teferra, B. G., Rueda, A., Samavi, R., Krishnan, S., Doyle, T., Rambhatla, S., DeJong, S., Sockalingam, S., Horsley, T., Hodges, B., & Bhat, V. (2025). Opportunities and barriers of generative artificial intelligence in the training of psychiatrists: A competencies-based perspective. *Academic Psychiatry, 49*(1), 25–30. https://doi.org/10.1007/s40596-024-02087-2

Pottle, J. (2019). Virtual reality and the transformation of medical education. *Future Healthcare Journal, 6*(3), 181–185. https://doi.org/10.7861/fhj.2019-0036

Ramesh, D., & Sanampudi, S. K. (2022). An automated essay scoring systems: A systematic literature review. *Artificial Intelligence Review, 55*(3), 2495–2527. https://doi.org/10.1007/s10462-021-10068-2

Randhawa, G. K., & Jackson, M. (2020). The role of artificial intelligence in learning and professional development for healthcare professionals. *Healthcare Management Forum, 33*(1), 19–24. https://doi.org/10.1177/0840470419869032

Raths, D. (2024). Research seeks to leverage AI, behavioral data to improve mental health. *Healthcare Innovation*. https://www.hcinnovationgroup.com/population-health-management/behavioral-health/news/55139634/research-seeks-to-leverage-ai-behavioral-data-to-improve-mental-health

Ray, A., Bhardwaj, A., Malik, Y. K., Singh, S., & Gupta, R. (2022). Artificial intelligence and psychiatry: An overview. *Asian Journal of Psychiatry, 70*, 103021. https://doi.org/10.1016/j.ajp.2022.103021
Sallam, M. (2023). ChatGPT utility in healthcare education, research, and practice: Systematic review on the promising perspectives and valid concerns. *Healthcare (Basel, Switzerland), 11*(6), 887. https://doi.org/10.3390/healthcare11060887
Sami, A., Tanveer, F., Sajwani, K., Kiran, N., Javed, M. A., Ozsahin, D. U., Muhammad, K., & Waheed, Y. (2025). Medical students' attitudes toward AI in education: perception, effectiveness, and its credibility. *BMC Medical Education, 25*(1), 82. https://doi.org/10.1186/s12909-025-06704-y
Sundara, K., & Narendran, N. (2023). The Digital Personal Data Protection Act, 2023: Analysing India's dynamic approach to data protection. *Computer Law Review International, 24*(5), 129–141. https://doi.org/10.9785/cri-2023-240502
Torous, J., Bucci, S., Bell, I. H., Kessing, L. V., Faurholt-Jepsen, M., Whelan, P., Carvalho, A. F., Keshavan, M., Linardon, J., & Firth, J. (2021). The growing field of digital psychiatry: Current evidence and the future of apps, social media, chatbots, and virtual reality. *World Psychiatry : Official Journal of the World Psychiatric Association (WPA), 20*(3), 318–335. https://doi.org/10.1002/wps.20883
Weisenburger, R. L., Mullarkey, M. C., Labrada, J., Labrousse, D., Yang, M. Y., MacPherson, A. H., Hsu, K. J., Ugail, H., Shumake, J., & Beevers, C. G. (2024). Conversational assessment using artificial intelligence is as clinically useful as depression scales and preferred by users. *Journal of Affective Disorders, 351*, 489–498. https://doi.org/10.1016/j.jad.2024.01.212
Williams, S. S. (2024). Fine-tuning postgraduate psychiatry training in South Asia. *Indian Journal of Psychological Medicine, 46*(5), 380–381. https://doi.org/10.1177/02537176241280284
World Health Organization. (2018). *Mental health atlas 2017*. World Health Organization. https://iris.who.int/handle/10665/272735

# Chapter 22
# Strengthening Psychiatry's Academic Core: Faculty Development and Leadership in Psychiatry in South Asia

**Satish Suhas, Venkata Lakshmi Narasimha, and Pratima Murthy**

**Abstract** South Asia faces a widening "training gap" in psychiatry, with the number of students and training institutions steadily rising while the pool of qualified faculty remains limited. This gap highlights the urgent need for robust faculty development initiatives that not only enhance teaching effectiveness and mentorship but also foster scholarly productivity. At the same time, cultivating leadership among psychiatry faculty has become critical, equipping them with the skills to manage services, influence policy, allocate resources, and lead interdisciplinary teams-whether in academic, public, or private sectors. In response to evolving educational paradigms, both global and regional efforts have emerged to address these needs. This chapter offers a comprehensive examination of faculty development and leadership in psychiatry across South Asia, drawing on current data, cross-country comparisons, and illustrative case studies. By spotlighting initiatives from countries such as Afghanistan, Bangladesh, Bhutan, India, Maldives, Nepal, Pakistan, and Sri Lanka, we explore context-sensitive strategies and pathways for building a stronger academic core in regional psychiatry.

**Keywords** Psychiatry · South Asia · Faculty development · Academic leadership · Competency-based education · Medical education · Mental health workforce · Teaching mentorship · Capacity building · Health professions education

S. Suhas
Department of Psychiatry, National Institute of Mental Health and Neurosciences (NIMHANS), Bengaluru, Karnataka, India

V. L. Narasimha
Centre for Addiction Medicine, Department of Psychiatry, National Institute of Mental Health and Neurosciences (NIMHANS), Bengaluru, Karnataka, India

P. Murthy (✉)
National Institute of Mental Health and Neurosciences (NIMHANS), Bengaluru, Karnataka, India



S. K. Kar et al. (eds.), *Teaching and Training in Psychiatry in South Asia*, South Asian Perspectives in Mental Health and Psychology, https://doi.org/10.1007/978-981-95-1845-6_22

# 1 Introduction

Psychiatric education and workforce development are critical priorities worldwide, especially in low- and middle-income regions where the mental health treatment gap remains large. South Asia, home to nearly a quarter of the global population, faces a shortage of psychiatrists and mental health professionals. According to recent data, almost all South Asian countries have far fewer than 1 psychiatrist per 100,000 population (Mia & Griffiths, 2022; Suhas et al., 2023). For example, Pakistan has only ~0.19 psychiatrists per 100,000 people (Main Thompson & Saleem, 2025) and Bangladesh around ~0.2 per 100,000 (roughly 350 psychiatrists for ~170 million people) (Hasan et al., 2021). India, trains larger number of doctors, and yet has only about 0.75 psychiatrists per 100,000 as of 2022, a figure far below the World Health Organization's recommended minimum of 3 per 100,000 (Arafat & Kar, 2024; Suhas et al., 2023). Furthermore, the number of psychiatry teachers remains low even as the number of students and training institutions continues to grow, widening the existing "training gap". This acute training gap underscores the urgency of strengthening faculty development in psychiatry. Scaling up training capacity requires not just more residency slots but also qualified educators and leaders to mentor the next generation of psychiatrists.

In the last decade, significant shifts in medical education paradigms have occurred to address the training gap and promote uniformity across institutions. In India and neighbouring countries, for example, competency-based medical education (CBME) has been introduced at the undergraduate level (alongside a new curriculum for bachelor's degree in medicine rolled out in 2019) and is being extended to postgraduate training (Sethi et al., 2024). This transformation moves away from time-based training towards ensuring that graduates attain specific competencies essential for effective clinical practice. Implementing such reforms places new demands on faculty, who must adopt modern teaching methods and assessment tools (e.g. workplace-based assessments) and take on mentorship roles for trainees (Gopalakrishnan et al., 2022). Yet, a persistent challenge in the region is the transition of senior residents to faculty positions. There are limited opportunities to transition to faculty roles (Buer et al., 2024). Additionally, there is lack of dedicated training and preparation for faculty roles as well. Upon assuming faculty roles, they are expected to automatically excel as teachers and academicians despite minimal formal training in those domains. Across countless departments, colleagues voice the same frustration: that new faculty arrive eager yet under-prepared because no clear induction or development pathway exists. Recognizing this weak link, many training centres now treat faculty and leadership development as parallel, mutually reinforcing priorities.

Faculty development focuses on the craft of teaching, the art of mentorship, and the steady production of high-quality scholarly work (Misky et al., 2023). Leadership cultivation, by contrast, trains psychiatrists to run services, negotiate policy, manage budgets, and inspire multidisciplinary teams, competencies equally valuable in government hospitals, private networks, or academic settings. The pipeline, therefore, ideally ought to open well before a psychiatrist earns a formal faculty badge. During residency, practical leadership experiences, running a quality-improvement audit, coordinating a small clinical team, and engaging in reflective supervision lay the first stones. Once an appointment is secured, more structured offerings such as executive coaching, health-systems management modules, or workshops in strategic communication can be layered on, creating an unbroken arc from trainee to leader.

Embedding leadership themes inside (but not limited to) conventional faculty-development courses ensures that every psychiatrist, whether bound for teaching, clinical service, or administration, acquires the vision, skills, and tools to shape mental-health care at multiple levels. In short, faculty development must stretch beyond better classroom technique: it should nurture future heads of department, grant-winning researchers, and persuasive advocates. Such leadership is urgently needed in South Asia, where psychiatry often sits low on the administrative pecking order. Without a cadre of confident psychiatric leaders, the field's voice in health-system planning will remain faint; with them, it can no longer be ignored (Williams, 2024). Although empowerment alone cannot guarantee outcomes, positioning psychiatric educators as leaders in universities, professional societies, and policy circles ideally equips the mental-health community to advocate more effectively for resources, reforms, and innovative models of training and care.

Effective medical leadership involves understanding team dynamics and being influenced by, and influencing, organizational culture. Good leaders must be authentic, principled, and capable of sharing their vision to unite and motivate teams (Sultan et al., 2019). Faculty development and leadership development are integral to strengthening psychiatry training and service delivery, particularly in regions like South Asia, where there is a critical shortage of mental health professionals. Over the past few decades, significant efforts have been made globally and locally to enhance the leadership abilities among faculty members. By empowering psychiatric educators as leaders in universities, professional societies, and policy forums, the mental health community can better advocate for resources, reforms, and innovation in training and care.

This chapter provides a comprehensive overview of faculty development and leadership in psychiatry in South Asia. We synthesize updated data and insights from global and regional sources, highlighting diversity across countries (Afghanistan, Bangladesh, Bhutan, India, Maldives, Nepal, Pakistan, and Sri Lanka). We examine case studies of successful initiatives from international programmes such as the leadership and professional skills course for early-career psychiatrists led by the National Institute of Mental Health and Neurosciences (NIMHANS), India (Naskar & Varadharajan, 2024). National programmes like India's competency-based curriculum rollout and Medical Education Units (MEUs) to grassroots innovations like TIPPS in India, as well as international collaborations (e.g. FAIMER fellowships (Yuan et al., 2024), World Psychiatric Association, and Royal College programmes). We address critical gaps and highlight cultural contextualization of training, incorporating trainee perspectives, promoting gender equity in academic psychiatry, and engaging the growing private sector in medical education. Throughout, we interweave relevant theoretical frameworks (adult learning principles, the Kirkpatrick model for training outcomes, and competencies such as CanMEDS) to ground our discussion in educational theory. We conclude with actionable recommendations and a future roadmap to cultivate a robust psychiatric education ecosystem in South Asia that can produce the next generation of skilled, compassionate, and visionary mental health professionals.

## 2 Importance of Faculty Development in Psychiatry

Faculty development refers to a range of institutional activities aimed at enhancing the knowledge, skills, and attitudes of academic staff. Psychiatry straddles biology, mind, and society, so its teachers need a skill set that stretches well beyond bedside diagnosis. The conventional Doctor of Medicine (MD) or Diplomate in National Board (DNB) pathway sharpens clinical judgement but seldom tackles the finer arts of supervising therapy, inventing fresh classroom methods, guiding novice researchers, leading cross-disciplinary teams, or running a department. Targeted faculty-development schemes close these gaps (Kallivayalil & Enara, 2021). They arm new consultants with the know-how to switch fluently between roles like clinician, lecturer, mentor, administrator, and public advocate. India's breakneck growth in medical colleges makes that support non-negotiable; without it, swelling numbers risk diluting standards. Well-designed programmes lift teaching quality, spark inventive learning approaches, and cultivate a culture of inquiry that benefits both staff and students.

## 3 Current Status of Psychiatry Faculty Development in South Asia

South Asia now houses about one quarter of humanity—2.08 billion people, approximately 25% of the world's population (TRIVEDI et al., 2007), and yet the subcontinent's seven mainland SAARC members together employ just over 10,000 psychiatrists (Garg et al., 2019; Grover, 2023). World-over, there are about 250,000 psychiatrists as per the World Psychiatric Association data on members of registered psychiatry bodies across the globe (About Us | World Psychiatric Association, 2025.). This implies that barely 4–5% of the world's psychiatrists are serving 25% of the entire humanity. These data point to the fact that a region containing one in every four people commands only a sliver of the world's specialist mental-health workforce. Expanding training seats alone cannot reverse that deficit; each new residency slot also needs a competent supervisor, a curriculum steward, and ultimately a psychiatrist-leader who can reshape services and policy. Faculty development and leadership development, therefore, sit at the fulcrum of mental health scale-up in the region. Until the mid-twentieth century, India had only a handful of diploma courses in mental health, and even those were patterned after colonial curricula with limited academic depth. Ambitious psychiatrists therefore pursued advanced qualifications such as the DPM or MRCPsych in London, Edinburgh, or Dublin, or completed residency and fellowship tracks in major U.S. centres. It was not until the 1960s–1970s, when institutes like NIMHANS, AIIMS, CIP-Ranchi, etc., established full MD and DNB programmes, that a robust, home-grown postgraduate pipeline truly took shape. Because formal psychiatric education in India took off relatively late, an entire generation of senior teachers earned their credentials overseas. Today's trainees, by contrast, can finish every stage of their learning at home. That historical lag is more than an interesting footnote; it is a reminder that faculty- and leadership-development programmes must move at a faster clip. They are not an optional polish; they are the structural scaffolding needed to build a home-grown tradition of psychiatric scholarship, service, and governance.

Over the past 20 years, similar conversations have echoed across South Asia. India, Pakistan, Sri Lanka, Bangladesh, Nepal, Bhutan, and the Maldives all face the familiar trio of too few trained teachers, uneven curricula, and scarce earmarked funds dedicated to this cause (Kallivayalil & Enara, 2021; Trivedi & Dhyani, 2007). Yet the region also enjoys powerful assets: closely intertwined cultures, shared histories, and an engaged diaspora that keep academic bridges and the room for collaborations open. Fostering research networks, bilateral training exchanges, and region-wide teaching initiatives are already showing how mental health care can rise when countries pull in the same direction. With its mix of clinical experience, cultural insight, and a receptive global climate, South Asia has every ingredient to craft a distinctive model of psychiatric leadership, one that could influence mental-health practice far beyond the subcontinent and set the stage for other low- and middle-income countries to follow suit (Williams, 2024).

Regulation and professional advocacy have provided much of the forward thrust in these areas. In India, the Indian Psychiatric Society continually updates educational benchmarks and conducts capacity-building workshops, while the shift to competency-based curricula under the Medical Council of India has prompted a re-examination of how teachers are trained and assessed. National Teacher Training Centres are now offered to faculty across the country, and the long-running FAIMER regional fellowships that are hosted in Ludhiana, Mumbai, Coimbatore, Manipal, and elsewhere have equipped hundreds of clinician-educators with modern pedagogy and an international peer network. FAIMER has also taken innovations forward, such as online role plays across South Asian countries for faculty development (Ladhani et al., 2011). Taken together, these efforts are knitting a vibrant community of psychiatric educators determined to raise standards across the region (ECFMG, 2022). These initiatives are designed to accomplish two objectives simultaneously i.e., refine the day-to-day teaching craft and cultivate the leadership instincts that good departments rely on, thereby alleviating the persistent shortage of seasoned medical educators. They usually roll out in ascending stages: an opening tier of guided reading or online modules, followed by hands-on workshops, and capped by immersive fellowships. Each step pushes participants a little further, there by sharpening lesson design, deepening dialogue with learners, and nurturing the habit of turning classroom experience into publishable scholarship.

**Key Developments in the Region** A pivotal turning point occurred in 2009, when the Medical Council of India (now renamed the National Medical Commission) introduced the National Faculty Development (NFD) programme to enhance teaching standards nationwide. Starting with eight regional training hubs, the scheme has since expanded to approximately 20 regional centres, supported by ten nodal centres located across the country. Through a calendar of tightly structured workshops, the NFD introduces faculty to contemporary teaching techniques, competency-based curricula, educational technology, and the nuts and bolts of research design; all of which are intended to raise the overall calibre of medical education. These workshops train faculty members to become more effective educators, administrators, researchers, and mentors. Despite its expansion, the NFD has faced challenges such as limited faculty participation and uneven distribution of centres (with fewer centres historically in Eastern and Northeastern regions), which has hindered its full potential.

Medical Education Units (MEUs) were introduced by the Medical Council of India (now the National Medical Commission) in the late 1990s and upgraded in 2009, to improve the teaching capabilities of medical faculty by providing training in modern educational strategies. Each medical college in India was mandated to establish an MEU to ensure that faculty members receive training in teaching methods and education technology (Vagha et al., 2023). A recent review suggests a significant increase in the proportion of medical teachers trained after 2009. However, the implementation of MEUs has faced challenges, as many institutions have not fully utilized or developed their MEUs. Although MEUs were intended to serve as hubs for faculty development and pedagogical innovation, many have remained under-resourced and underutilized, limiting their impact on the quality of medical education as compared to their original vision. There are currently efforts ongoing to revitalize MEUs through better funding and integration into faculty promotion criteria.

Another positive development is the emergence of dedicated centres for psychiatric education. Institutions such as NIMHANS in Bengaluru have carved out dedicated units that drive curriculum innovation, run faculty-training programmes, and spearhead research on psychiatric education (Narasimha et al., 2024). NIMHANS' Digital Academy offers web-based courses that provide mental-health training to clinicians in hard-to-reach regions, while its on-campus workshops regularly refine faculty members' teaching techniques and deepen their understanding of research ethics (India, 2023). Dedicated centres act as nerve centres for educational innovation, experimenting with new training formats and serving as gathering points for faculty development. Cross-border partnerships widen the horizon even further. Collaborations with bodies such as the World Psychiatric Association and the Royal College of Psychiatrists have paved the way for exchange placements, visiting-scholar posts, and structured knowledge-sharing schemes. The WPA's early-career arm, for example, has repeatedly organized student and faculty exchanges alongside regional workshops on teaching methods and leadership.

Yet sizeable shortcomings persist. Many departments still run on a skeletal teaching staff, and ongoing professional development is rarely compulsory. Funding streams and career advancement criteria continue to reward research output far more generously than excellence in the classroom. Training syllabi also lean heavily towards clinical proficiency, leaving pedagogy and leadership skills undernourished. In short, although the trajectory is encouraging, South Asia still needs to embed faculty development more deeply and consistently within psychiatric education systems.

## 4 Need for Leadership Development

Leadership training is too often treated as an afterthought, yet it is indispensable to the professional maturation of psychiatric faculty. In addition to their duties as clinicians and teachers, psychiatrists must oversee academic programmes, drive curriculum reform (Suhas et al., 2022b), set research priorities, and speak for mental health interests in policy arenas (Williams, 2024). These responsibilities are especially complex in South Asia, where administrative constraints, cultural diversity, and social inequality intersect. Faculty-development programmes refine an individual's teaching and scholarly skills; leadership training, by contrast, equips psychiatrists to influence departments, institutions, and health systems as a whole.

Structured leadership training is no longer optional for psychiatry faculty. A limited cadre of seasoned administrators means many professors step into roles such as department chair or programme director without prior grounding in finance, strategic planning, or organizational management, relying on trial-and-error learning that blunts their impact (Narasimha et al., 2024). Succession gaps are common, with few medical schools cultivating clear pipelines, leaving unprepared juniors to fill sudden voids upon retirements. Leaders must also navigate local beliefs, stigma patterns, and traditional healing practices, tailoring services so mental-health programmes resonate with the communities they serve. In addition, psychiatrists who can negotiate effectively with ministries, funders, and NGOs are crucial for securing resources and shaping legislation that elevates mental health on national agendas (Kestel, 2022). Leadership content, therefore, belongs in core faculty-development programmes, covering management, negotiation, and advocacy alongside teaching skills, while faculty should be encouraged to practise these competencies through committee work, professional societies, and community projects. Cultivating these abilities will yield a generation of psychiatrists ready to steer academic departments and drive broader mental-health reforms.

In psychiatry, leading therefore goes far beyond routine administration. It also includes energizing teams, defending mental-health rights, and charting the discipline's future. Core leadership domains, thus, include:

- *Strategic Vision:* Understanding long-term trends in mental health care and education, and planning training programmes to meet future needs (for example, anticipating the need for more community psychiatry training as deinstitutionalization progresses).
- *Policy Advocacy:* Engaging with government bodies, non-governmental organizations, and international agencies to advocate for mental health priorities and resource allocation.
- *Team stewardship:* Cultivate and steer multidisciplinary groups in classrooms and clinics alike, drawing on clear communication, deft conflict-resolution, inspired delegation, and the knack for keeping colleagues motivated.
- *Innovation and change leadership:* Drive syllabus overhauls, weave in emerging tools such as tele-psychiatry and simulation, and champion fresh clinical services or research ventures (Parate et al., 2024; Satish et al., 2023).
- *Cultural and Ethical Leadership:* Upholding ethical standards and cultural sensitivity in all aspects of psychiatric practice and teaching, and modelling these values for trainees.

Leadership capability can be built in several complementary ways. Formal routes span everything from intensive workshops to multi-month fellowships or certificate courses in health-care management. Experience on the ground matters just as much, whether a junior consultant is asked to spearhead a curriculum overhaul, chair a task force, or spend a term shadowing a hospital administrator. Pairing rising psychiatrists with seasoned mentors provides steady guidance, while short stints at overseas leadership institutes broaden perspective.

In South Asia, psychiatry is only beginning to make this training a priority. The World Psychiatric Association and various national bodies have begun incorporating leadership modules into existing faculty development workshops. The Indian Psychiatric Society's Early Career Psychiatrist programme, for example, now runs a webinar series on leadership skills, and Bangladesh dedicated its first conference session to leadership in mental health in 2022. These are encouraging signs, but a more coordinated, longitudinal strategy is still required to shape the next generation of psychiatric leaders. A structured approach to leadership development would span a faculty member's career stages. Junior faculty could receive an introduction to leadership principles and project management basics (so they can effectively lead a small research project or a curriculum committee subtask). Mid-career faculty may receive training in strategic planning, human resource management, and financial stewardship, as these areskills essential for leading a department or managing a grant or programme. Senior faculty might focus on advocacy skills, influencing policy and high-level institutional leadership (preparing them for roles like hospital director or national advisor). This pipeline approach ensures sustainability and helps reduce leadership gaps in the future by grooming successors.

## 5 Models and Approaches for Faculty Development in Psychiatry- With Select Examples

Faculty development can be approached through several models that combine adult learning principles, reflective practice, and competency-based progression (Van Schalkwyk et al., 2024). In South Asia, these models must be adapted to local needs, resource limitations, and institutional cultures. Below, we outline some key models and strategies the strengths of which are detailed following the examples in Table 22.1.

1. *Workshop-Based Model:* Workshops are a popular and effective method for delivering faculty development content. They can be short (1–2 days) or

**Table 22.1** Features and examples of existing models of faculty and leadership development

| Model | Key features | Illustrative South Asian examples |
|---|---|---|
| Workshop-based model | Short 1- to 2-day or longitudinal formats; interactive methods (case discussions, role-play, micro-teaching, and simulation); hands-on practice in feedback, OSCE design, curriculum building. | Indian Psychiatric Society national workshops; Basic Course in Medical Education Technology; similar initiatives in Pakistan and Sri Lanka. |
| Mentorship model | Formal pairing of junior faculty with senior mentors; structured career planning, teaching, research, and leadership guidance; boosts confidence in hierarchical settings. | Indian Teachers of Psychiatry (IToP) forum with scholarships, CME events and research seed grants |
| Train-the-trainer Programmes | Intensive up-skilling of a core group who then train peers, creating a multiplier effect; useful where resources are scarce. | WPA-backed CBME and psychotherapy-supervision trainer cohorts disseminating modern methods in home institutions. |
| E-learning and blended models | Self-paced or synchronous digital courses; bridges geographic and curricular gaps; mainly knowledge-focused to date. | NIMHANS Digital Academy & Virtual Knowledge Network; ECHO-style case-based courses; NAMAH resilience initiative; postgraduate digital primers |
| Dedicated centres for faculty development | Institutional units that organize training, craft curricula, conduct education research, and act as regional hubs. | NIMHANS initiative for Psychiatric Faculty Development, Post-graduate Institute of Medicine (Colombo) |
| Leadership & professional skills training | Condensed executive-style courses on CV building, grant writing, team leadership, media skills; alumni networks for continued growth. | Annual 3-day Leadership & Professional Skills Course at NIMHANS, guided by Prof. Norman Sartorius and senior South-Asian faculty |
| Communities of practice and peer learning | Informal, tech-enabled educator networks sharing resources and solving problems in real time; low-cost, sustainable. | TIPPS national chat-and-webinar platform; eJCIndia online journal club; Sri Lanka national trainee social media groups. |

longitudinal (spread over weeks or months with periodic sessions). Key features include interactive learning (e.g. case discussions, role plays, and micro-teaching exercises), hands-on practice of educational skills (such as giving feedback, developing OSCE stations, or designing curricula), and exposure to innovations in psychiatry education (e.g. simulation-based learning). Workshops have been instrumental in India, Pakistan, and Sri Lanka for promoting new teaching methodologies, as seen in national training programmes endorsed by the Indian Psychiatric Society. The basic course in medical education in technology is another workshop-based model that has been explored (Bembade et al., 2025).

2. *Mentorship Model:* Pairing junior faculty with experienced mentors fosters skill development in a personalized manner. A structured mentorship programme supports career planning, development of teaching and research skills, leadership skill-building, and provides psychosocial support. In South Asia's traditionally hierarchical academic culture, establishing formal mentorship programmes can help junior faculty navigate the system more confidently. Structured mentoring improves faculty skills, job satisfaction, and productivity. Emphasizing mentorship is especially important in work environments where informal guidance might otherwise be limited by senior–junior gaps or other resource constraints. The Indian Teachers of Psychiatry (IToP) forum offers a home-grown, excellent template that unites psychiatry educators, supplies tailored training resources, and seeds educational research (Kishor & Isaac, 2024). IToP has also introduced scholarships for academic research in addition to regularly organizing national conferences and continuing medical education programmes for Indian teachers and students of psychiatry (Verma et al., 2024).
3. *Train-the-Trainer Programmes:* Train-the-Trainer programmes involve training select faculty members who then become trainers for their peers, creating a multiplier effect (Bansal & Supe, 2007; Seethamraju et al., 2021). This approach is valuable when resources are limited, where a core group of faculty champions can extend the reach of faculty development. Examples include programmes supported by the WPA and national institutions where select psychiatrists were intensively trained in modern teaching methods (such as CBME and psychotherapy supervision techniques) and then tasked with disseminating this knowledge at their home institutions.
4. *E-Learning and Blended Models:* The rapid proliferation of online education platforms presents extensive opportunities for postgraduate training and faculty development in psychiatry. Psychiatry training in India and other South Asian countries exhibits considerable heterogeneity across institutions, often resulting in gaps in the acquisition of essential knowledge and skills during postgraduate education. E-learning platforms offer a promising solution by enabling self-paced, focused learning that can effectively bridge these gaps. The National Institute of Mental Health and Neurosciences (NIMHANS), Bengaluru, has been a pioneer in technology-enabled training through the establishment of the NIMHANS Digital Academy (NDA) and the Virtual Knowledge Network (VKN) (https://nda.nimhans.ac.in, https://vknnimhans.in). These platforms have facilitated the development of numerous courses and self-paced digital primers

in the fields of mental health and addiction psychiatry. The current suite of self-paced primers covers essential topics, including tobacco cessation, motivational interviewing, and relapse prevention, enabling flexible and accessible learning for mental health professionals (https://nimhanselearning.org). In addition, online courses based on the Extension for Community Healthcare Outcomes (ECHO) model have been introduced. These courses utilize a fully digital, case-based learning approach, featuring expert-led discussions within an "all-teach, all-learn" framework. Initially focused on alcohol use disorders, the model has since expanded to encompass a broad range of mental health conditions (Kumar et al., 2020; Mahadevan et al., 2020). This approach has successfully addressed geographic barriers and knowledge disparities, extending its impact beyond medical doctors to include psychologists, social workers, counsellors, and dentists. Evaluative studies have affirmed the effectiveness of these programmes in enhancing professional competencies. Psychiatrists also play a pivotal role in promoting institutional mental health and supporting the well-being of healthcare professionals. In this context, NIMHANS has launched an innovative programme titled NAMAH (https://www.namahnimhans.in), designed to enhance the mental health and well-being of doctors (Parate et al., 2024). This initiative aims to build individual and institutional capacity to support physician mental health and has demonstrated effective outcomes in improving the resilience and well-being among healthcare providers. Beyond clinical skill-building, several e-learning programmes are aligned with postgraduate curricula, offering targeted content for academic revision and examination preparedness (Suhas et al., 2022a). A notable digital teaching and learning initiative in India has shown how virtual platforms can enrich psychiatric education by promoting academic discourse, mentorship, and skill development. The high enrolment and completion rates of these courses highlight the growing demand for such initiatives. However, most existing programmes predominantly address the knowledge domain, with limited offerings in research methodology and leadership development. This gap points to the urgent need for faculty to acquire competencies in digital pedagogy to train the next generation of mental health professionals effectively. Alongside national initiatives, global platforms such as Coursera, edX, and Udemy provide extensive resources in mental health, addiction medicine, and general medical education. Given the shortage of trained faculty, the heterogeneity of psychiatry training, and persistent knowledge gaps, particularly in South Asian contexts, these e-learning platforms represent an essential component of faculty development, especially in remote or underserved areas.

5. *Development of Dedicated Centres for Faculty Development:* Establishing departments or centres devoted to medical education within institutions can anchor faculty development. These centres can organize regular training, develop curricula, and conduct educational research. As mentioned, NIMHANS in India has a dedicated academic section focusing on educational development, and similarly, the Postgraduate Institute of Medicine at the University of Colombo has units that support faculty training. Such dedicated centres provide sustained resource and policy attention to improving teaching and therefore often become

centres of excellence that train faculty not only from their own institution but across the region as well. NIMHANS is also working towards a centre for faculty training and development dedicated to Psychiatrists (Narasimha et al., 2024).

6. *Dedicated Leadership and Professional Skills Training:* Leadership training is fast becoming a staple within faculty-development schemes, frequently delivered through partnerships with hospital management schools or condensed executive courses. Typical offerings include hands-on workshops in management, team-leadership simulations, and sponsored places on recognized healthcare-leadership programmes. A flagship example is the annual Leadership & Professional Skills Course for Early-Career Psychiatrists run by NIMHANS, which attracts participants from across India and neighbouring South Asian nations. Helmed by NIMHANS under the visionary guidance of Professor Norman Sartorius, President of the Association for the Improvement of Mental Health Programmes (Sartorius, 2013, 2023), this initiative unites the region's foremost mental-health scholars; Professor Mohan K. Isaac, Professor Santosh K. Chaturvedi, Professor Pratima Murthy, and Professor Prabha S. Chandra, together with dynamic mid-career faculty such as Professor Arun Kandasamy, Professor Krishna Prasad M., and Dr Suhas Satish, who coordinate and lead its sessions. Participants from across South Asia- mainly from Bangladesh, India, Nepal, and Sri Lanka apply for this prestigious course, with 16 participants being finally selected to attend the 3-day course. Across the three demanding days, participants transform their professional toolkit: they tighten CVs, craft persuasive motivation letters, polish slide decks, and collaborate on grant-writing sprints. They also learn to chair meetings, handle media inquiries, mediate conflicts, and even campaign in a mock election. Poster walks, anonymized proposal reviews, and priority-setting drills sharpen critical appraisal and resource-allocation skills, while rapid feedback loops and evening group tasks lock in every lesson. By the end, each delegate leaves with a refined CV, a nearly submission-ready grant proposal, several presentation credits, and a tailored plan for sustained leadership growth—momentum now inspiring national psychiatric bodies to create new fellowships and recognition awards. Guided by accomplished senior faculty, the course emphasizes real-time practice over passive lectures, ensuring every skill is road-tested before participants depart. Small-group dynamics foster peer mentoring and camaraderie, creating a support network that often endures long after the workshop ends. An alumni forum introduces past graduates who share post-course successes and open doors to collaborative research across continents. Evening debriefs encourage self-reflection, helping attendees link fresh insights to their personal leadership style and career ambitions. Many participants report renewed confidence when pitching ideas, moderating difficult discussions, or steering multidisciplinary teams. Collectively, the programme functions as an incubator for the next generation of mental-health leaders, spreading best practices throughout hospitals, universities, and policy circles worldwide(Naskar & Varadharajan, 2024).
7. *Communities of Practice, Capacity Building, and Peer Learning:* Informal peer networks can rival formal courses in influence. When teachers swap tips, ideas,

and lecture slides in a shared space, they form what educational theorists call a "community of practice". On the ground this often means simple WhatsApp or Facebook groups where psychiatry lecturers crowd-source solutions in real time. India's Training Initiative for Psychiatry Post-Graduates (TIPPS) shows the idea in action. Launched in 2015 by a handful of early-career psychiatrists alarmed by the gulf between elite centres and outlying colleges, TIPPS uses chat groups, webinars, and crowdsourced reading lists to spread journal-club culture and case-conference know-how to programmes that previously had none. In doing so, it levels the playing field for trainees, no matter how remote their campus. To bridge this gap, the founders created an online portal (eventually named "TIPPS-Excel") which offers concise summary notes on key psychiatry topics (covering both practical clinical points and exam-focused material), a discussion forum where residents can post questions (answered by peers or expert moderators), regular live webinars on important themes, and an archive of past examination questions and tips. This initiative essentially created a virtual national classroom for psychiatry trainees. Initially, some faculty viewed TIPPS as a student-driven supplement rather than a faculty development tool. However, over time, faculty began to engage with TIPPS; for example, by moderating discussions or delivering webinars, and found value in it. Seeing the types of questions residents ask on TIPPS has given faculty insight into common gaps and misconceptions, which they can then address in their local teaching. During the COVID-19 lockdowns, when in-person classes were halted, TIPPS usage surged as weekly virtual case discussions and online journal clubs were organized. Faculty who participated had to adapt to engaging learners virtually (using polls, chat discussions, etc.), which built their digital pedagogy skills. TIPPS also fostered a community of practice among psychiatric educators: the moderators (often young faculty or senior residents) gained leadership experience in steering discussions, curating content, and managing an online learner community (Suhas et al., 2022a). A byproduct has been cross-institutional collaboration where trainees and faculty who met on TIPPS have later collaborated on multi-centre research and academic projects. The success of TIPPS hints at an important strategy for faculty development: leveraging bottom-up, peer-led networks to complement top-down formal programmes. E-Journal club of India (eJCIndia), launched in 2015, is India's first online psychiatry journal club, created to strengthen research and teaching skills nationwide. Now it is over 10 years old; it hosts roughly 100 activities a year for 400-plus psychiatrists and trainees-ranging from article critiques and reviewer training to study-design consultations. The discussions have already generated about 20 published papers and even launched a multi-centre research project. Because members can join from anywhere and revisit archived threads, the model overcomes time-zone, workload, and geographic barriers. Its success shows that online journal clubs may be the quickest, most economical way to build research capacity in resource-spread settings (Thakurdesai et al., 2018). Notably, analogous initiatives have emerged elsewhere: a similar concept was trailed in Sri Lanka via a WhatsApp group that included all psychiatry trainees nationally, moderated occasionally by faculty for Q&A. Although not as elaborate as TIPPS, it improved the sharing of learning resources. In many countries, the young Psychiatrists forums across social media exist formally and informally, which facilitate discussion of clinical cases and exam preparation tips, which many faculty quietly observe to gauge trainee difficulties and step in with guidance when needed. These examples show that empowering trainees and junior faculty to connect/network across institutions can directly and indirectly serve faculty development by highlighting blind spots or weaknesses and encouraging senior faculty to stay updated while mentoring or serving beyond their own institution for a larger cause.

## 6 Theoretical Frameworks and Iterative Agile Learning

In the South Asian context, faculty development and leadership must move beyond imported or rigidly structured models to embrace frameworks that allow for local adaptability, cultural sensitivity, and institutional diversity. Theoretical grounding remains vital to lend coherence and direction, but it must be complemented by an iterative, agile learning approach that recognizes the evolving realities of psychiatric education in the region. Many institutions face shifting faculty roles, constrained resources, and wide variations in training capacity, factors that demand flexibility rather than prescriptive programming. Agile learning enables institutions to experiment with small-scale interventions, such as mentorship circles, digital teaching logs, or interdisciplinary teaching modules, and refine them through real-time feedback and local reflection. This approach also empowers faculty to co-create their development trajectories, fostering ownership and relevance. Over time, such iterative cycles of action and reflection help build institutional memory, adapt educational practices to the sociocultural milieu, and create sustainable models of leadership that are grounded in South Asia's unique academic and service challenges. At the heart of any sustainable faculty-development and leadership programme lies an agile, iterative learning cycle: every workshop, mentoring session, or toolkit is treated as a prototype that is tested, measured, and refined in real time. Adult learning theory gives the cycle its learner-centred focus; the Kirkpatrick hierarchy provides milestones for tracking change from initial reaction to organizational impact; and competency frameworks such as CanMEDS define the end-point behaviours against which progress is judged. By feeding rapid feedback loops; pre- and post-tests, reflective check-ins, peer observations-directly back into programme design, we avoid static, one-off interventions and instead build a living curriculum that continually recalibrates to learners' needs, institutional goals, and emerging evidence. In this way, evaluation is not an afterthought but the engine that drives "what we do next", ensuring each iteration delivers sharper skills, wider leadership reach, and measurable improvements in mental-health outcomes. The sections that follow illustrate these principles through two representative exemplars: the Kirkpatrick evaluation model and the CanMEDS competency framework. Before turning to region-specific initiatives, it is essential to anchor the discussion in the conceptual scaffolding that guides effective faculty and leadership programmes. Without a clear theoretical lens, trainings risk becoming a patchwork of well-meaning workshops whose impact is hard to gauge or replicate (Van Schalkwyk et al., 2024). Adult learning principles help us match content to the self-directed, experience-rich learner; the Kirkpatrick model reminds us to evaluate not just satisfaction, but behaviour change and organizational benefit; frameworks such as CanMEDS clarify the competencies a modern psychiatrist must embody. By briefly mapping these models, we establish a common vocabulary and a set of quality benchmarks against which local innovations-whether in South Asia or elsewhere, can be designed, adapted, and judged. These frameworks provide a foundation for designing programmes and evaluating their impact.

**Adult Learning Theory** Unlike children, adults learn best when education is self-directed, problem-centred, and directly relevant to their work. Malcolm Knowles' principles of adult learning (andragogy) emphasize that adult learners need to know the purpose of learning something, bring their own rich experiences into the process, are ready to learn things that help solve real-life problems, prefer task-oriented learning, and are driven more by internal motivation than external rewards. In faculty development, this means programmes should be learner-centred and practical. For example, workshops should use the faculty's own teaching challenges as case studies, encourage experience-sharing among participants, and focus on skills that can be immediately applied (designing a curriculum, giving feedback, etc.). Moving away from didactic lectures to interactive techniques (small-group discussions, role plays simulating classroom scenarios, peer feedback on teaching presentations, and project-based assignments) not only increases engagement but also models the learner-centric pedagogy we want faculty to adopt with their students.

**Kirkpatrick's Model for Training Evaluation** A common framework to evaluate educational interventions is Kirkpatrick's four-level model (Fig. 22.1) (Kirkpatrick, 1959). It assesses: Level 1-participants' reactions (satisfaction and perceived value of the training), Level 2-learning (acquisition of knowledge or skills, measured, for instance, by pre- and post-tests or self-assessment of confidence), Level 3-behaviour change (whether participants apply new skills on the job, such as adopting a new teaching method in their classes), and Level 4-results (broader outcomes, such as improved student performance, better patient outcomes, or other organizational impacts resulting from the training). Faculty development programmes are increasingly designed with these outcomes in mind (Rouse, 2011). For example, after a workshop on psychotherapy teaching, organizers might measure Level 2 by testing knowledge of psychotherapy supervision principles, then measure Level 3 by observing whether faculty implement regular supervision sessions in their clinics 3 months later. Achieving Level 4 outcomes is challenging (it is difficult to attribute improved exam scores or patient outcomes solely to faculty development), but aligning faculty programmes with institutional goals (like improving residency pass rates or patient satisfaction) helps maintain focus on relevant results. Using Kirkpatrick's model encourages a results-oriented approach-faculty development is

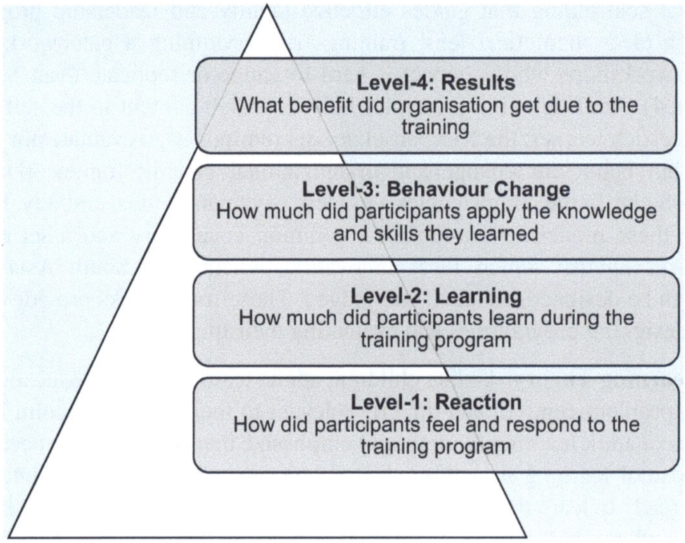


**Fig. 22.1** Kirkpatrick's model for training evaluation

not just an academic exercise, but something that should tangibly improve teaching quality and, ultimately, trainee competencies and patient care.

**Competency Frameworks (CanMEDS and Others)** Modern medical education is grounded in competency frameworks that define the roles and abilities required of physicians. One widely adopted example is the CanMEDS framework by the Royal College of Physicians and Surgeons of Canada (Fig. 22.2). CanMEDS defines seven core roles for physicians: Medical Expert, Communicator, Collaborator, Leader (formerly "Manager"), Health Advocate, Scholar, and Professional (Royal College of Physicians and Surgeons of Canada, 2024). Embracing such frameworks in faculty development ensures that training is comprehensive. For instance, a faculty development curriculum in psychiatry might include modules corresponding to these roles, not only covering medical expertise (clinical knowledge) and teaching (scholar role) but also training faculty in collaboration (working in multidisciplinary teams or co-supervising multidisciplinary research), leadership (as discussed, managing programmes or advocating for services), and professionalism and advocacy (ethics, wellness, and public education). Residency programmes across South Asia are inching towards competency-based assessment, and faculty development benefits from the same discipline. Tying workshops and mentoring to explicit competencies turns a scatter of initiatives into a unified strategy that can be tracked for real gains in teaching finesse and leadership reach. Grounding these efforts in established educational frameworks keeps planners true to three essentials: a learner-centred approach, a focus on demonstrable outcomes, and coverage of every hat a psychiatrist-educator must wear.

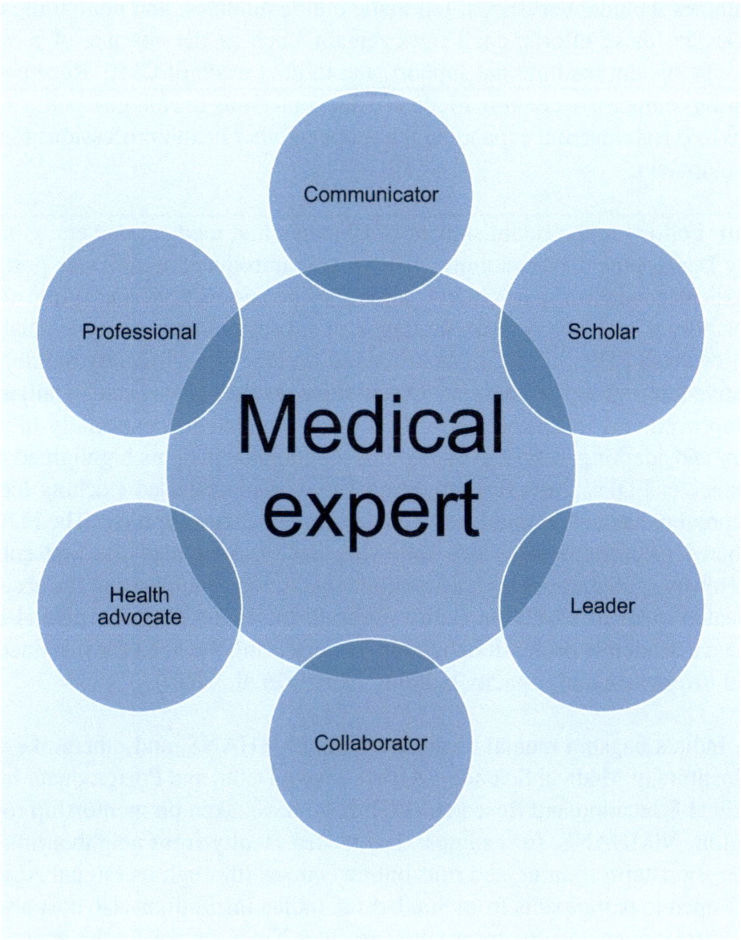


**Fig. 22.2** CanMEDS framework with seven roles of a physician

## 7 Regional and International Initiatives and Innovations

There have been few country-specific efforts in South Asia, some of which are highlighted below. Hearteningly, there have been growing regional collaborations and innovative programmes that transcend national boundaries in the recent decades as well.

**Bangladesh** Faculty development programmes in Bangladesh aim to enhance the personal and professional competencies of medical educators, including teachers, clinicians, and administrators (Uddin et al., 2016). Initiatives began in the 1980s with the establishment of the Centre for Medical Education (CME), which now conducts training, curriculum development, and quality assurance. Various programmes include workshops, seminars, online modules, and continuing education. Despite these efforts, challenges remain, such as the absence of a national policy, insufficient institutional support, and limited reach of CME. Recent recommendations emphasize creating Medical Education Units in colleges, policy reform, incentivized training, and expanding the scope to other health professions for holistic development.

**Bhutan** Following the establishment of Bhutan's first medical university in 2012, Faculty Development Programmes (FDPs) were introduced to enhance postgraduate medical education, particularly among clinician-teachers managing multiple responsibilities amid workforce shortages. A mixed-methods study evaluated the impact of these FDPs, involving a structured training for 18 faculty members and qualitative focus group discussions. Quantitative results showed statistically significant improvements in teacher self-efficacy and competency, especially in subject delivery and adapting to system constraints. Qualitative insights highlighted greater acceptance of FDPs, shifts from traditional to workplace-based teaching methods, and improvements in communication and professional development. The FDPs also contributed to curriculum reform following the graduation of the first cohort in 2018. However, challenges included limited institutional support and the absence of a dedicated medical education centre. Overall, the FDPs played a pivotal role in early-stage academic professionalization, underscoring the need for sustained institutional investment and capacity building (Tenzin et al., 2019).

**India** India's flagship mental health institute, NIMHANS, and others like the All India Institute of Medical Sciences (AIIMS), New Delhi, and Postgraduate Institute of Medical Education and Research (PGIMER) have taken on mentorship roles for the region. NIMHANS, for example, has hosted faculty from neighbouring countries for short-term training and runs online courses (through its Digital Academy) that are open to participants from South Asia. Indian institutions also host observerships where young faculty from countries like Nepal or Sri Lanka spend a few weeks observing teaching methods and academic practices. These initiatives help disseminate best practices regionally.

**Pakistan** Faculty development in medical institutions across Pakistan is progressing, highlighting both advancements and challenges (Mukhtar & Chaudhry, 2010). While institutions have started offering training programmes, mostly focused on teaching and communication skills, these efforts are still not uniform or widespread. The presence of medical education departments seems to play a key role in whether such programmes exist and how effective they are. Although more faculty members are getting involved, participation is still uneven, especially among senior faculty. Several barriers, such as limited motivation, lack of recognition, and insufficiently trained educators to lead sessions, were identified. Overall, the published data indicate a need for better planning, institutional support, and incentives to build stronger, more consistent faculty development systems that can raise the quality of medical education in the country (Mukhtar & Chaudhry, 2010).

**Sri Lanka** The Sri Lankan College of Psychiatrists (SLCPsych) Continuing Professional Development (CPD) programme, launched in 2015, was the first national initiative to promote ongoing education among psychiatrists in Sri Lanka (Kathriarachchi, 2016). It included two planning and six content workshops focused on skill and personal development, attitude change, reflective learning, and knowledge enhancement. Topics ranged from couple therapy and leadership to psychopharmacology and medico-legal issues. Tailored to the needs of psychiatrists, especially those in peripheral areas, the programme aimed to update clinical knowledge and promote gender-sensitive and reflective practices.

**International Collaboration: South Asian Networks** Several regional collaborative efforts have emerged, involving institutions from India, Bangladesh, Nepal, and Bhutan (and sometimes extending to other neighbouring countries). Cross-border faculty exchanges have also been facilitated across global (with North–South and South–South partnerships) (Breuer et al., 2016; Sharma & Razzaque, 2017; Suhas et al., 2021; Suhas et al., 2024b). The Journal of the South Asian Association for Regional Cooperation (SAARC) in Psychiatry and the South Asian Forum for mental health training are platforms that foster knowledge sharing; expanding these to practical training collaborations could reduce duplication of effort and elevate smaller programmes by linking them with larger centres. Additionally, global partnerships continue to play a role. WHO's regional office and the WPA have occasionally sponsored training programmes that bring multiple South Asian countries together.

All these efforts illustrate an encouraging trend: a move from isolated, institution-bound faculty development to a more collaborative, region-wide approach where resources and expertise are shared.

## 8 Challenges to Faculty and Leadership Development in South Asia

Despite considerable progress, numerous challenges continue to hinder the optimal development of faculty and leadership capacity in psychiatry across South Asia:

1. *Resource Constraints:* The availability of training programmes is significantly limited compared to the substantial demand from educators requiring training (Mondal, 2025). Many institutions lack financial and infrastructural support for faculty development activities. Organizing workshops, mentorship programmes, and leadership trainings requires sustained funding and administrative commitment, which are often missing in low- and middle-income settings. Budgetary constraints make it difficult to hire full-time medical education experts or invest in technologies (e.g. e-learning platforms or simulation labs) that support faculty training.

2. *Shortage of Trained Faculty and Protected Time:* The existing senior faculty cadre is often overstretched with clinical, administrative, and teaching duties, leaving little time for their own professional development or for mentoring junior faculty. Faculty development might be viewed as a luxury when service delivery needs are pressing (Cintra et al., 2023). Thus, even where faculty development programmes exist, major needs like ensuring protected time for teachers, establishing mentoring systems, and building teaching skills often remain unmet. Funding shortages and heavy clinical workloads pose significant barriers to an academic career focus, as faculty struggle to balance multiple responsibilities.
3. *Lack of Institutional Incentives:* Academic advancement in the region is still primarily tied to clinical experience and research publications rather than teaching excellence or educational leadership. There are limited rewards or recognition for faculty who excel in teaching or take on educational administrative roles. The absence of promotion criteria that value educational contributions means faculty have little extrinsic motivation to invest time in improving teaching skills.
4. *Cultural and Organizational Barriers:* Hierarchical institutional cultures can discourage open dialogue, critical feedback, and innovation-all of which are crucial for educational improvement. In many traditional settings, junior faculty may feel unable to critique or introduce new teaching methods in the presence of seniors. A resistance to change is often observed, with some faculty being accustomed to traditional didactic methods and hesitant to adopt newer pedagogical models such as interactive learning or online education. This cultural resistance can slow the implementation of CBME or modern assessment tools.
5. *Fragmentation and Lack of Standardization:* There is significant variability in psychiatry training across the region and even within countries (for instance, between older institutions and newer private medical colleges). Faculty development initiatives are often ad hoc or localized, without standardized curricula or accreditation. One medical college might have an excellent faculty-training programme, while another has none. The lack of national guidelines or certification for medical teachers means quality is uneven.
6. *Faculty Workload and Burnout:* Psychiatry faculty commonly face substantial clinical and administrative loads (especially in countries where psychiatrists are very few). Teaching and academic activities may be seen as secondary, and faculty may experience burnout that reduces their engagement in development programmes. With urgent patient care duties, it can be challenging to get faculty to attend workshops or complete courses. This overload also means new faculty often do not get mentored properly, as their seniors have limited time.
7. *Limited Leadership Opportunities:* Even though leadership training is important, many institutions do not have structured pathways for faculty interested in educational leadership (Lieff et al., 2012). For example, there may be no roles such as "director of medical education" or "curriculum coordinator" in some schools, or those roles may exist but with no training or dedicated time. Without clear opportunities, faculty may focus on clinical or research tracks where advancement is more defined.

Addressing these challenges is essential to sustain and accelerate progress in faculty development.

## 9 Intermediate Roadmap to Enhance Faculty and Leadership Development

To catalyse lasting transformation in psychiatric education across South Asia, a phased approach is essential. In the short term, initiatives should focus on strengthening foundational engagement-this includes structured faculty orientation programmes for new entrants, formal recognition of teaching contributions in appraisal and promotion processes, and the nurturing of peer-led communities of practice that encourage mutual learning and mentorship. As institutions mature in their academic commitment, medium-term goals should aim to institutionalize protected time for educational duties, implement individualized leadership development plans for faculty, and establish regional platforms that foster collaboration, curriculum innovation, and cross-border exchange. In the long run, the vision must coalesce into a sustained regional strategy, anchored in a South Asian consortium for faculty and leadership development, that promotes shared capacity building, resource pooling, and contextually grounded scholarship across the region.

Given the above challenges, a strategic multi-pronged approach is needed to strengthen faculty and leadership development in psychiatry across South Asia. Key strategies include:

1. *Institutional Commitment:* Leadership at the level of universities, medical colleges, and health ministries must prioritize faculty development as part of their core mission. This involves allocating dedicated budgets, providing facilities (like skills labs or e-learning studios), and assigning personnel to coordinate faculty development. Establishing formal departments or centres for medical education (or specifically for psychiatric education) can significantly enhance outcomes. NIMHANS's dedicated faculty development programme, for example, could be emulated by other institutions. High-level endorsement also helps create a culture where teaching is valued.
2. *Integration into Career Pathways and Promotions:* Faculty development activities should be formally integrated into faculty appraisal, promotion criteria, and career advancement pathways. For instance, completing certain teacher-training courses or demonstrating educational innovation could be made essential prerequisites for promotion to associate professor. Recognizing and rewarding excellence in teaching and educational leadership, through awards, grants, or accelerated promotions, would incentivize faculty to engage in development programmes. Academic institutions might introduce titles or roles (such as "Education Coordinator" or "Director of Postgraduate Training") to acknowledge those contributions. There must be a structured and inclusive approach to recognizing academic contributions that extends beyond the narrow confines of

traditional scholarly research, valuing excellence in teaching, mentorship, curriculum innovation, and educational leadership as integral to academic advancement.

3. *Collaboration and Networking:* Enhanced collaboration at national and regional levels can maximize resources. National collaboration could mean psychiatry departments across a country sharing faculty development resources, conducting joint workshops, or agreeing on a common faculty development curriculum (so that a workshop done at one institution is recognized elsewhere). International partnerships with global bodies like the WPA, WHO, and academic institutions abroad can bring in global best practices and resources. For example, the WHO's regional office might assist in developing standard faculty training modules, or a partnership with a university in Australia might allow exchange visits for faculty trainees. South–South collaborations (e.g. between South Asian and South-East Asian countries through APEC or SEARO networks) can also be beneficial, given similar context and challenges.
4. *Customized Programmes to Local Needs:* Faculty development must be context sensitive. Programmes should be adapted to local realities, considering language (Suhas et al., 2024a), culture, patient population, and health system needs. Modules on cultural psychiatry, community mental health, or stigma reduction are highly relevant in South Asia and should be incorporated. Similarly, training in low-resource teaching techniques (like using role-play when high-fidelity simulators are not available) is important. One size does not fit all: urban tertiary hospitals and rural medical colleges may have different needs.
5. *Blended and Flexible Learning:* Online faculty development programmes for health professions educators in low- and middle-income countries can effectively enhance professional and interpersonal skills when structured around active, community-based engagement. Well-designed online learning environments that foster interaction and reflection, though evidence on generalizability remains limited (Keiller et al., 2022). Leveraging e-learning can help overcome geographical barriers. Developing short online modules or "just-in-time" learning resources allows busy faculty to engage in development at their convenience. National tele-education platforms (like India's NTEL for medical education or similar programmes) could host psychiatry-specific teacher training content. Massive open online courses (MOOCs) and webinars can complement in-person workshops and ensure continuity (for example, a series of follow-up online sessions after an initial face-to-face workshop to reinforce learning).
6. *Building a Research Culture:* Encouraging and supporting educational research among psychiatry faculty can have long-term benefits. When faculty investigate their own teaching methods and student outcomes, they adopt a scholarly approach to education. Providing seed grants for education research, creating communities of practice for education scholars, and offering guidance on publishing in medical education can help. This will not only improve teaching practices based on evidence but also promote academic scholarship and can attract institutional recognition (since publications and grants in education contribute to a university's profile).

7. *Structured Leadership Development:* Leadership training should be a deliberate, structured process beginning early in a psychiatrist's career. As described earlier, offering tiered leadership development (introductory leadership workshops for junior faculty, advanced training or administrative internships for mid-career, etc.) will create a pipeline of capable leaders. Mentoring in leadership-pairing emerging leaders with experienced administrators is another approach. Countries could also consider formal leadership fellowships in mental health (perhaps a 6-month programme where selected faculty spend time in health administration settings or undergo management training). By making leadership development an expected part of career progression (rather than something one learns informally), the system will gradually populate itself with faculty who have both the vision and the skills to advance psychiatric education and services.

Over the next 5 years, faculty development and academic leadership in psychiatry will require a tiered and integrated approach across policy, institutional, programmatic, and individual levels. Regulatory frameworks must move beyond symbolic endorsements to enforce accountability; linking accreditation and promotions to demonstrable engagement in teaching and leadership training. Institutions, in turn, should reconfigure faculty roles by structurally allocating time and resources for academic work and embedding leadership preparation into professional development from the outset. At the training programme level, nurturing future educators through structured peer learning and reflective practice will help embed academic values early. For individual faculty members, sustained engagement through planning, scholarly output, and inter-institutional mentorship can ensure personal growth aligns with broader system goals. This layered strategy creates alignment between macro policy and micro practice, paving the way for a culture where academic excellence is cultivated, recognized, and sustained. By implementing these strategies, South Asian countries can create an ecosystem that continuously develops and empowers its psychiatric faculty. Some of the priority action points towards these strategies are summarized in Table 22.2. The goal is a sustainable model where each generation of teachers is better prepared than the last, and where educational excellence and leadership are part of the professional of psychiatrists.

## 10 Conclusion

Robust faculty and leadership development sit at the heart of any plan to expand mental health care in South Asia. When educators acquire up-to-date teaching, mentoring, and managerial skills, the benefit multiplies with every resident they train. This chapter has underscored the region's stark contrasts: acute shortages of specialists and patchy training on one hand; on the other, imaginative home-grown projects such as TIPPS and a growing web of regional collaborations.

Progress from here demands concerted action on three fronts: Governments must create the infrastructure and incentives that make systematic faculty training

**Table 22.2** Actionable blueprint for improving faculty development programmes

| Level | Priority actions (next 5 years) |
|---|---|
| Policy/ Regulator | Mandate documented Faculty and Leadership Development hours for promotion; tie college accreditation to functional MEUs; micro-grant scheme for education research. |
| Institution | Protect ≥20% faculty time for education; embed Leadership Development modules in faculty induction; sponsor such training exercises. |
| Programme (residency) | Residents-as-teachers curricula; peer-mentoring circles; digital portfolios with reflection prompts mapped to CanMEDS. |
| Individual faculty | Annual faculty development plan; publish at least one educational-scholarship output every 2 years; seek cross-institution coaching. |

possible. Universities and teaching hospitals need to reward educational excellence and cultivate leadership potential, rather than measuring success by research metrics alone. Individual psychiatrists must embrace a career-long commitment to honing their teaching and leadership craft.

Though still a relatively new focus, purposeful programmes, mentoring schemes, and targeted support can transform the journey from trainee to teacher to leader into a deliberate, well-supported progression. By closing existing gaps and scaling proven models, South Asian nations can assemble a strong corps of psychiatric educators and leaders who will not only train the next generation but also champion policy reform and service innovation. The next decade should see isolated national efforts knitted into a coherent regional framework; one that guarantees every trainee learns from skilled faculty and that the profession is steered by leaders with the vision to elevate mental-health care. With shared resolve, psychiatry's traditional neglect in the region can become a historical footnote, replaced by an era defined by educational excellence and decisive leadership.

South Asia's mental-health ambitions hinge on a robust cadre of psychiatrist-educators who can also steer teams, budgets, and policy dialogues. The region now possesses a lattice of training hubs (MEUs, FAIMER, and Digital Academies) and a growing slate of leadership incubators. What remains is to knit these into a coherent, monitored pipeline that carries a trainee from resident-teacher to a junior faculty, to a education scholar, and towards becoming a system leader. Nations that align promotion rules, funding, and cultural incentives with that pipeline will shrink the treatment gap faster and build mental-health systems resilient to future crises. Prioritizing faculty development and leadership training is not a luxury but a necessity for South Asia. Strategic investment in this area will yield dividends in the form of better-trained psychiatrists, more effective mental health services, and stronger advocacy for resources and rights. International organizations and regional bodies should continue to support these efforts, but local ownership is crucial. Finally, ongoing research and evaluation should guide these initiatives by measuring what works, the region can refine its approaches and serve as a model for other low-resource settings in building capacity through faculty and leadership development.

## References


*About Us | World Psychiatric Association*. (2025). WPA. Retrieved June 25, 2025, from https://www.wpanet.org/about-wpa

Arafat, S. M. Y., & Kar, S. K. (2024). Epidemiology of psychiatric disorders and overview of access to mental health care in South Asia. In S. M. Y. Arafat & S. K. Kar (Eds.), *Access to mental health care in South Asia: Current status, potential challenges, and ways out* (pp. 1–15). Springer Nature. https://doi.org/10.1007/978-981-99-9153-2_1

Bansal, P., & Supe, A. (2007). Training of medical teachers in India: Need for change. *Indian Journal of Medical Sciences, 61*(8), 478–484.

Bembade, S., Rathod, P. G., Sharma, S. K., Narlawar, U., Ajaya Krishnan, P., Rath, D., Pogula, P., & Mohajir, M. F. (2025). Enhancing teaching competence through a faculty development program: Impact of the basic course in medical education technology (BCME) program in a tertiary medical institution. *Cureus, 17*(4). https://doi.org/10.7759/cureus.82972

Breuer, E., De Silva, M. J., Shidaye, R., Petersen, I., Nakku, J., Jordans, M. J. D., Fekadu, A., & Lund, C. (2016). Planning and evaluating mental health services in low- and middle-income countries using theory of change. *The British Journal of Psychiatry, 208*(Suppl 56), s55–s62. https://doi.org/10.1192/bjp.bp.114.153841

Buer, T. S., Kutzler, M. A., Salcedo, A., Overholser, B., Pollart, S. M., & Spector, N. D. (2024). Revisiting a faculty career management life cycle model: Anticipating and navigating career transitions in academic medicine. *Journal of Clinical Psychology in Medical Settings, 31*(4), 648–658. https://doi.org/10.1007/s10880-024-10054-0

Cintra, K. A., Borges, M. C., Panúncio-Pinto, M. P., de Almeida Troncon, L. E., & Bollela, V. R. (2023). The impact and the challenges of implementing a faculty development program on health professions education in a Brazilian Medical School: A case study with mixed methods. *BMC Medical Education, 23*, 784. https://doi.org/10.1186/s12909-023-04754-8

ECFMG. (2022, August 3). FAIMER fellow becomes medical education leader in India. *Storytellers*. https://www.intealth.org/storytellers/2022/08/03/ecfmgfaimer-storytellers-8/

Garg, K., Kumar, C. N., & Chandra, P. S. (2019). Number of psychiatrists in India: Baby steps forward, but a long way to go. *Indian Journal of Psychiatry, 61*(1), 104–105. https://doi.org/10.4103/psychiatry.IndianJPsychiatry_7_18

Gopalakrishnan, S., Catherine, A. P., Kandasamy, S., & Ganesan, H. (2022). Challenges and opportunities in the implementation of competency-based medical education – A cross-sectional survey among medical faculty in India. *Journal of Education and Health Promotion, 11*, 206. https://doi.org/10.4103/jehp.jehp_1130_21

Grover, S. (2023). Status of mental health in South Asian countries. *Journal of SAARC Psychiatric Federation, 1*(1), 1. https://doi.org/10.4103/jspf.JSPF_15_23

Hasan, M. T., Anwar, T., Christopher, E., Hossain, S., Hossain, M. M., Koly, K. N., Saif-Ur-Rahman, K. M., Ahmed, H. U., Arman, N., & Hossain, S. W. (2021). The current state of mental healthcare in Bangladesh: Part 1 – An updated country profile. *BJPsych International, 18*(4), 78–82. https://doi.org/10.1192/bji.2021.41

India, N. (2023). *NIMHANS Digital Academy*. NIMHANS DIGITAL ACADEMY(NDA). https://nda.nimhans.ac.in/

Kallivayalil, R. A., & Enara, A. (2021). Education and training in psychiatry in South Asian countries. *Asia-Pacific Psychiatry, 13*(4), e12494. https://doi.org/10.1111/appy.12494

Kathriarachchi, S. T. (Ed.). (2016). *Continuing Professional Development for Psychiatrists in Sri Lanka (First)*. The Asia Foundation.

Keiller, L., Nyoni, C., & van Wyk, C. (2022). Online faculty development in low- and middle-income countries for health professions educators: A rapid realist review. *Human Resources for Health, 20*(1), 12. https://doi.org/10.1186/s12960-022-00711-6

Kestel, D. (2022). Transforming mental health for all: A critical role for specialists. *World Psychiatry, 21*(3), 333–334. https://doi.org/10.1002/wps.21030

Kirkpatrick, D. L. (1959). Techniques for evaluation training programs. *Journal of the American Society of Training Directors, 13*, 21–26.

Kishor, M., & Isaac, M. (2024). Can subject specific teacher's forum transform medical education in India? The IToP Model. *Indian Journal of Psychiatry, 66*(12), 1081–1082. https://doi.org/10.4103/indianjpsychiatry.indianjpsychiatry_1060_24

Kumar, C. N., Chand, P. K., Manjunatha, N., Math, S. B., Shashidhara, H. N., Basavaraju, V., Thirthalli, J., Manjappa, A. A., Parthasarathy, R., Murthy, P., Ibrahim, F. A., Jagtap, N., Jyrwa, S., Reddy, S., Arora, S., Hawk, M., Kumar, S., Egan, J., & McDonald, M. (2020). Impact evaluation of VKN–NIMHANS–ECHO model of capacity building for mental health and addiction: Methodology of two randomized controlled trials. *Indian Journal of Psychological Medicine, 42*(6 Suppl), S80–S86. https://doi.org/10.1177/0253717620969066

Ladhani, Z., Chhatwal, J., Vyas, R., Iqbal, M., Tan, C., & Diserens, D. (2011). Online role-playing for faculty development. *The Clinical Teacher, 8*(1), 31–36. https://doi.org/10.1111/j.1743-498X.2010.00401.x

Lieff, S., Baker, L., Mori, B., Egan-Lee, E., Chin, K., & Reeves, S. (2012). Who am I? Key influences on the formation of academic identity within a faculty development program. *Medical Teacher, 34*(3), e208–e215. https://doi.org/10.3109/0142159X.2012.642827

Mahadevan, J., Shukla, L., Chand, P. K., Komaromy, M., Murthy, P., & Arora, S. (2020). Innovative virtual mentoring using the Extension for Community Healthcare Outcomes model for primary care providers for the management of alcohol use disorders. *The Indian Journal of Medical Research, 151*(6), 609–612. https://doi.org/10.4103/ijmr.IJMR_1851_18

Main Thompson, A., & Saleem, S. M. (2025). Closing the mental health gap: Transforming Pakistan's mental health landscape. *Frontiers in Health Services, 4*. https://doi.org/10.3389/frhs.2024.1471528

Mia, M. A., & Griffiths, M. D. (2022). Can South Asian countries cope with the mental health crisis associated with COVID-19? *International Journal of Mental Health and Addiction, 20*(4), 1923–1932. https://doi.org/10.1007/s11469-021-00491-5

Misky, G. J., Sharpe, B., Weaver, A. C., Niranjan-Azadi, A., Gupta, A., Rennke, S., Ludwin, S., Piper, C., Mlis, Sun, V. K., Brotman, D. J., & Frank, M. (2023). Faculty development in academic hospital medicine: A scoping review. *Journal of General Internal Medicine, 38*(8), 1955–1961. https://doi.org/10.1007/s11606-023-08089-4

Mondal, H. (2025). Unique challenges and potential solutions in faculty development programs in India. *Medical Teacher*, *0*(0), 1–1. https://doi.org/10.1080/0142159X.2025.2458275

Mukhtar, F., & Chaudhry, A. M. (2010). Faculty development in medical institutions: Where do we stand in Pakistan? *Journal of Ayub Medical College Abbottabad, 22*(3), 210–214.

Narasimha, V. L., Suhas, S., Kishor, M., Dixit, A., & Murthy, P. (2024). Advances in psychiatry training and faculty development in India. *Indian Journal of Psychological Medicine, 46*(5), 391–399. https://doi.org/10.1177/02537176241284348

Naskar, C., & Varadharajan, N. (2024). Beyond the couch: Empowering psychiatrists to be leaders—A brief report from a leadership and skills training course for psychiatrists in India. *Journal of Psychosocial Rehabilitation and Mental Health, 11*(1), 135–138. https://doi.org/10.1007/s40737-023-00384-x

Parate, N., Manjunatha, B., Sanchitha, R., Narasimha, V. L., Mahadevan, J., Chand, P., Murthy, P., & Arora, S. (2024). NAMAH—An innovative tele-ECHO mentoring program to foster well-being among physicians. *Indian Journal of Psychological Medicine*, 02537176241287839. https://doi.org/10.1177/02537176241287839

Rouse, D. N. (2011). Employing Kirkpatrick's evaluation framework to determine the effectiveness of health information management courses and programs. *Perspectives in Health Information Management, 8*(Spring), 1c.

Royal College of Physicians and Surgeons of Canada. (2024). *CanMEDS*. https://www.royalcollege.ca/en/standards-and-accreditation/canmeds.html

Sartorius, N. (2013). Acquiring leadership skills: Description of an international programme for early career psychiatrists. In *Leadership in psychiatry* (pp. 226–232). Wiley. https://doi.org/10.1002/9781118569948.ch19

Sartorius, N. (2023). Leadership for early career psychiatrists – A rough guide on theory, practice and what to avoid. *European Psychiatry, 66*(S1), S56. https://doi.org/10.1192/j.eurpsy.2023.206

Satish, S., Narayana, M., Naveen Kumar, C., & Suresh, B. M. (2023). Navigating telepsychiatry: Unveiling practices and regulations in the Indian context. In *Indian psychiatric update—Digital psychiatry* (Vol. 8, pp. 17–29). Indian Psychiatric Society South Zonal Branch. https://ipsszb.org/wp-content/uploads/2024/07/Digital-Psychiatry-2024-1.pdf

Seethamraju, R. R., Stone, K., & Shepherd, M. (2021). Evaluation of a simulation faculty training workshop in a low-resource setting: A qualitative study. *BMJ Simulation & Technology Enhanced Learning, 7*(6), 478–486. https://doi.org/10.1136/bmjstel-2020-000829

Sethi, S., Tekkalaki, B., Shah, N., Smitha, C. A., & Kumar, R. (2024). Undergraduate psychiatry CBME curriculum revision: The process and the way ahead. *Indian Journal of Psychiatry, 66*(11), 1066. https://doi.org/10.4103/indianjpsychiatry.indianjpsychiatry_821_24

Sharma, M., & Razzaque, B. (2017). Research capacity strengthening in South Asia: Based on the experience of South Asian Hub for Advocacy, Research and Education on Mental Health (SHARE). *Global Mental Health (Cambridge, England), 4*, e9. https://doi.org/10.1017/gmh.2017.5

Suhas, S., Arvind, B. A., Sukumar, G. M., Banandur, P. S., Nirisha, L. P., Kumar, C. N., Benegal, V., Rao, G. N., Varghese, M., & Gururaj, G. (2023). A bird's eye view of the mental health systems in India. *Indian Journal of Psychiatry, 65*(12), 1214–1222. https://doi.org/10.4103/indianjpsychiatry.indianjpsychiatry_845_23

Suhas, S., Basavarajappa, C., Korwar, M., Shamanna, V., Mittal, A., Kumar, N., Bg, K., Harbishettar, V., Ghadigaonkar, D. S., Manjunatha, N., & Math, S. B. (2024a). Clinical linguistic proficiency program: An innovation to bridge language incompatibility in the training of psychiatric residents. *Indian Journal of Psychological Medicine, 46*(5), 480–484. https://doi.org/10.1177/02537176241273749

Suhas, S., Chithra, N. K., Nair, S., Huddar, S., Naik, S. S., Lakshmanan, S., Mahadevan, J., Kumar, V., Kandasamy, A., Desai, G., Kesavan, M., & Murthy, P. (2021). Psychotherapy across epochs and methods NIMHANS – TAVISTOCK Psychotherapy conference. *Asian Journal of Psychiatry, 56*, 102459. https://doi.org/10.1016/j.ajp.2020.102459

Suhas, S., Chougule, A., Innamuri, R., Nayok, S. B., Sheth, S., Nagendrappa, S., Patel, K. G., Shetty, S. B., Nagendra, B., Bhaumik, U., Pugalenthi, S., Uppal, G., Babu, G. N., Rao, N. P., & Behere, R. V. (2022a). Training initiative for psychiatry post-graduate students (TIPPS)-a unique early career psychiatry training initiative in india and its response to the COVID-19 pandemic. *Academic Psychiatry, 46*(6), 763–768. https://doi.org/10.1007/s40596-021-01570-4

Suhas, S., Gangadhar, B., Vanikar, A. V., Malik, Y., Girish, N., Kumar, V., & Math, S. B. (2022b). Undergraduate medicine curriculum in India: Untying the Gordian knot. *Indian Journal of Preventive & Social Medicine*. http://imsear.searo.who.int/handle/123456789/224002

Suhas, S., Reddy, P. V., Arasappa, R., Viswanath, B., & Kesavan, M. (2024b). BDICON 24: Bipolar disorder international conference organized at NIMHANS, India. *Asian Journal of Psychiatry, 101*, 104218. https://doi.org/10.1016/j.ajp.2024.104218

Sultan, N., Torti, J., Haddara, W., Inayat, A., Inayat, H., & Lingard, L. (2019). Leadership development in postgraduate medical education: A systematic review of the literature. *Academic Medicine, 94*(3), 440. https://doi.org/10.1097/ACM.0000000000002503

Tenzin, K., Dorji, T., Choeda, T., & Pongpirul, K. (2019). Impact of faculty development programme on self-efficacy, competency and attitude towards medical education in Bhutan: A mixed-methods study. *BMC Medical Education, 19*(1), 468. https://doi.org/10.1186/s12909-019-1904-4

Thakurdesai, A., Ghosh, A., Menon, V., Sahoo, S., Tripathi, A., Harshe, D., & Andrade, C. (2018). Electronic journal clubs for capacity building: A case study in psychiatry as a model for medical disciplines in developing countries. *Asian Journal of Psychiatry, 34*, 93–97. https://doi.org/10.1016/j.ajp.2018.04.026

Trivedi, J. K., & Dhyani, M. (2007). Undergraduate psychiatric education in South Asian countries. *Indian Journal of Psychiatry, 49*(3), 163–165. https://doi.org/10.4103/0019-5545.37314

Trivedi, J. K., Goel, D., Kallivayalil, R. A., Isaac, M., Shrestha, D. M., & Gambheera, H. C. (2007). Regional cooperation in South Asia in the field of mental health. *World Psychiatry, 6*(1), 57–59.

Uddin, M. M., Yusuff, S. M., Mitra, T., Awal, A., & Chowdhury, A. A. (2016). Faculty development in medical education. *Journal of Chattagram Maa-O-Shishu Hospital Medical College, 27*(1), 11–16.

Vagha, S., Mishra, V., & Joshi, Y. (2023). Reviving medical education through teachers training programs: A literature review. *Journal of Education and Health Promotion, 12*(1), 277. https://doi.org/10.4103/jehp.jehp_1413_22

Van Schalkwyk, S., Amaral, E., Anakin, M., Chen, R., Dolmans, D., Findyartini, A., Fobian, N., Leslie, K., Muller, J., O'Sullivan, P., Ramani, S., Sorinola, O., Vakani, F., Yang, D., & Steinert, Y. (2024). Disentangling faculty development: A scoping review towards a rich description of the concept and its practice. *Medical Teacher*, 1–22. https://doi.org/10.1080/0142159X.2024.2429612

Verma, N., Gupta, S., & Shatadal, P. (2024). Research in psychiatry medical education through "MUST Enrich Grant": A scoping review. *Indian Journal of Psychological Medicine, 46*(5), 382–390. https://doi.org/10.1177/02537176241265742

Williams, S. S. (2024). Fine-tuning postgraduate psychiatry training in South Asia. *Indian Journal of Psychological Medicine, 46*(5), 380–381. https://doi.org/10.1177/02537176241280284

Yuan, S., Rahim, A., Kannappan, S., Dongre, A., Jain, A., Kar, S. S., Mukherjee, S., & Vyas, R. (2024). Success stories: Exploring perceptions of former fellows of a global faculty development program for health professions educators. *BMC Medical Education, 24*(1), 1072. https://doi.org/10.1186/s12909-024-05823-2

# Index





S. K. Kar et al. (eds.), *Teaching and Training in Psychiatry in South Asia*, South Asian Perspectives in Mental Health and Psychology ,
https://doi.org/10.1007/978-981-95-1845-6

MIX
Papier aus verantwortungsvollen Quellen
Paper from responsible sources
FSC® C105338

If you have any concerns about our products,
you can contact us on
**ProductSafety@springernature.com**

In case Publisher is established outside the EU,
the EU authorized representative is:
**Springer Nature Customer Service Center GmbH**
**Europaplatz 3, 69115 Heidelberg, Germany**

Printed by Libri Plureos GmbH
in Hamburg, Germany